An Occupational Therapist's Guide *to* Sleep *and* Sleep Problems

by the same author

Sleep
Multi-Professional Perspectives
Edited by Andrew Green and Alex Westcombe
With Ved Varma
Foreword by David Nutt
ISBN 978 1 84905 062 3
eISBN 978 0 85700 257 0

of related interest

The Core Concepts of Occupational Therapy
A Dynamic Framework for Practice
Jennifer Creek
Foreword by Anne Lawson-Porter
ISBN 978 1 84905 007 4
eISBN 978 0 85700 362 1

Sleep Difficulties and Autism Spectrum Disorders
A Guide for Parents and Professionals
Kenneth J. Aitken
ISBN 978 1 84905 259 7
eISBN 978 0 85700 550 2

Sleep Better with Natural Therapies
A Comprehensive Guide to Overcoming Insomnia,
Moving Sleep Cycles and Preventing Jet Lag
Peter Smith
ISBN 978 1 84819 182 2
eISBN 978 0 85701 140 4

An Occupational Therapist's Guide *to*

SLEEP

and

SLEEP PROBLEMS

EDITED BY ANDREW GREEN AND CARY BROWN

Foreword by Professor Michael Iwama

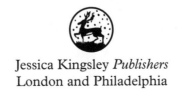

Jessica Kingsley *Publishers*
London and Philadelphia

The Bristol Sleep Profile in Appendix 8.2 is reprinted by kind permission of Sue Wilson.

First published in 2015
by Jessica Kingsley Publishers
73 Collier Street
London N1 9BE, UK
and
400 Market Street, Suite 400
Philadelphia, PA 19106, USA

www.jkp.com

Copyright © Andrew Green and Cary Brown 2015
Foreword copyright © Michael Iwama 2015

Library of Congress Cataloging in Publication Data
An occupational therapist's guide to sleep and sleep problems / edited by Andrew Green and Cary Brown ; foreword by Michael Iwama.
    p. ; cm.
 Includes bibliographical references and index.
 ISBN 978-1-84905-618-2 (alk. paper)
 I. Green, Andrew, 1957 February 4- , editor. II. Brown, Cary (Professor), editor.
 [DNLM: 1. Sleep. 2. Occupational Therapy. 3. Sleep Disorders. WL 108]
 RC547
 616.8'498--dc23

2014033343

British Library Cataloguing in Publication Data
A CIP catalogue record for this book is available from the British Library

ISBN 978 1 84905 618 2
eISBN 978 1 78450 088 7

Printed and bound in the United States

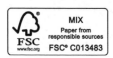

Dedicated to the memory of
Rosemary Barnitt (1943–2011)

CONTENTS

FOREWORD

There is a well-known Japanese proverb – 'todai moto kurashi' (燈台下暗し), which, translated literally, means 'Living at the foot of a lighthouse'. It implies that even though a truth is there in front of you, that does not mean you will notice and appreciate it. The guiding light emanating from the top of the lighthouse can be seen and appreciated by those from a distance, but it is less appreciated – or even less noticed – by those who abide at its base. Such is the matter of 'sleep' to the field of occupational therapy. Though most occupational therapists may agree that sleep qualifies as an occupation in itself, and one that supports and affects other essential and valued occupations of daily life, sleep has been under-represented and largely overlooked in occupational therapy discourse, education and practice.

'Man, through the use of his hands, as energized by mind and will, can influence the state of his own health.' This iconic quote, attributed to Professor Mary Reilly, is familiarly employed by occupational therapists worldwide as the *raison d'etre* for their profession and a unifying tenet for its core concept: occupation. The use of one's hands energized by mind and will, doing and acting with purpose, flowing through life's circumstances, participating in activities in which we want or need to participate and so forth, among a plethora of definitions for occupation, form the common grand narrative that runs up and down the columns of this great profession. Sleep, as important as it is, as an occupation as well as an essential support of occupations in general, has taken a back seat to other occupations and issues deemed worth knowing about among occupational therapists. By placing our emphases on agency, action, participation and 'doing', what have we done about our understanding of the essential occupation of sleep?

The idea of occupational therapy, having originated in the Western world, has traditionally favoured ideologies of human well-being grounded in pragmatism and individual agency. Much emphasis has been placed on individual ability, independence, skill development and enhancing functional capacity. Perhaps this privileging of individual doing and participating has resulted in the matter of sleep being relegated to the rear of our occupational imaginations. The essentiality of sleep and its role in enhancing occupational performance become more than apparent when occupational therapy clients experience deprivation of (or an excess of) sleep. Thus, if we earnestly want to understand human occupation and performance, occupational therapists should take a corresponding interest in the matter of sleep.

The magnificent promise of occupational therapy can be simply stated as: 'to enable people from all walks of life to engage and participate in meaningful activities and processes of daily life'. Though this promise is simply stated, it is actually very complex and challenging to fulfil. The authors of this landmark book take us closer toward delivering on this magnificent promise. Cary Brown, Andrew Green and colleagues, through *An Occupational Therapist's Guide to Sleep and Sleep Problems*, bring us out from below the 'lighthouse' toward 'knowing' sleep and comprehending its complexities as an essential and supportive component of human occupation.

Michael Iwama PhD OT(C)
Department Chair and Professor, Department of Occupational Therapy,
Georgia Regents University, Augusta, GA, USA
March 2014

PREFACE

Andrew Green: My clinical interest in sleep and sleep problems began in 1999 with participation in a therapy group for people with insomnia – leading the session on relaxation in the first instance. This gradually developed into an increasing amount of work with sleep disorders, and to an opportunity to participate in a research project. It was in the writing of an article reporting part of that project that I became aware that, with regard to sleep, the occupational therapy literature was limited and inconsistent. I therefore carried out a more thorough survey of the literature and the result was a further article. To say that in response to that I was deluged with correspondence would be an exaggeration, but I did receive a lot of messages, one of which led to the eventual publication of a book. Other messages included requests for information from students embarking on research projects and from clinicians with client groups experiencing sleep problems – more than I would have expected. For each person sending a message it might be assumed that there are many more with an interest who do not make contact, which suggested a substantial interest in sleep among occupational therapists. This book is a response to that interest, and a reassuring thing is that in the process of planning it, we found so many others in the profession who are investigating sleep and how to improve the sleep of their patients/clients. Therefore, the book that was first conceived as a single-authored book, and then a co-authored book, has become the edited work that it now is. An important part of that transition was the involvement of Cary Brown.

Cary Brown: I was so pleased when Andrew Green approached me to be involved in this book. I first became aware of the importance of sleep through my teaching and research in the area of chronic pain. I am firmly convinced that occupational therapy has much to offer in this long-neglected personal and public health issue. The more evidence I explored and the more clients, caregivers, parents and health care providers I spoke with, the greater became my conviction that occupational therapists were needed in the prevention and management of sleep problems. The importance of restorative sleep for occupational therapy clients became such an integral belief for me that I quite clearly remember being at a loss for words when once asked, 'Why would sleep be an occupation?' The question came after a presentation I did during the interview process for an academic post. Of course, I had travelled across six time zones for the interview and was significantly sleep deprived at the time. So perhaps the word loss was not all related to the question!

Over the past 10 years I have focused on knowledge exchange research to explore how best to get evidence-based, non-pharmacological sleep intervention and practice knowledge to the people who need it. This journey has spanned from children to military personnel and from persons with enduring musculoskeletal pain to older adults with dementia. Currently my team and I are exploring the outcome of pre-bedtime transitional activities (like self-massage) based on neurophysiological theories suggesting that we are only able to fully attend to one task at a time. If this is the case, we may be able to help people decrease sleep-interfering ruminations. We are also studying educational strategies to promote sleep-friendly environmental modifications in the bedroom – a very relevant occupational therapy intervention. I have been fortunate to meet so many passionately concerned therapists during the course of my teaching and research. Everyone is hungry for resources and I am pleased to have been involved in creating a book that will go a long way to help fill that gap.

AG: As ever, a book like this is only possible with the help and cooperation of many people. The contributors to each chapter are acknowledged in their place, but many have assisted in advising on other chapters and it is impossible to record all their extra efforts. We are grateful to them all. Particularly helpful have been members of the 'sleep community' in Bristol for practical assistance in proofreading, for example, and for general support. Special mentions of Dietmar Hank and, as always, Sue Wilson for sharing encyclopaedic knowledge so freely and advising on technical details, are well deserved. Thanks are also due to Drs Johanna Herrod and Fiona Pattison (of, and formerly of, respectively, the North Bristol neuropsychiatry service) for helpful advice. Lastly, I would like to offer special thanks to Eva Nakopoulou for her unswerving enthusiasm and support for the project, as well as all the practical help.

This book is dedicated to the memory of Rosemary Barnitt, who I feel privileged to have known when she was joint supervisor of my research at the University of Southampton. A very helpful piece of her practical wisdom was that the advantage of having two supervisors is that the student can choose which advice to take. The same might be said of a book like this with many authors and perspectives. We have tried to ensure that there is no conflicting information, but some choices for the reader may remain.

Notes

- Items in the glossary are denoted by an asterisk*.
- The case examples and vignettes in this book are derived from the clinical experience of the chapter authors. Most of them are an amalgam of several cases and in the others no identifying information has been included.

1

INTRODUCTION

Andrew Green and Cary Brown

Sleep disturbance is a clinical feature of nearly all psychiatric conditions and sleep is disrupted by symptoms of many physical conditions, for example by pain or discomfort caused by the condition itself or by its treatment. Sleep disturbance is a clinical feature of some neurological conditions, such as Parkinson's disease, and often accompanies others, such as multiple sclerosis. Furthermore, worry about a serious illness – or an illness perceived as serious – is likely to impact further on sleep. It is also possible to have a sleep disorder that co-exists with other conditions.

It is likely therefore that most patients or clients seen by occupational therapists could have sleep problems, and many *will* have sleep problems, but do we routinely ask about them? If we do ask, are we then able to offer any help? If we do offer help, how well informed is any advice that we give? Do we consider whether, or how much, sleep and activity have an effect on each other?

There was certainly no discussion of sleep or sleep problems in training in occupational therapy on the national diploma of the College of Occupational Therapists in the UK in the 1980s, and it is doubtful that there has been much change if occupational therapy training reflects medical training. For example, Peile (2010) notes that in the US the average amount of teaching time on sleep in a 4-year medical school curriculum is less than 2 hours. Stores and Crawford (1998) reported that in the UK the median time of teaching on sleep and sleep disorders in undergraduate medical training was 5 minutes, and Stores (2007) observes that 'there is no reason to believe that the situation has improved since then' (p.1293). Noting that there are similar shortcomings in the training of nurses and clinical psychologists, Stores (2007) suggests that 'in theory, [they] are well placed to identify and, in some instances, treat sleep disorders' (p.1293). The same could be said of occupational therapists.

It may be a matter for debate whether or how much it is the business of occupational therapists to involve themselves in managing sleep disorders, or sleep problems, but the reality is that there is insufficient capacity in sleep clinics, in the UK at least, to deal adequately with sleep disorders such as insomnia – hence suggestions of stepped care (Espie 2009; Vincent and Walsh 2013) and online interventions (Espie *et al.* 2012). If patients with sleep difficulties in the context of other conditions were all referred to sleep clinics, the clinics would be overwhelmed. As this book shows, sleep problems are widespread and it would seem to be the responsibility of all health professionals to respond – not least occupational therapists. The skill mix and professional ethos of occupational therapists, focusing on prevention, maintenance and rehabilitation throughout the lifespan, from both the individual patient and public health perspectives, position them to assume a wider role in promoting good sleep.

The purpose of this book is to provide a comprehensive and accessible resource for therapists. It argues that therapists should be aware of sleep difficulties, routinely screen for them and be able to offer advice for the management of many problems. Furthermore, as occupational therapists we should be more aware of the relationships between sleep and daytime activity.

The book consists, essentially, of two sections, if Chapter 2 is considered an extension of this introductory chapter. In the first section sleep and sleep disorders are explored from a general perspective, drawing on research from the sciences and other disciplines. The chapters in the second section, on managing sleep difficulties in different circumstances or in different client groups, are written by occupational therapists from a variety of backgrounds.

The extent to which sleep relates to occupational therapy and to occupational science has been discussed by Green (2008). Chapter 2 continues that discussion and traces the place of sleep in occupational therapy from its early years to the present. It is commonly suggested that since sleep was cited by Adolf Meyer in the early 1920s as one of the four factors necessary for balance and health, occupational therapy has lost sight of the restorative occupations of rest and sleep. However, it is argued in the chapter that occupational therapy never actually gave serious consideration to sleep until the 1990s, when occupational science began to take an interest. Since that time, sleep has been increasingly covered in the occupational therapy literature and now is included in some standard occupational therapy textbooks. Finally, it is argued that there are now good reasons for occupational therapists to become involved in managing sleep problems.

To be able to give advice on managing a sleep problem, it is necessary to have some grounding in the science of sleep: a well-informed client is much more likely to accept advice and a well-informed therapist is better placed to give it. Chapter 3 examines elements of sleep science that underpin any advice that might be given, although many aspects of sleep remain a mystery and it is only possible here to consider the essentials and correct some misconceptions. For example, natural sleep is not a single unbroken state in which a person must spend a set amount of time each night; sleep consists of several stages and there is considerable variation between individuals in the amount of sleep that they need and in the time that they take it. However, science is only part of the picture. Chapter 4 explores the social context of sleep and how the 'rules' of sleep discussed in the previous chapter are broken. Sleep patterns have been different in history, they can vary between cultures and there are variations within cultures and society – for example, between men and women. But society is changing and there are competing demands for our time. This has always been the case to some degree (as for centuries people have used the night hours for social activity or studying, for example), but there is now so much more opportunity to delay or curtail sleep with modern technology and with the advent of the World Wide Web. The chapter therefore also considers how we make choices about sleep, noting the increasing pressure of other activity.

At the simplest level other activity can impact on sleep if less time is therefore allocated for sleep, but the relationship between sleep and activity is more complex. It might be tempting to think of sleep as 'downtime' but, although we do not know the precise functions of sleep, we do know what happens if we do not get enough sleep. As Chapter 5 shows, sleep is most certainly not downtime and essential processes continue during sleep and permit optimum performance of waking activity. In discussing the consequences of poor sleep it has become a tradition, almost a cliché, to list major incidents that have occurred as a result of, or been attributed to, sleep deficit – either because people worked too long without sleep or because of working at a time when naturally they should have been asleep. But apart from the large-scale or high-profile incidents there are countless 'near misses' and smaller incidents that do not make the headlines where, for example, a sleepy driver dies alone in the small hours of the morning. It is impossible to review the expansive range of evidence on the effects of sleep loss, and so the main focus of the chapter is on two important areas of occupational performance and executive function: driving, and memory and learning. Two key messages from the literature in these areas are that without adequate sleep our ability to drive, or to carry out other tasks that carry risks, can be negatively affected, to the extent that it would be by the consumption of alcohol, and that unless we sleep, learning can be compromised.

The other side of the reciprocal relationship between sleep and activity is considered in Chapter 6, which looks at the way that our daytime occupations – what we do and when we do it – can affect the amount and quality of our sleep at night. Research evidence shows the importance of physical activity as a means of improving sleep at all ages and especially for older people. Also, in old age it can be important to maintain regular routines and to remain engaged in activity. It is suggested that interaction with the environment is one of the factors that maintains the drive to sleep, and to have deep sleep, but a further benefit of activity is proposed. Daytime activity is the backdrop against which sleep occurs: it provides the 'behavioural contrast' that is necessary before winding down at night to sleep. It is argued that, therefore, occupational therapists could assume a more influential role in promoting better sleep, particularly among people whose daytime activity is restricted by their condition or circumstances (for example, some people in residential care).

Following the discussion of normal sleep in the first chapters, Chapter 7 turns to sleep disorders. An occupational therapist is unlikely to be asked to assist in the management of a less common sleep problem, but in most cases it is helpful to be aware of signs and symptoms of sleep disorders. Patients will, in the context of other interventions, often mention things to therapists or nurses that they might feel they cannot trouble a doctor with, or things that they had not even thought to talk about before. Armed with the basic information on sleep disorders, a therapist should know whether it is something that a patient needs to be concerned about and when it is necessary to advise referral to a specialist clinic. For example, phenomena such as sleep paralysis and hypnic jerks (described in Chapter 7) occurring on their own are harmless and should present no serious problem. There are some conditions where the advice that an occupational therapist might give can be considered 'fail-safe' in that it would be good advice for anyone, and common-sense rules might apply; however, in other cases, such as suspected obstructive sleep apnoea, restless leg syndrome or rapid eye movement (REM) sleep behaviour disorder, referral to the appropriate specialist service is needed.

Chapter 8 goes on to look in more detail at an area where an occupational therapist can make a difference and explores the management of insomnia in particular. It is stressed that reading an explanation of cognitive behavioural therapy for insomnia (CBT-I) methods here does not qualify readers to become 'sleep therapists', but the level of detail included should inform the reader of the evidence-based physiological rationale for seemingly straightforward advice such as not staying too long in bed or maintaining a regular rising time. It should also prevent the giving of unhelpful advice (such as to go to bed early to allow for extra sleep, or to go to bed at a regular time – because it can be unwise to go to bed unless one is sleepy). Management of excessive sleep is less well researched and the issue can be confused when fatigue is involved (discussed later), but there are some principles that can be applied and therapists should be aware of the possibilities.

The remainder of the book considers the particular sleep-related challenges faced by different sections of the population, or by people with a variety of conditions, and the sleeping conditions of people in particular circumstances. The sleep of children is especially important if it is assumed that sleep is essential for growth and development and for learning: children's sleep is also important for family harmony and the well-being of parents who need time to wind down before their own sleep. However, children's sleep differs in significant ways from the sleep of adults. First, it is to a great extent controlled by others: young children have limited influence over their environment and the timing of sleep. Second, they are less likely than an adult to realize that they have a sleep problem or to complain about it. Third, their sleep problems differ from adult sleep problems: there is the variation that exists between adults and children in all areas of medicine, but also some disorders of childhood sleep are culturally influenced. Furthermore, childhood sleep problems present a 'moving target' (Kuhn 2011, p.241): for example, it can be difficult to diagnose excessive sleepiness in a child of an age where daytime napping is the norm. Chapter 9 therefore reviews the physical, environmental and social components that contribute to sleep deficiency in young people. A case study of a young girl with cerebral palsy is woven through the chapter to illustrate the application of theory and evidence to occupational therapy practice. Assessment tools and non-pharmacological interventions are discussed, and the Model of Human Occupation (MoHO) is applied to illustrate how well-established occupational therapy theory can guide practice in this area.

At the other end of the age spectrum, the sleep of older adults is affected by, or changes as a part of, the ageing process. There are life changes and differences in roles and routines in later life along with the increasing possibility of infirmity and its consequences. The evidence shows a clear relationship between sleep deficiency and the risk for diabetes, falls, cardiovascular conditions and dementia. It is therefore important that occupational therapists working with older adults understand that addressing sleep problems is an essential component of any treatment plan. A particular barrier to dealing with sleep problems among older adults is the popular misconception that poor sleep is just a part of ageing, and to be expected; this might deter an elderly person from asking for help or might cause a professional to assume that nothing can be done. Chapter 10 challenges that assumption and, again, using the MoHO to help to make sense of the complex set of factors affecting sleep in older adults, presents an illustrative case study guiding the reader through aetiology, assessment and intervention. The intervention focus in this chapter is particularly on the range of evidence-based, pragmatic, easy-to-achieve environmental modifications that can be made in the home setting or in residential facilities to promote better sleep.

Like children, and some older adults in residential care, many people with a learning disability, or intellectual disability, might have less control over their environment, and their conditions can also have a negative impact on sleep. Figures show that sleep problems are very common for people with a learning disability, but (as with the elderly) it is probable that many health professionals assume that little or nothing can be done to help, or they may not ask about sleep problems. Research in this area is limited, but Chapter 11 draws on what evidence there is and on the authors' experience to make recommendations for measures to improve sleep. It is evident that a good balance of daytime activity can promote healthy night-time sleep, and therefore a challenge for all services is to encourage greater engagement.

Illness can interfere with sleep at any stage in the life cycle. It has been observed already that sleep disruption is associated with most mental illnesses, something that was noted by Emil Kraepelin in 1883 (Wulff *et al.* 2010). Furthermore, as noted by Spiegelhalder *et al.* (2013), disturbed sleep is a risk factor for many psychiatric disorders. The relationship between anxiety and insomnia is so close that it may not be clear which precedes the other. Early waking is a feature of depression, whereas in hypomania sleep is often reduced; in schizophrenia the timing of sleep may be disturbed.

In the case of post-traumatic stress disorder, chronic sleep deficiency is a risk factor for the development of the condition, while insomnia is a common symptom of it. Members of the armed services, police officers and firefighters experience a high rate of sleep problems as an outcome of traumatizing experiences in job situations with ongoing exposure to harmful and stressful events. The majority of sleep research in trauma-exposed workers involves members of the military. This research demonstrates that social values, workplace cultures and role expectations of endurance – to the extent that seeking help for sleep deficiency could be seen as a weakness – all contribute to sleep problems being under-assessed and under-treated in this group. Chapter 12 therefore draws heavily on the evidence base as it relates to sleep and military personnel, but occupational therapists can use the information presented as a basis to understand the sleep difficulties of their patients in similarly stressful, trauma-exposed work settings.

Chapter 13 considers sleep problems in the wider context of psychiatric disorders, including dementias. It would be easy, from a medical perspective, to target sleep problems with medication alone, just as it would be to suggest that cognitive behavioural strategies are the exclusive answer. Rather, this chapter takes a wider perspective and considers the concept of well-being. Sleep is not just something we do at night to pass the time: it is part of a bigger picture and many aspects of change to our waking activity can impact on it. It is therefore important to work towards a healthy and balanced lifestyle. The 'Sound Sleep' course is included in the appendices of the chapter. It is much 'slower' than a CBT-I course, as is appropriate for the client group who may have multiple problems; however, the course could be adapted for use in a range of settings and with a range of other client groups.

The evidence shows a close relationship between sleep problems and psychiatric disorder and also between sleep problems and neurodegenerative disease: as Wulff *et al.* (2010) point out, sleep disturbance is the most commonly reported sign preceding the onset of such conditions. Other neurodegenerative conditions are considered in Chapter 15, but sleep problems in the context of dementia, principally Alzheimer's disease, are discussed in Chapter 14. Dementia is an increasing problem as the population ages and also has implications on the sleep of carers. Wulff *et al.* (2010) observe that timed activities and social cues are useful in regulating sleep, adding further support to the suggestion that there is a role for occupational therapists in managing sleep problems.

Sleep might be disturbed by symptoms of any physical illness, from the common cold to cancer, but there are particular effects in some neurological conditions, such as Parkinson's disease, multiple sclerosis (MS), brain injury and stroke, where it is not only discomfort or pain that disrupts sleep. Chapter 15 describes some of the complications in sleep experienced by people with such conditions. For example, restless legs syndrome, which appears to be related to MS, can disrupt night-time sleep, leading to daytime sleepiness, which in turn complicates the experience of fatigue that is common in MS. In other cases there is the possibility of damage to sleep-wake or circadian systems. However, there appears to be a significant gap in the medical knowledge when it comes to sleep problems in the context of neurological conditions and therefore a consequent lack of evidence for management. The chapter suggests that, having intensive and/or ongoing contact with neurological patients, occupational therapists are in a position to investigate the management of their sleep difficulties.

Occupational therapists are also accustomed to dealing with patients with chronic pain and patients with chronic fatigue; in both cases sleep is frequently compromised and, in turn, disrupted sleep makes worse the experience of the other problem. Chapter 16 outlines the relationship between sleep and pain. Advances in neuroscience indicate that pain and sleep mechanisms share many neural pathways and neurotransmitters, which in the coming years might bring important developments in treatment. It is common, as observed by Ashworth, Davidson and Espie (2010), that sleep problems are often attributed to pain, and for chronic-pain patients to believe that only when pain is relieved will their sleep improve. It is a common-sense view, but Ashworth *et al.* (2010) suggest that people might therefore fail to use effective strategies to manage sleep. There is, in fact, much that can be done to improve sleep, especially interventions that promote self-efficacy and align with the principles of self-management, demonstrated to be influential in pain management programmes. The research indicates that sleep and pain appear to have a reciprocal relationship such that it is reasonable to assume that when clients with chronic pain have improved sleep, a lessening of pain symptoms will also follow.

Chronic fatigue is another symptom where occupational therapists are frequently involved in self-management programmes, and occupational therapy may be the profession with the greatest representation in specialist services for chronic fatigue syndrome/myalgic encephalomyelitis. As Chapter 17 indicates, sleep problems are commonly associated with it: insomnia, excessive sleep and disruption of sleep patterns are all common. Despite the main feature being fatigue, chronic fatigue syndrome is not caused by sleep deprivation nor is it 'cured' by sleep. A particular difficulty, however, is that the experiences of fatigue and need for sleep are closely related. One possible way in which disruption to sleep patterns occurs is when an individual rests because of tiredness and begins to sleep for longer periods, and for periods during the day. It is also likely that, as in other cases, it is difficult to keep to the healthy routines that help to maintain a regular pattern of sleep.

It is very easy to give advice to adjust bedtimes and rising times, to turn the heating up or down, or to encourage exercise as a means of improving sleep; however, that would be to assume that there is always individual choice. It can be difficult for anyone to incorporate new things into their routines, and harder still if that has an impact on a partner or on children, but for some people restrictions of their particular living conditions impose constraints that can make change extremely difficult. In Chapter 18 the environmental conditions necessary for sleep are revisited since investigation of the 'normal' provides the necessary background for looking at three particular situations where other priorities do not always allow the creation of conditions ideal for sleep: hospital, correctional institutions and residential care. This is another area where the evidence is thin: there is very little research on which to draw, especially in relation to prisons where only a small number of occupational therapists work. It may not be realistic to make wholesale changes to conditions in acute hospital wards or prisons, for example, but with enhanced understanding of sleep and its relationship to daytime occupation and to the environment, occupational therapists can advise on modifications to environment or routines that could lead to improved sleep.

A contention of this book is that occupational therapists need to understand sleep. If occupation has a close relationship with use of time, as suggested by Farnworth (2004) and Finlay (2004), occupational therapists have been overlooking a major occupation for too long. Sleep is essential for health and well-being, and occupational therapists can contribute to improved sleep in four ways. First, they can be active in the prevention of sleep problems by raising awareness of the complex associations between sleep and many health-related issues. Second, they can be involved in the screening of patients and clients for treatable sleep problems. Third, they can help to improve sleep by applying basic principles of 'sleep therapy' as well as by encouraging participation in the exercise and activity that promote good sleep, especially in those whose opportunities might be more limited. Finally, they can be advocates for the organizational changes in living environments, school settings, care facilities and workplaces that are required to reduce the risk of sleep deficiency.

This book cannot provide all the answers: as noted above, there is still so much that is unknown about sleep. Furthermore, although the pharmacological and cognitive behavioural management of sleep disorders have been well researched, the principles of other non-pharmacological and environmental sleep management have yet to be widely studied. Additionally, we need better understanding of the sleep problems that occur in the context of other biopsychosocial problems, psychiatric or neurological, or in childhood or old age. Occupational therapists are well-established practitioners in all these circumstances: they understand how illness affects our daily activity and, crucially, how our actions can influence our health. They are perfectly positioned to take on the assessment of sleep problems in their patients and clients. Furthermore, if they do not take more responsibility in terms of helping with the management of sleep problems, it is not clear who else will.

References

Ashworth, P.C.H., Davidson, K.M. and Espie, C.A. (2010) 'Cognitive-behavioral factors associated with sleep quality in chronic pain patients.' *Behavioral Sleep Medicine 8*, 1, 28–39.

Espie, C.A. (2009) '"Stepped care": a health technology solution for delivering cognitive behavioural therapy as a first line insomnia treatment.' *Sleep 32*, 12, 1549–1558.

Espie, C.A., Kyle, S.D., Williams, C., Ong, J.C. *et al.* (2012) 'A randomized, placebo-controlled trial of online cognitive behavioural therapy for chronic insomnia disorder delivered via an automated media-rich web application.' *Sleep 35*, 6, 769–781.

Farnworth, L. (2004) 'Time Use and Disability.' In M. Molineux (ed) *Occupation for Occupational Therapists.* Oxford: Blackwell.

Finlay, L. (2004) *The Practice of Psychosocial Occupational Therapy*, 3rd edn. Cheltenham: Nelson Thornes.

Green, A. (2008) 'Sleep, occupation and the passage of time.' *British Journal of Occupational Therapy 71*, 8, 339–347.

Kuhn, B.R. (2011) 'BSM Protocols for Pediatric Sleep Disorders: Introduction.' In M. Perlis, M. Aloia and B. Kuhn (eds) *Behavioral Treatments for Sleep Disorders: A Comprehensive Primer of Behavioral Sleep Medicine Interventions.* London: Elsevier.

Peile, E. (2010) 'A Commentary on Sleep Education.' In F.P. Cappuccio, M.A. Miller and S.W. Lockley (eds) *Sleep, Health, and Society: From Aetiology to Public Health.* Oxford: Oxford University Press.

Spiegelhalder, K., Regen, W., Nanovska, S., Baglioni, C. and Riemann, D. (2013) 'Comorbid sleep disorders in neuropsychiatric disorders across the life cycle.' *Current Psychiatry Reports 15*, 6, 364.

Stores, G. (2007) 'Clinical diagnosis and misdiagnosis of sleep disorders.' *Journal of Neurology, Neurosurgery and Psychiatry 78*, 12, 1293–1297.

Stores, G. and Crawford, C. (1998) 'Medical student education in sleep and its disorders.' *Journal of the Royal College of Physicians of London 32*, 2, 149–153.

Vincent, N. and Walsh, K. (2013) 'Stepped care for insomnia: an evaluation of implementation in routine practice.' *Journal of Clinical Sleep Medicine 9*, 3, 227–234.

Wulff, K.L., Gatti, S., Wettstein, J.G. and Foster, R.G. (2010) 'Sleep and circadian rhythm disruption in psychiatric and neurodegenerative disease.' *Nature Reviews Neuroscience 11*, 8, 589–599.

2

SLEEP AND OCCUPATION

Andrew Green

2.1 Introduction

It is suggested in Chapter 1, and argued throughout this book, that occupational therapists could take a greater part in managing the sleep difficulties of their patients and clients. It is proposed that from a more practical perspective there is a strong argument that they are well placed to assume a positive role; occupational therapists are 'on the ground' and already working in practical ways with patients – looking at the intricacies of their daily lives and encouraging personal independence. Adding the management of sleep problems to their portfolio would not be a big step in reality; however, the chief purpose of this chapter is to investigate the more theoretical case for occupational therapists taking an interest in promoting good sleep. It outlines the place of sleep in occupational therapy from early times to the present, traces the recent growth of interest in sleep in occupational therapy and occupational science, and concludes by making the case for occupational therapists to be involved in managing sleep problems.

2.2 Sleep in occupational therapy, from the early years

It is often observed that Adolf Meyer (neuropsychiatrist and early proponent of occupational therapy) stressed the importance for health of the balance between the 'big four': work, play, rest and sleep (Meyer 1922). In exploring the concept of rest, Howell and Pierce (2000) note how rest and sleep were largely ignored, in spite of being among Meyer's primary categories of occupation; they state that in Meyer's time 'both work and sleep were newly freed from the age-old tempo of daylight and dark by the advent of electricity' thereby 'plung[ing] humans into chronic and culture-wide sleep-debt' (p.68). They suggest that the oversight of the restorative qualities of occupation by occupational therapy is 'striking' and that Meyer's argument in favour of balance should have led to greater interest in restorative occupation. They observed that 'despite the current research in sleep medicine, sleep has received very little attention from occupational science. This is remarkable…' (Howell and Pierce 2000, p.69). However, on reflection, it is perhaps not surprising that occupational therapists did not pay much attention to sleep in the early years of the profession, and it is likely that in approaching the question of balance from different angles, and in different eras, Meyer and Howell and Pierce place a different emphasis on things. Howell and Pierce, writing in present times, argue from a perspective that suggests that we are insufficiently rested, and they reasonably support restorative occupations (or 'doing' less), whereas Meyer was arguing for his patients to be more active and to do more.

Although Meyer argued reasonably for balance, there is no evidence that he proposed that occupational therapists should do anything to promote sleep when he named his 'big four…which our organism must be able to balance'. He continued: 'The only way to attain balance in all this is *actual doing, actual practice*, a program of wholesome living' (Meyer 1922, p.6; original emphasis). While Meyer was arguing for balance, it seems clear that he perceived the missing element for his patients to be work:

> Man learns to organize time and he does it in terms of *doing* things, and one of the many good things he does between eating, drinking and wholesome nutrition generally and the flights of fancy and aspiration, we call *work and occupation*. (Meyer 1922, p.9; original emphasis)

Indeed, earlier in his address (to the National Society for the Promotion of Occupational Therapy in 1921) he quoted from a report on 'the employment of the insane', dated 1882: 'Employment of some sort should be made obligatory for all able-bodied patients' (Meyer 1922, p.2). The difficulty was the presence of private patients who, presumably, could not be compelled to work.

In Meyer's time, and in the context of institutional care, the lack of opportunity for sleep was not the problem. Therapy was *occupation* and the emphasis would naturally be on activity, as opposed to the inactivity that might otherwise be evident in asylums or hospital wards: nurses could be expected to take care of patients' need for sleep and rest. Sleep was therefore never likely to be part of occupational therapy's role in the very early years. As Koketsu (2013) observes, it could be that occupational therapists are so busy attending to patients' needs in areas of waking occupations that focusing on sleep might not be prioritized. Furthermore, as Iwama notes in the foreword of this book, occupational therapy has its roots in the Western world where work is particularly valued – a point also made by Howell and Pierce (2000) (see also Chapter 4). This emphasis on activity and work persisted in most occupational therapy practice.

In his foreword, Iwama also draws attention to Reilly's frequently quoted, but untested, hypothesis that it is the use of our *hands* that influences health (Reilly 1962). In her 1961 lecture she states that the 'duty of an organism is to grow and be productive…

If it were not desirable to be productive, the skills and practices of occupational therapy would be irrelevant' (p.5). She claims that 'the logic of occupational therapy rests upon the principle that man has a need to master his environment, to alter and improve it' (p.6), and throughout the lecture she discusses work – drawing on a range of perspectives, as is clear from her bibliographical notes. Reilly makes no more than a passing mention of sleep in her lecture; like Meyer, she recognizes its importance for self-preservation but, also like Meyer, she gives no indication that occupational therapists should pay any attention to it.

Two decades after Reilly, following a fascinating account that traced the origins of occupational therapy, Bing (1981) reminded his audience that 'occupational therapy is the only major health profession whose focus centers upon the total human organism's involvement in *tasks* – a *making* or *doing*' and that 'any differentiation between ourselves and other health providers must have as its major theme *occupation and leisure*' (p.515). Again, the focus remained more on doing, and not on sleeping.

A year before Bing (1981) gave his lecture, Kielhofner and Burke (1980) noted that occupational therapy lacked 'a universal conceptual foundation to shape its identity and guide its practice' (p.572) and unveiled their Model of Human Occupation (MoHO), which has since become a major influence in the profession. A search of digital copies of that article, and the subsequent three articles that introduced the model, confirms that the word 'sleep' does not appear to be used anywhere – not even in the context of balance as Meyer (1922) and Reilly (1962) used it. Of course, Kielhofner and Burke did discuss balance, as Christiansen (1996) notes, and also nod towards Meyer in discussing habits, as follows: 'While the adult generally has habits organized around requirements for productivity, habits must also allow time for rest, play and sleep' (Kielhofner and Burke 1985, p.29).

Forsyth and Kielhofner (2011) note that the MoHO provides a theory to account for occupation and the occupational problems that are associated with illness and disability, and they claim that it is the most evidence-based, occupation-focused model. Accordingly, Lee *et al.* (2008) found in a survey of 1000 therapists in the US that over 80% of respondents reported using the MoHO at least some of the time. The latest adaptation of the model (Kielhofner 2008) also makes little mention of sleep yet, despite that, the case studies in four chapters of this book draw upon the model in discussion of the management of sleep problems. The omission of sleep is not a criticism of the MoHO, but it is a testament to the strength of the model that it can be applied anyway.

The MoHO is consistent with other occupational therapy models in not emphasizing sleep, although some do, of course, acknowledge it. For example, among the intrinsic factors comprising the Person-Environment-Occupation-Performance (PEOP) model (Baum, Bass-Haugen and Christiansen 2005) are physiological factors which include sleep. The authors note that 'people cannot be truly well if they cannot participate fully in their lives' (Christiansen, Baum and Bass 2011, p.96). They could have added that people cannot participate fully in their lives if they do not regularly get adequate sleep; however, although Christiansen has much more to say on sleep, in relation to balance, the PEOP model says no more. Other models also acknowledge balance without much reference to sleep. (For more information on occupational therapy models see, for example, Duncan 2011.)

It has been shown that there is a long history of occupational therapy being concerned with doing: quite recently, Lee *et al.* (2008) confirmed that 'contemporary scholars in occupational therapy agree that *occupation* should be the central construct underlying the field and its practice' (p.106; emphasis added). It is therefore not surprising that occupational therapy models have overlooked sleep. It is not known whether this relates to the uncertain status of sleep as an occupation (see Green 2008), but there does seem to have been a shift in emphasis. Whereas Kielhofner and Burke (1985) could state that 'occupational behaviour' is 'activity in which persons engage during most of their *waking* time' (p.12; emphasis added), the American Occupational Therapy Association (AOTA) now clearly places sleep among categories of occupation (AOTA 2008, 2014), and Wilcock and Townsend (2014) have stated that 'occupation is used to mean all the things people want, need, or have to do…and is inclusive of sleep and rest' (p.542). This upsurge of interest is discussed in the following section.

2.3 Recent interest in sleep among occupational therapists

In the previous section it is suggested that the focus of occupational therapy has been occupation (that is, more active occupation as opposed to restorative occupation), but that is not to imply that occupational therapists have been wilfully negligent in not focusing on sleep. It has been noted previously (Green 2008) that standard occupational therapy textbooks overlooked sleep, and that coverage of the issue was patchy in more specialized texts. A search of the electronic index of the *American Journal of Occupational Therapy* between 1980 and 2013 revealed one article with 'sleep' in the title (a brief report relating to infant sleep and play positioning). A search for the word in the abstract of articles during the same period yielded nine occurrences, mostly related to older adults or to children; however, one article (Krupa *et al.* 2003) referred to sleep in relation to time use (see below).

It is uncertain why interest in sleep has grown in occupational therapy in recent years. Articles on sleep appeared in the occupational therapy literature in the UK during the first decade of the new century (Green 2008; Green *et al.* 2005; Green, Hicks and Wilson 2008).[1] At the same time, between 2002 and 2008, the AOTA upgraded 'sleep and rest' to a separate occupational performance area in successive versions of its Occupational Therapy Practice Frameworks (AOTA 2002, 2008). Accordingly, new editions of two major textbooks have chapters on sleep (Boyt Schell, Gillen and Scaffa

2014; McHugh Pendleton and Schultz-Krohn 2013), and occupational therapists are beginning to publish on aspects of sleep: in Canada the first article on sleep in an occupational therapy publication appeared in 2009 (Fjeldsted and Hanlon-Dearman 2009), and Brown and colleagues have published in a New Zealand occupational therapy journal (Brown *et al.* 2012) as well as various interdisciplinary journals (Brown *et al.* 2013; Brown, Berry and Schmidt 2013).

Engel-Yeger and Shochat (2012) conducted what appears to be the first quantitative study relating to sleep to be published in an occupational therapy journal – adding to qualitative studies by Green *et al.* (2008) and O'Donoghue and McKay (2012). They investigated the relationship between sleep quality and sensory processing patterns in healthy adults using existing psychometric assessments. They found that poor sleep quality was predicted by the increased avoidance of sensory stimuli, specifically auditory stimuli, and that 'it appears that poor sleepers not only exhibit a low-sensory threshold (i.e. are hypersensitive), but actively try to fend off or avoid disturbing sensations in their environment' (p.139). They suggest that, 'together with their clients, therapists may create environmental accommodations that will fit these sensory needs' (p.139). They conclude that occupational therapists' assessments and interventions should include information about sleep quality, especially where the individual has sensory processing difficulties.

More recently, another Canadian team (Fung *et al.* 2013) proposed that the assessment of sleep (and wakefulness) should be routine in occupational therapy practice and point to the AOTA (2008) practice framework that includes sleep (as noted above). They argue that occupational therapists are in a position to provide education and interventions to modify behaviours to optimize sleep. In order for such assessment and intervention to occur, Fung *et al.* (2013) advocate the inclusion of education on sleep and wakefulness in occupational therapy curricula and in post-qualification professional development.

A possible reason for this increased interest in sleep is the growth of occupational science. As noted elsewhere (Green 2008), during the 1990s Charles Christiansen, with others, and Ann Wilcock started to become influential in exploring the relationship between sleep and occupation. Basing her comments on the study of sleep science, Wilcock (1998) stressed the importance of sleep for the performance of occupations and suggested the possibility of a relationship between sleep patterns and regular occupation. Subsequently, Wilcock (2003) placed sleep firmly in the 'occupation cycle' (p.171). Perhaps sleep has to be considered in this context: if occupational scientists are studying human occupation and/or time use, it would make no sense to stop observations when people go to bed. Similarly, if sleep is one of the factors that affects occupational performance, it would seem to be a legitimate, even essential, area of concern for occupational scientists.

Christiansen (1996) appears to have two starting points in exploring sleep: first, balance – beginning with Meyer and noting his emphasis on work – and, second, time use, stating that 'to consider activity patterns is to contemplate how we allocate or "budget" time' (p.434). In reviewing the influences on chronological balance, Christiansen (1996) inevitably discusses biological rhythms, including circadian rhythms and the sleep-wake cycle, or rest-activity cycle. He noted the importance of environmental and social factors (known as zeitgebers*; see Chapter 3) in regulating circadian rhythms. On reviewing social factors he concluded prophetically: 'While being out of balance with our internal rhythms is seldom considered as a performance factor in occupational therapy, it may well be substantially more important than we realize' (p.445); see Chapters 5 and 6 for further discussion.

Working with Kathleen Matuska, Christiansen has explored further the concept of lifestyle balance (Christiansen and Matuska 2006; Matuska and Christiansen 2008). Lifestyle balance is defined by Christiansen and Matuska (2006) as 'a consistent pattern of occupations that results in reduced stress and improved health and well-being' (p.50). They note that imbalance may be experienced, among other things, as fatigue or drowsiness as a result of insufficient sleep, and they suggest that certain conditions 'that reflect atypical occupational patterns…should be considered *de facto* indicators of lifestyle imbalance' (p.56). Among these conditions they include insomnia and sleep disorders (as well as workaholism, burnout and obesity).

Matuska and Christiansen (2008) proposed a model of lifestyle balance. The first dimension of the model is 'biological health and physical safety', and it is noted that the needs of biological health, security and safety are generally accepted as a given, despite a lack of research on how best to meet these needs. However, Matuska and Christiansen (2008) observe that cumulative research is convincing on the health benefits of 'good nutrition, exercise, safety practices…adequate sleep and avoiding addictive substances' (p.12). They note that health and safety needs were clearly identified by Maslow (1943), for example, but that they are not emphasized because they are generally accepted as being health-promoting (that is, 'everyone knows'). However, their model gives prominence to these needs and Matuska and Christiansen (2008) conclude that 'without good health, the likelihood of sustaining occupations to meet other critical needs is diminished' (p.12). In explaining the fifth dimension of the model ('organize time and energy to meet important personal goals and personal renewal') they note that in contemporary Western society time may be seen as a commodity, and that 'routine demands of living exceed the time available for them' (p.14) and they stress the importance of regular routines for health.

The clearest indication of the importance of sleep is given by Matuska and Christiansen (2009) in reviewing factors that can disrupt balance, which also include obesity and circadian desynchronosis (jet lag). They discuss insomnia and sleep disorders and note a clear association between stress and sleep, stating that 'because sleep is such a major and necessary daily occupation, its disturbance almost by definition constitutes an imbalance in time use and lifestyle' (p.157). They go on to point out that the literature shows a relationship between sleep quality and what people do in the day.

The work of Christiansen and Matuska is a welcome reminder of the importance of balance and looking after physiological needs, although they trace the concept of balance back to well before Meyer and Maslow (to ancient Greece, Chinese medicine and Native American healing, for example). The difference is perhaps that in contemporary Western society the pressures have changed. Although the majority of us are not confronted by the pressures of war and famine in the way that our ancestors were, for example, we are under different pressures, perhaps of our own making but which are hard to escape from and cause us to try to fit ever more into our time.

In examining how people make use of time (see also Chapter 4) it is inevitable that occupational therapists will start considering sleep – not least in working out how to differentiate daytime sleep from rest and sedentary activity (see Green 2012). For example, a number of studies published in the UK and US occupational therapy literature in the first decade of this century indicate that, for example, people with enduring mental health problems in the community, or in forensic units, tend to spend more time inactive or sleeping than the general population (Farnworth, Nikitin and Fossey 2004; Krupa *et al.* 2003; Shimitras, Fossey and Harvey 2003; Stewart and Craik 2007).

2.4 Why should occupational therapists be involved with sleep problems?

It is argued so far in this chapter that, first, throughout the evolution of occupational therapy the emphasis has been on occupation (i.e. doing) to the exclusion of more restorative occupations and sleep. Second, in the past two decades there has been a growing interest in sleep which appears to derive from the contribution of occupational science. However, it was not a failure of occupational therapy in neglecting sleep in its early years: as noted, the focus was understandably on activity, but at the time that Meyer was writing (and Reilly and even Bing decades later) sleep science was barely advanced,[2] and little evidence-based advice was available for busy therapists to give to their patients, assuming they had considered it their role to offer such advice. Furthermore, even doctors, as noted in Chapter 1, had – or have – very little education on sleep and sleep problems. It has only been since the 1980s that sleep medicine has really become established (for example, the British Sleep Society was formed in 1988), and understanding of many sleep disorders and their management followed many years later.

Research in sleep science and sleep medicine now confirms the importance of sleep, not only for daytime performance but also for long-term health. The effects of sleep loss on concentration and on memory and learning are considered in Chapter 5, but the associations of poor sleep with a number of psychiatric and medical conditions (for example, diabetes and obesity) make it the business of all health professionals to encourage good sleep habits in the same way that they should, for example, discourage smoking or promote regular exercise.

It is not only scientific knowledge that has changed: society has transformed in the century since Meyer cared for his institutionalized patients. Meyer died in 1950 and even then could not have conceived the changes that would occur with the revolutionary technological advances and globalization of the second half of the twentieth century and, importantly, their effects on people. Just two examples illustrate the changes: in post-war Britain, most people lived close to where they worked or made a relatively short journey by train or bus, on foot or by bicycle, but it is not uncommon now for people to drive an hour or more each way, or to have a 2-hour train journey to work; others might commute by air each week to another country. In post-war Britain, television was in its infancy and the telephone was expensive and far from universal; the opportunities now for entertainment and communication seem limitless and we can stay up all night watching films, playing games or chatting with friends. In the past, occupational therapists (or others) would not need to advise anyone to take time to wind down before sleep; the 'worst' that people did would be to take work home or to get too engrossed in a good book at bedtime.

It seems obvious that someone has to do something about sleep problems. Occupational therapists are used to looking at the way people live their lives, at their routines and at their environment. It is a relatively small extension of practice to take account of sleep. Whether sleep is or is not an occupation is perhaps an academic question, but the relationship that sleep has with occupation, as can be seen in Chapters 5 and 6, is beyond doubt. A substantial body of research, coupled with everyday experience, tells us of the importance of sleep: research is increasingly suggesting that what we do in the day – our occupations – can affect our sleep. Given that, it is difficult to see how occupational therapy can fail to pay attention to sleep.

2.5 Conclusion

Occupational therapy has overlooked sleep for much of its history, focusing instead on more active occupation. More recently, interest in sleep has grown, perhaps under the influence of occupational science. Scientific knowledge of sleep has also increased and we now understand better the associations between sleep and health. Furthermore, society has changed and increased the pressure on individuals to curtail sleep. All health professionals should encourage good sleep, but occupational therapists are particularly well placed to do so because of their understanding of environment and the routines of their patients, as well as their understanding of occupation, which is both affected by and affects sleep.

Notes

1   It is fair to say that my interest in sleep did not develop from any theoretical standpoint or review of the literature. As so often, it was through a series of random events: first, being asked to be involved in the insomnia group programme, and then just adapting to meet the needs of patients referred from the sleep clinic. My interest in sleep grew simply because sleep is so interesting. What happened then is that I became concerned that it could be suggested that it is not the place of an occupational therapist to be involved in managing sleep problems. My strategy to establish the case for involvement started with a simple tactic: if articles on sleep were published in a peer-reviewed occupational therapy journal, it must be a legitimate concern for an occupational therapist. In the process of publishing I became aware that some colleagues in my profession lacked understanding of sleep and I therefore set out to investigate further what was known – the eventual result being this book.

2   For an overview of the state of sleep science at that time see Bruce (n.d.) or Sumner (1923).

Acknowledgements

Thanks to Jennifer Garden of Capilano University, British Columbia, and Mallory Watson of the University of Alberta for contributions to a previous draft of this chapter.

References

American Occupational Therapy Association (2002) 'Occupational Therapy Practice Framework: Domain and Process.' *American Journal of Occupational Therapy 56*, 6, 609–639.

American Occupational Therapy Association (2008) 'Occupational Therapy Practice Framework: Domain and Process, 2nd edn.' *American Journal of Occupational Therapy 62*, 6, 625–683.

American Occupational Therapy Association (2014) 'Occupational Therapy Practice Framework: Domain and Process, 3rd edn.' *American Journal of Occupational Therapy 68*, Suppl. 1, S1–S48.

Baum, C.M., Bass-Haugen, J. and Christiansen, C.H. (2005) 'Person-Environment-Occupation-Performance: a Model for Planning Interventions for Individuals and Organizations.' In C.H. Christiansen, C.M. Baum and J. Bass-Haugen (eds) *Occupational Therapy: Performance, Participation and Well-being*, 3rd edn. Thorofare, NJ: Slack Incorporated.

Bing, R.K. (1981) 'Occupational therapy revisited: a paraphrastic journey.' *American Journal of Occupational Therapy 35*, 8, 499–518.

Boyt Schell, B.A., Gillen, G. and Scaffa, M.E. (eds) (2014) *Willard & Spackman's Occupational Therapy*, 12th edn. Philadelphia, PA: Lippincott Williams & Wilkins.

Brown, C.A., Berry, R. and Schmidt, A. (2013) 'Sleep and military members: emerging issues and nonpharmacological intervention.' *Sleep Disorders*. doi: 10.1155/2013/160374.

Brown, C.A., Berry, R., Tan, M., Khoshia, A., Turlapati, L. and Swedlove, F. (2013) 'A critique of the evidence-base for non-pharmacological sleep interventions for persons with dementia.' *Dementia: The International Journal of Social Research and Practice 12*, 2, 174–201.

Brown, C., Swedlove, F., Berry, R. and Turlapati, L. (2012) 'Occupational therapists' health literacy interventions for children with disordered sleep and/or pain.' *New Zealand Journal of Occupational Therapy 59*, 2, 9–17.

Bruce, H.A. (n.d.) *Sleep and Sleeplessness.* Kila, MT: Kessinger Publishing. (Original work published in 1915.)

Christiansen, C.H. (1996) 'Three Perspectives on Balance in Occupation.' In R. Zemke and F. Clark (eds) *Occupational Science: The Evolving Discipline.* Philadelphia, PA: F.A. Davis.

Christiansen, C., Baum, C. and Bass, J. (2011) 'The Person-Environment-Occupation-Performance (PEOP) Model.' In E.A.S Duncan (ed) *Foundations for Practice in Occupational Therapy*, 5th edn. Edinburgh: Churchill Livingstone.

Christiansen, C.H. and Matuska, K.M. (2006) 'Lifestyle balance: a review of concepts and research.' *Journal of Occupational Science 13*, 1, 49–61.

Duncan, E.A.S. (ed) (2011) *Foundations for Practice in Occupational Therapy.* Edinburgh: Churchill Livingstone.

Engel-Yeger, B. and Shochat, T. (2012) 'The relationship between sensory processing patterns and sleep quality in healthy adults.' *Canadian Journal of Occupational Therapy 79*, 3, 134–141.

Farnworth, L., Nikitin, L. and Fossey, E. (2004) 'Being in a secure forensic psychiatric unit: every day is the same, killing time or making the most of it.' *British Journal of Occupational Therapy 67*, 10, 430–438.

Fjeldsted, B. and Hanlon-Dearman, A. (2009) 'Sensory processing and sleep challenges in children with fetal alcohol spectrum disorder.' *Occupational Therapy Now 11*, 5, 26–28.

Forsyth, K. and Kielhofner, G. (2011) 'The Model of Human Occupation.' In E.A.S Duncan (ed) *Foundations for Practice in Occupational Therapy*, 5th edn. Edinburgh: Churchill Livingstone.

Fung, C., Wiseman-Hakes, C., Stergiou-Kita, M., Nguyen, M. and Colantonio, A. (2013) 'Time to wake up: bridging the gap between theory and practice for sleep in occupational therapy.' *British Journal of Occupational Therapy 76*, 8, 384–386.

Green, A. (2008) 'Sleep, occupation and the passage of time.' *British Journal of Occupational Therapy 71*, 8, 339–347.

Green, A. (2012) 'A Question of Balance: The Relationship Between Daily Occupation and Sleep.' In A. Green and A. Westcombe (eds) *Sleep: Multiprofessional Perspectives.* London: Jessica Kingsley Publishers.

Green, A., Hicks, J., Weekes, R. and Wilson, S. (2005) 'A cognitive-behavioural group intervention for people with chronic insomnia: an initial evaluation.' *British Journal of Occupational Therapy 68*, 11, 518–522.

Green, A., Hicks, J. and Wilson, S. (2008) 'The experience of poor sleep and its consequences: a qualitative study involving people referred for cognitive-behavioural management of chronic insomnia.' *British Journal of Occupational Therapy 71*, 5, 196–204.

Howell, D. and Pierce, D. (2000) 'Exploring the forgotten restorative dimension of occupation: quilting and quilt use.' *Journal of Occupational Science 7*, 2, 68–72.

Kielhofner, G. (2008) *Model of Human Occupation: Theory and Application*, 4th edn. Philadelphia, PA: Lippincott Williams & Wilkins.

Kielhofner, G. and Burke, J.P. (1980) 'A Model of Human Occupation, Part 1: Conceptual framework and content.' *American Journal of Occupational Therapy 34*, 9, 572–581.

Kielhofner, G. and Burke, J.P. (1985) 'Components and Determinants of Human Occupation.' In G. Kielhofner (ed) *A Model of Human Occupation: Theory and Application.* Baltimore, MD: Williams and Wilkins.

Koketsu, J.S. (2013) 'Sleep and Rest.' In H. McHugh Pendleton and W. Schultz-Krohn (eds) *Pedretti's Occupational Therapy: Practice Skills for Physical Dysfunction*, 7th edn. St Louis, MO: Elsevier Mosby.

Krupa, T., McLean, H., Eastabrook, S., Bonham, A. and Baksh, L. (2003) 'Daily time use as a measure of community adjustment for persons served by Assertive Community Treatment teams.' *American Journal of Occupational Therapy 57*, 5, 558–565.

Lee, S.W., Taylor, R., Kielhofner, G. and Fisher, G. (2008) 'Theory use in practice: a national survey of therapists who use the Model of Human Occupation.' *American Journal of Occupational Therapy 62*, 1, 106–111.

Maslow, A.H. (1943) 'A theory of human motivation.' *Psychological Review 50*, 4, 370–396.

Matuska, K.M. and Christiansen, C.H. (2008) 'A proposed model of lifestyle balance.' *Journal of Occupational Science 15*, 1, 9–19.

Matuska, K. and Christiansen, C.H. (2009) 'A Theoretical Model of Life Balance and Imbalance.' In K. Matuska and C.H. Christiansen (eds) *Life Balance: Multidisciplinary Theories and Research.* Thorofare, NJ: Slack Incorporated.

McHugh Pendleton, H. and Schultz-Krohn, W. (2013) *Pedretti's Occupational Therapy: Practice Skills for Physical Dysfunction*, 7th edn. St Louis, MO: Elsevier Mosby.

Meyer, A. (1922) 'The philosophy of occupational therapy.' *Archives of Occupational Therapy 1*, 1, 1–10.

O'Donoghue, N. and McKay, E.A. (2012) 'Exploring the impact of sleep apnoea on daily life and occupational engagement.' *British Journal of Occupational Therapy 75*, 11, 509–516.

Reilly, M. (1962) 'Occupational therapy can be one of the great ideas of the 20th century.' *American Journal of Occupational Therapy 16*, 1, 1–9.

Shimitras, L., Fossey, E. and Harvey, C. (2003) 'Time use of people living with schizophrenia in a North London catchment area.' *British Journal of Occupational Therapy 66*, 2, 46–54.

Stewart, P. and Craik, C. (2007) 'Occupation, mental illness and medium security: exploring time-use in forensic regional secure units.' *British Journal of Occupational Therapy 70*, 10, 416–425.

Sumner, K. (1923) 'The secret of sound sleep.' *American Magazine 95*, 14–15, 98–104. Available at www.sidis.net/soundsleep.htm, accessed on 11 April 2014.

Wilcock, A.A. (1998) *An Occupational Perspective of Health.* Thorofare, NJ: Slack.

Wilcock, A.A. (2003) 'Occupational Science: The Study of Humans as Occupational Beings.' In P. Kramer, J. Hinjosa and C. Brasic Royeen (eds) *Perspectives in Human Occupation: Participation in Life.* Philadelphia, PA: Lippincott Williams & Wilkins.

Wilcock, A.A. and Townsend, E.A. (2014) 'Occupational Justice.' In B.A. Boyt Schell, G. Gillen and M. Scaffa (eds) *Willard and Spackman's Occupational Therapy*, 12th edn. Philadelphia, PA: Lippincott Williams & Wilkins.

3

THE REASON OF SLEEP
Sleep Science

Andrew Green and Sue Wilson

3.1 Introduction

This chapter focuses on normal sleep and therefore forms a foundation for other chapters. As noted in Chapter 1, much about sleep remains unknown, despite the rapid growth of research since the first sleep laboratory investigations of the 1950s (see Hudson 2012 and, for a detailed history of sleep research, Kroker 2007). Probably still the biggest mystery is what sleep is really for but, as described here, it is known to serve many functions. The chapter also considers the timing and duration of sleep and some of the possible consequences of insufficient sleep, as well as the structure of sleep and the ways in which sleep changes through life. It is only by understanding normal sleep and its variations that we can identify problems in sleep. Furthermore, many people may find it reassuring that what they might perceive as a problem with sleep is actually a natural phenomenon.

3.2 Definition and functions of sleep

There are many definitions of sleep and the following are two recent examples:

> Sleep can be defined as a state of immobility with greatly reduced responsiveness, which can be distinguished from coma or anaesthesia by its rapid reversibility. An additional defining characteristic of sleep is that when it is prevented, the body tries to recover the lost amount. (Siegel 2005, p.1264)

> Sleep is a reversible behavioural state of perceptual disengagement from, and unresponsiveness to, the environment. It is also true that sleep is a complex amalgam of physiologic and behavioral processes. Sleep is typically (but not necessarily) accompanied by postural recumbence, behavioural quiescence, closed eyes, and

all the other indicators one commonly associates with sleeping. (Carskadon and Dement 2011, p.16)

Whatever the definition, everyone knows what sleep is and most people are likely, if asked, to say that it is for rest and recovery; however, the functions of sleep are not really known – or cannot be specified with certainty – and debate about the purposes of sleep continues. In fact, the function of sleep has been questioned since at least the time of Aristotle (384–322 BCE) who suggested that sleep relates to the cardinal humours (blood, phlegm, black bile and yellow bile) and to changes in body temperature that result from eating and digestion (Aristotle 2011, first published around 350 BCE). In the mid-seventeenth century the pioneering neuroscientist Thomas Willis held that emotions were caused by spirits flowing through the nervous system; however, they could not flow without rest – hence the need for sleep (Zimmer 2005). By the early twentieth century Addington Bruce asserted that sleep 'is an active, positive function, a protective instinct of gradual evolution…its object being not so much the recuperation of the organism…as to save [it] from the destructive consequences of uninterrupted activity' (Bruce n.d., pp.8–9, first published in 1915).

The idea that sleep is for recuperation was challenged by Meddis (1977). He highlighted the wide variation in the sleep of animals and suggested that the 'sleep instinct merely seems to schedule the activity-inactivity periods of an animal' (p.130). He argued that 'scientists have been misled by the similarity between the feelings of fatigue which follow exercise and those that precede sleep' (p.131). This line of argument was supported more recently by Rial *et al.* (2007) who observe that sleep shares features with the resting state of animals whose body temperature fluctuates with environmental temperature ('cold-blooded' animals or *poikilotherms*). They conclude simply that 'waking is important: sleep is what animals do when they have nothing to do' (p.318) and that 'mammalian sleep has no function apart from the rest of simple organisms' (p.322).

Rattenborg *et al.* (2007) argue against the view that sleep has such a trivial function and note that despite risks from predators, or the need for continuous activity in the case of aquatic mammals (cetaceans), animals continue to sleep. They suggest that there must therefore be an essential function of sleep that outweighs the risks of having it and they note that various mechanisms have evolved to minimize those risks. Cetaceans continue to swim and surface in order to breathe while one hemisphere of the brain shows activity consistent with deep sleep and the other hemisphere appears to be awake. Birds are able to sleep with one eye open: mallard ducks sleeping at the edge of a group 'direct the open eye away from the other birds, as if watching for approaching predators' (Rattenborg *et al.* 2007, p.407). Many large herbivores can have deep sleep while standing, although (because of muscle atonia; see below) they must lie down for rapid eye movement (REM) sleep* (see below) which then makes them highly vulnerable to predators. Rattenborg *et al.* (2007) observe that survival of REM sleep, despite the risks, suggests that there is an important function beyond just rest. How human sleep compares with that of a variety of other species can be seen in Figure 3.1, and for more on the sleep of animals see Lacrampe (2003) and Paterson (2012).

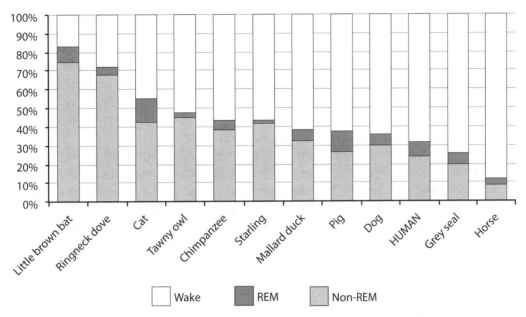

FIGURE 3.1 COMPARATIVE SLEEP TIMES (AS A PERCENTAGE OF 24 HOURS)
FOR A SELECTION OF MAMMALS AND BIRDS
Data from Lesku et al. (2008) and Roth et al. (2006).

In testing a 'null hypothesis' that 'sleep is just one of a repertoire of available behaviours that is useful without being essential' Cirelli and Tononi (2008, p.1605) argue that if that were the case, there would be three corollaries; however, in examining the evidence for each of them, they conclude that (a) there is no clear evidence of an animal species that does not sleep; (b) animals need recovery sleep on staying awake longer (that is, sleep is homeostatically regulated; see below); and (c) lack of sleep has negative consequences. Tononi and Cirelli (2006, 2012) propose a theory that deep sleep is needed for the reestablishment of synaptic homeostasis in the brain; plasticity in wakefulness has a cost in the brain's resources and cannot be sustained indefinitely, and therefore it may be necessary for the system to reset itself offline. They suggest that sleep is 'the price we have to pay for plasticity the previous day' (Tononi and Cirelli 2006, p.56).

The synaptic homeostasis hypothesis (described in Box 3.1) is complex but attractive, although it remains a hypothesis – that is, unproven (see Frank 2012, for example). However, it is reasonable to sum up the general discussion on the function of sleep with the words of Allan Rechtschaffen (who was involved in identification and classification of the stages of sleep; see below): 'If sleep does not serve an absolute vital function, then it is the biggest mistake the evolutionary process ever made' (Rechtschaffen 1971, p.88).[1]

BOX 3.1 The synaptic homeostasis hypothesis

According to this hypothesis we interact with our environment during wakefulness and acquire information which is stored through potentiation of synaptic strength (that is, synapses are strengthened and new synapses appear). This increase in synaptic strength to allow plasticity in wakefulness has a cost in terms of the energy and space required, and gradually the capacity to learn becomes saturated.

In sleep, we are virtually disconnected from the environment and changes in the brain trigger slow oscillations of electrical potential identified by electroencephalogram (EEG)* as slow-wave activity. This slow-wave activity causes the downscaling of the synapses, which decrease in strength back to a baseline level. Sleep therefore enforces synaptic homeostasis, saving space and energy. On wakening, the neural circuits retain a trace of previous experience but remain efficient at a recalibrated level.

The synaptic homeostasis hypothesis 'states that the homeostatic regulation of SWA is tied to the amount of synaptic potentiation that has occurred during previous waking' (Tononi and Cirelli 2006, p.52), that is, the amount of deep sleep is related to the response in the brain to what the individual has done during wakefulness.

It is suggested that without the recalibration that goes on during sleep, the brain could not continue to allow synaptic weight to increase without loss of plasticity. Sleep is needed to prevent synaptic overload and keep the brain working efficiently. Furthermore, it is suggested that connections between strongly correlated neurons survive while others are eliminated – essentially, clearing out unnecessary information. It is argued that a neuron can only assess its synaptic input objectively when it is offline during sleep and not responsible for action of any kind.

It makes evolutionary sense for an organism to 'go offline' and reset itself in an organized and systematic fashion, as in sleep. Where there is sleep deprivation there could be synaptic overload, which could account for the cognitive deficits that are known to accompany sleep loss. If the system is not allowed an orderly shutdown, it is possible that parts of the system will go offline independently – which could explain lapses of attention or word-finding problems, for example, when we are tired and in need of sleep.

Source: Tononi and Cirelli (2006)

A more recent summary of possible purposes of sleep was set out in a teachers' guide produced by the US National Institutes of Health (NIH) (2003):

- restoration and recovery of body systems

- energy conservation

- memory consolidation

- protection from predation

- brain development

- discharge of emotions through dreaming.

The same source notes that sleep is an active process – it needs a specific signal to prevent sensory input – and that 'there is no evidence that any major organ or regulatory system in the body shuts down during sleep' (NIH 2003, p.20). While this reinforces the idea that sleep is not just for when there is nothing better to do, the above theories have flaws: most, for example, do not explain why sleep is more effective than simply resting while awake (NIH 2003). It is unclear that sleep does offer protection from predation when it could equally increase vulnerability and, if the last of the suggestions above were to offer an explanation of the function of sleep in all species, it would imply that all animals dream and have emotions that can be discharged through dreaming.

For our purposes here, however, in the absence of a definitive answer to the question 'What is sleep for?' it is reasonable to take a common-sense view. We know how we feel if we do not sleep and experience tells us that sleep is essential for rest and recovery and to be alert and able to concentrate. Sleep also has a less tangible function for humans in that it punctuates time (as reflected in the question 'How many sleeps until Christmas?'). Furthermore, as Meddis (1977) argued, it is pleasant to switch off and have a break from responsibility, while Ballard (2006, first published in 1957) suggested that it is necessary to have 'eight hours off a day just to get over the shock of being yourself' (p.69).

3.3 Duration of sleep

It is accepted that we must sleep, but how much sleep do we actually need? The question is answered reasonably, but unhelpfully for readers wanting a precise figure, by Paterson (2012) who says that 'we simply need enough sleep to feel refreshed and to be able to perform our daily tasks satisfactorily' (p.19). A 20-page review by

Ferrara and De Gennaro (2001), which cites 100 papers, concludes: 'The best way to determine an *individual* sleep need is to go to bed when tired and sleepy, and to get up in the morning when feeling refreshed, without any alarm' (p.175). This may be difficult for a busy person to achieve with any consistency, and all but impossible in studies involving large numbers. In a study of circadian rhythms that aimed to assess the response of 15 young adults (20–36 years) to daily 14-hour periods of darkness over the course of 4 weeks, Wehr *et al.* (1993) found that sleep stabilized at an average of about 8.25 hours ± 50 minutes.

Larger surveys tend to measure how much sleep people have (or say that they have). For example, in the 'Sleep in America' poll (National Sleep Foundation 2002), respondents reported an average of 6.9 hours of sleep on weekdays and 7.5 hours on weekends (an average of about 7.1 hours per night over the week as a whole). Although 8 hours is the commonly cited figure for sleep need (and the one on which we base the assumption that we sleep for a third of our lives), the poll found that 70% of Americans slept for less than 8 hours a night and that 40% slept for less than 7 hours. Figures from another source (Kripke *et al.* 2002; see Figure 3.2a) are similar, and compared with an earlier study (Kripke *et al.* 1979; see Figure 3.2b), they show a slight tendency to sleep less. In the 2002 survey fewer people were sleeping for 8–9 hours and more were sleeping 6–7 hours. A similar slight tendency is also reflected in successive National Sleep Foundation polls (Swanson *et al.* 2006).

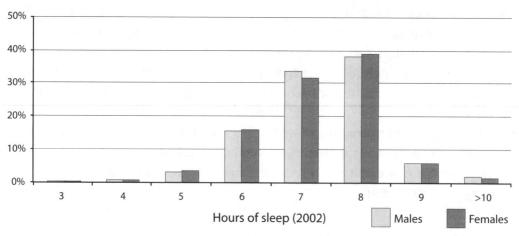

FIGURE 3.2A HOURS OF SLEEP OBTAINED PER NIGHT
Data from the responses of 1.1 million American adults over the age of 30 years (Kripke et al. 2002).

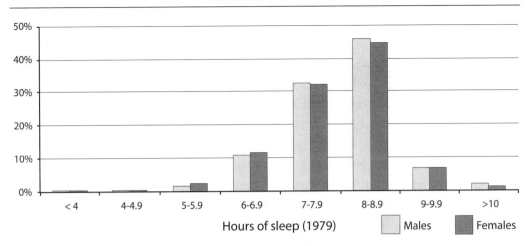

FIGURE 3.2B HOURS OF SLEEP OBTAINED PER NIGHT
Data from the responses of 0.82 million American adults over the age of 30 years (Kripke et al. 1979).

Whereas most people probably sleep for something between 7 and 8 of the 24 hours (and if sleep is curtailed by work or school commitments during the week, more at weekends), there is still wide individual variation. That variation relates to a number of factors, depending on the person and their age, and to some extent, their choices (as well as factors imposed by their individual circumstances and responsibilities). According to Carskadon and Dement (2011) volitional control is one of the most significant factors against the background of the genetic need for sleep (see below). Landolt and Dijk (2011) note that sleep duration shows a large variation among healthy individuals. They explore the genetic origins of this (among other aspects of sleep) and draw attention to the conclusion of a study by Aeschbach *et al.* (2003) which suggests that the differences between long sleepers and short sleepers relate to innate differences in tolerance of, and sensitivity to, signals in the brain to sleep and wake.

A more observable determinant of sleep duration is age, although there is still wide variation within age groups. A recent survey in the UK by Blair *et al.* (2012) shows how the sleep of children decreases, on average, from 13 hours and 12 minutes (in 24 hours) during infancy to 9 hours and 49 minutes at 11 years; however, the averages mask substantial individual differences, with totals between 10 and 17 hours in early infancy and a range of 8.5–11 hours at 11 years. As the authors note, these figures are rather less than figures in earlier studies, raising the possibility of a trend toward reduction in childhood sleep. If this is the case, it is a matter of some concern; for example, one problem attributed to short sleep in childhood is obesity (see below).

A commonly cited average total sleep duration for newborns is 16–18 hours (NIH 2003). During adolescence about 9 hours of sleep is needed, although teenagers are prone to get less than they need. It has been pointed out that 'being able to stay up late is not the same as requiring less total sleep' (NIH 2003, p.M1.2a). Sleep duration

(6–8 hours) decreases slightly during adulthood, but it is notable that the need for sleep of people over 70 years is not very different from the need of younger adults. The more disrupted night-time sleep of the elderly may be compensated by daytime naps. (Variation throughout life of the structure of sleep is discussed in section 3.7, and for more on the sleep of young children see Chapter 9 and also Jones and Ball 2012.)

Reflecting the observation that we might stay up late and deny ourselves sleep, there has been debate over whether or how much we can choose how long we sleep (see also Green 2012a). Horne (2010) argues that we need 'core sleep' of about 6.5 hours and that beyond that we can take 'optional sleep' in much the same way that we can continue eating after hunger is satisfied. This contrasts with the contention of Bonnet and Arand (1995) who suggest that we are sleep deprived to the extent of more than an hour per night – an argument backed by Martin (2003) who argues that in the West we live in a 'sleep-sick society' (p.5) where sleep is devalued. Of course, it is tempting to think that we can manage on less sleep and achieve more, but as Van Dongen *et al.* (2003) show, persistent sleep restriction of 6 hours or less per night leads to deficits in cognitive performance equivalent to what would be expected after two nights of total sleep deprivation (see also Chapter 5). Van Someren (2010) concludes: 'for now, doing with less sleep remains a dream' (p.16004). Although there has to be some short-term flexibility in sleep duration, at the same time there are limits to how much we can restrict our sleep.

3.4 The importance of sleep

Whether or not we choose to restrict our sleep, having enough of it is important, and this is not just because of how we feel and perform without it: it is also because of its relationship with our health. It is difficult to establish whether too little (or too much) sleep is dangerous to health because disruption of sleep patterns could itself be a result of ill health. However, as Wallander *et al.* (2007) observe, sleep could be seen as an important indicator of health status: accordingly, in a survey of over 12,000 primary care patients in the UK they found that those with a newly diagnosed sleep disorder were more likely to have co-morbid conditions. There were strong associations with prior psychiatric disorder, prior gastrointestinal disorder (including gastro-oesophageal reflux disease and irritable bowel syndrome) and prior circulatory conditions such as coronary heart disease, heart failure and transient ischaemic attack (Wallander *et al.* 2007).

The traditional view has been that there are no long-term seriously harmful consequences of short sleep. Phillips and Mannino (2005) confirmed that conditions such as hypertension, pulmonary disease and heart disease are associated with an increased risk of complaints of insomnia but concluded that insomnia confers no increased risk of death. Similarly, Ohayon (2005) notes that while insomnia is detrimental to health and quality of life, and may be a first symptom of a more severe condition, '[it] will not kill you and treating insomnia [with medication] will not kill you either' (p.1044). However, research into short and long sleep and mortality has suggested associations. Gale and Martin (1998), for example, found that spending more than 8 hours in bed was linked with increased mortality, while Kripke *et al.* (2002) found an increased risk of mortality among those sleeping for more than 8 hours or less than 6 hours – a finding supported by a meta-analysis by Cappuccio *et al.* (2010).

There is also evidence from recent systematic reviews relating to sleep duration and specific conditions. For example, Nielsen, Danielson and Sørensen (2011) found an association between short sleep and the development of obesity in children and young adults: the association was less consistent in older adults (see also Taheri 2006). Knutson (2010) found a similar link in cross-sectional studies between short sleep (less than 6 hours) and obesity, as well as an association with diabetes and hypertension; she also reported a link between longer sleep (over 8 hours) and cardiometabolic disease. She notes that despite some evidence in prospective studies of associations between short sleep and diabetes, hypertension and cardiovascular disease, further research is necessary to establish cause.

In one prospective study over about 16 years, Chien *et al.* (2010) hypothesized that short or long sleep duration and frequent insomnia predispose to a greater risk of all-cause deaths and cardiovascular events. Having asked 3430 people over the age of 35 years in Taiwan about habitual sleep duration and insomnia, they found that in the follow-up period 420 participants developed cardiovascular disease and 901 participants died. They concluded that an optimal sleep duration of 7–8 hours and infrequent insomnia predicted fewer events of cardiovascular disease and less death. This finding was supported by a meta-analysis of 13 prospective studies which concluded that insomnia is associated with a greater risk of developing cardiovascular disease (Sofi *et al.* 2014; see also Cappuccio *et al.* 2011).

While the direction of causality is unclear in the case of sleep duration and physical illness, the negative consequences of sleep deprivation on cognitive performance are well established (as discussed more fully in Chapter 5). Briefly, the more we go without sleep, the more sleepy we become; that is, subjective sleepiness increases, as does objective sleep propensity that can be measured in a sleep laboratory. While lack of sleep simply makes it harder to stay awake and focus on a task, sleep is also necessary for various cognitive processes to take place in wakefulness, in particular memory and learning. Although it seems clear that sleep deprivation affects performance in the short and medium term, it is not known whether there are any cognitive consequences of reduced sleep in the longer term, and it would be neither practical nor ethical to find out.

3.5 The timing of sleep

Like sleep duration, *when* we sleep is affected by genetic makeup. As Foster and Kreitzman (2005) explain, we each have an individual inherent preference, or chronotype, that varies from one person to the next. Some people are larks, who work best late in the morning and are most alert around midday. On the other hand, owls work better in the afternoon and are most alert at around 6 p.m. Larks tend to be older, whereas in adolescents and young adults sleep is naturally delayed. This is something that parents might prefer their teenaged children not to know, although Worthman and Melby (2002) suggest that it is advantageous for a community where some people (the more elderly) are vigilant in the early morning while adolescents with later sleep onset and offset are vigilant at the other end of the day. About 10% of people are 'extreme owls' and 10% are 'extreme larks', whereas the majority of people are something in between. According to Foster and Kreitzman (2005) 'this evening/morningness is less a matter of choice than it is of genetics' (p.188) and is not related to willpower or how much sleep someone has had. At the very ends of the spectrum people are considered to have a circadian rhythm disorder (see Chapter 7). Foster and Kreitzman (2005) observe that larks might adopt 'a smug moral superiority based on Benjamin Franklin's maxim "Early to bed and early to rise makes a man healthy, wealthy and wise"' (p.188) but note that there are no grounds for Franklin's assertion. Following up a 1970s UK Department of Health survey after more than 20 years, Gale and Martin (1998) found no evidence that early bedtimes and rising times are linked with any 'health, socioeconomic, or cognitive advantage [and] if anything, owls were wealthier than larks' (p.1677) (although no healthier or wiser). An idea of how sleep fits into people's lives can be gained from time-use surveys. Chapter 4 gives some examples; it also illustrates that there is no right or wrong about exactly when we sleep apart from our biological needs: people's sleep patterns have varied during the course of history and are different around the world.

The regulation of an individual's sleep is dependent on two interacting processes: the homeostatic recovery process (S) and the circadian process (C) – together known as the two-process model of sleep (see Figure 3.3; Borbély 1982). The homeostatic process (S) relates simply to time since the last sleep: the drive to sleep increases in relation to the time awake, that is, it is a self-regulating process, much like satisfying hunger. When someone has had insufficient sleep, the drive to sleep will be higher, whereas after a long afternoon nap, or after sleeping late in a long morning lie-in, the drive will be diminished and it may be harder to get to sleep at the desired bedtime.

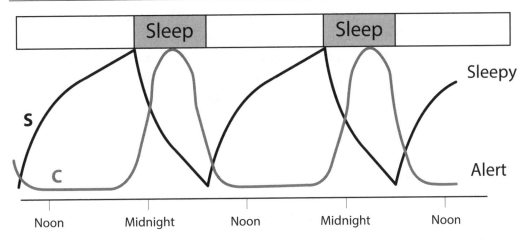

FIGURE 3.3 THE TWO-PROCESS MODEL

This figure shows how the need to sleep changes during the 24-hour cycle in response to circadian and homeostatic processes. C is the circadian sleep drive which reaches a maximum around 4 a.m. and tails off in the morning, keeping us alert until early evening. S is the homeostatic sleep propensity which reaches a maximum after about 16 hours of wakefulness and declines rapidly during sleep.

Whereas the homeostatic process is relatively intuitive, the circadian process is more complex. The literal meaning of the word 'circadian' (from the Latin *circa diem*) provides the clue: 'about a day'. The solar day is 24 hours, whereas the period of the human's natural rhythm is only *about* 24 hours. It is not certain why we should have evolved to have a different period; various figures are found in the literature, but Czeisler *et al.* (1999) suggest it is about 24 hours and 10 minutes in humans. The average human free-running period, when a person is isolated from natural rhythms of light and dark, is often cited as being higher (typically up to about 25 hours). The difference relates to the experimental conditions in which the period is measured (see Eastman *et al.* 2012).

Whatever the figure, elaborate mechanisms have evolved to ensure that we can entrain to the solar cycle (and accommodate seasonal variation). Entrainment to the solar day relies on environmental cues known as zeitgebers ('time givers') which regulate the body's master clock. This clock resides in a group of cells in the suprachiasmatic nucleus (SCN) of the hypothalamus and acts as a pacemaker. The SCN is directly linked to cells in the retina which detect light. These cells are quite distinct from the rod and cone cells which are involved in vision and therefore are important in allowing sightless people with eyes to entrain to daily rhythms.

In regulating sleep, one of the chief roles of the SCN is in the daily variation of the synthesis of the hormone melatonin, which is produced by the pineal gland. This variation is light dependent (made possible by the link via the SCN from the retina) and, as noted by Wulff (2012), serum concentration of melatonin at night exceeds daytime levels by 50 times. Melatonin (therefore known as 'the darkness hormone') is a precursor to sleep, among other functions, and its production is suppressed by light. This accounts for the importance of controlling light to promote sleep. In a person who regularly sleeps at night (in the dark) the circadian process sees production of melatonin commencing about 3 hours before sleep and then rising sharply around normal bedtime; it reaches a maximum about an hour after the midpoint of sleep, and then declines rapidly as soon as the eyes are open and daylight is seen in the morning. Cortisol is low in the evening and starts to rise at the melatonin maximum and temperature minimum. Despite being known as the stress hormone, cortisol is part of the body's defence and is necessary for many metabolic processes; it shows a sharp rise when one gets up and starts to move around. Like melatonin, it appears to be important in maintaining entrainment to the 24-hour cycle (see Figure 3.4; Van Someren and Riemersma-van der Lek 2007). For further information on chronobiology see, for example, Foster and Kreitzman (2005), Roenneberg (2012) and Wulff (2012).

Ideally, the homeostatic and circadian processes interact to produce sleepiness at the biologically appropriate time to sleep, in the evening, followed by wakening in the morning (see Figure 3.3); however, it is possible to override the circadian process and remain awake late into the night despite the homeostatic drive continuing to produce increased sleepiness. If the individual is able to withstand the pressure to sleep, come morning the circadian process will promote wakening and sleepiness (as opposed to tiredness) will diminish. The person will be able to get on with daytime activity (although they may also be aware of being tired and more or less aware that their capacity is impaired). The particularly troublesome time is likely to be in early afternoon when the circadian process allows for an afternoon sleep, and resisting sleep after, say, more than 30 hours awake might be very difficult. It should be added that the 'afternoon dip' has nothing to do with having eaten a midday meal: we do not doze off easily after breakfast or an evening meal. Maas (1998) suggests that 'lunch…simply unmasks the physiological sleepiness that is already in your body' (p.131), because this tendency to sleep in the early afternoon is a natural mechanism that permits the siesta in warm climates (see Chapter 4). For getting off to sleep at night we need to take advantage of the two processes and, as well as that, be in a state of low arousal, that is, be physically comfortable and not unduly anxious, angry or excited.

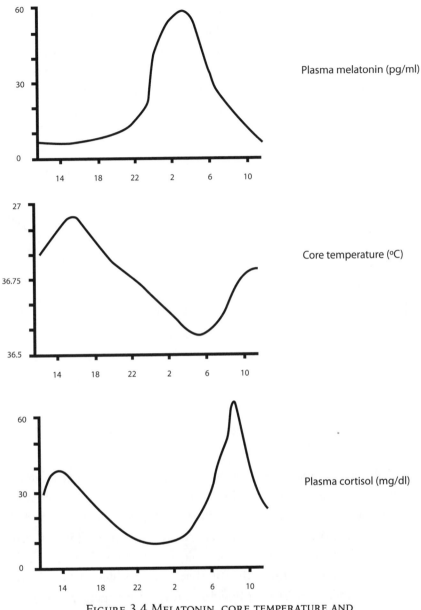

FIGURE 3.4 MELATONIN, CORE TEMPERATURE AND
CORTISOL RHYTHMS DURING THE 24-HOUR PERIOD

3.6 Stages of sleep

When asked to chart their ideal sleep (on a graph plotting of 'depth of sleep' against time), people with little or no previous knowledge of sleep science[2] tend to produce something like a cross-section of a wide 'U'-shaped valley – with a gentler slope on the morning side (see Figure 3.5). Indeed, it is usually (in the absence of insomnia) our *experience* that we spend a short time 'on the level' (awake in bed) before dipping into drowsiness and then 'falling over the edge' into sleep where we remain for the night; perhaps in the early morning there is an awareness of lighter sleep – including dozing after the alarm goes off. People are mostly surprised, however, by the reality, for as indicated above, sleep is not a single continuous state and comprises two states: REM sleep and non-REM (NREM) sleep. NREM sleep consists of three or four stages. These stages and REM normally occur in several cycles throughout the night and tend to be separated by short awakenings.

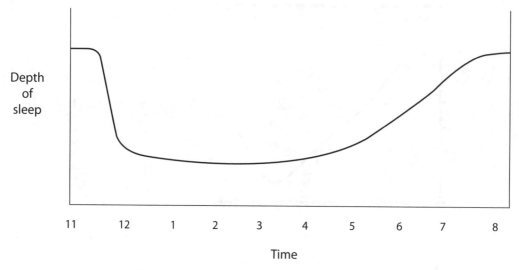

FIGURE 3.5 IDEALIZED 'GOOD NIGHT'S SLEEP'

Whether NREM sleep is subdivided into three or four stages is an academic question best left to diagnosticians and researchers, but for the consumer of research, or the therapist, it is sufficient to know that the different classifications exist and how they relate to each other. REM sleep was first identified in the early 1950s (Aserinsky and Kleitman 1953) and the stages of non-REM sleep were first classified in the 1960s when stages I to IV were identified (Rechtschaffen and Kales 1968). Subsequently, in the American Academy of Sleep Medicine's revised manual, the two stages that comprise deep sleep (stages III and IV) were amalgamated (see Table 3.1; Iber *et al.* 2007). The stages are distinguished by differences in brainwave patterns (in conjunction with other factors, such as movement) recorded in an overnight EEG as part of a process known as polysomnography (PSG) (see Hudson 2012 for further explanation). The newer terms (N1 to N3) are used here and they also relate to experience. To some extent we are aware of these stages – or having been in them – or we might observe them in others, whereas we could not distinguish between stages III and IV.

Table 3.1 Stages of sleep

Terms – 1968	Terms – 2007	Sleep (%)[*]	Description
I	N1	2–5	Transitional stage/drowsiness
II	N2	45–55	Light sleep
III	N3	3–8	Deep (slow-wave) sleep; also known as delta sleep
IV		10–15	
REM	REM	20–25	Dream sleep

[*]Proportions relate to the sleep in a normal young adult without sleep problems and who has a conventional sleep-wake pattern. Wakefulness might account for up to 5% of the night (figures from Carskadon and Dement 2011).

Stage N1 is very light sleep – a drowsy transition from wake to sleep in which very little time is spent during the night, usually lasting between 1 and 7 minutes on first going to sleep. It is associated with slow eye-rolling movements and may be experienced during the day. It is something that is familiar to most people when it may be hard to attend to an afternoon talk or meeting, when voices begin to seem distant. On being roused from stage N1, which occurs easily, a person is likely to deny having been asleep. Stage N2 is also quite light sleep and is the stage in which a person spends about half of the night. It is relatively easy to wake someone from stage N2 and they will quickly be oriented. Characteristic features of the EEG in stage N2 sleep, which are often mentioned in the literature, are patterns known as K complexes and sleep spindles. The sleep spindle is an EEG feature that is unique to sleep (De Gennaro and Ferrara 2003). They are involved in memory consolidation, suggesting an important role for stage N2 sleep (see, for example, Mednick *et al.* 2013).

Stage N3 is deep sleep (also known as slow-wave sleep [SWS] because of the characteristic pattern of the waves on the EEG) in which a young adult spends about 20% of the night (older people have less; see below). Heart rate and breathing have both slowed down by this stage. It is much harder to rouse someone from stage N3 and, on being woken, the person will be disoriented for a short time. Stage N3 is thought to be restorative sleep and tends to occur early in the night – as if it is given priority; indeed, if a person misses a whole night's sleep (although they will not sleep for double the time on the following night), they will sleep for longer and will have a longer-than-normal period of SWS. Slow-wave sleep is therefore an indicator of sleep need because it increases depending on the duration of wakefulness prior to sleep and decreases as sleep goes on, but it also appears to be linked to what we do in wakefulness. In early experiments extra SWS was also found after extreme exertion (Shapiro *et al.* 1981) and after a full day of novel experiences (Horne and Minard 1985). More recently, in researching the mechanisms that control SWS, Huber, Tononi and Cirelli (2006) found that laboratory rats would have more SWS when they had been allowed to spend more time in exploratory behaviour than when awake for a similar period engaged in grooming or quiet wakefulness. Such evidence suggests that our daytime activity has some influence on night-time sleep (see Chapter 6).

REM sleep represents an entirely separate state of being from both non-REM sleep and wakefulness, and it is associated with dreaming. It is also known as paradoxical sleep because in most respects the brain activity resembles that of wakefulness. The key difference from wakefulness is the muscle atonia which prevents the individual acting out their dreams – something that would present great danger to both the individual and those around them. The muscles controlling eye movement are unaffected; circulation continues and the diaphragm maintains respiration while intercostal muscle tone is reduced. The importance of continuing vital functions is plain, but we do not know why the eyes move; maybe we are scanning dream scenes, although activation in scans during REM sleep is in the visual association area and memory-related limbic areas, whereas the primary visual cortex is not active (see Maquet *et al.* 2000).

Dreaming is normal and everyone does it, but usually a dream is only recalled, although often just fleetingly, if an individual wakes from the dream. Much has been written on the meaning of dreams over the years; dreaming is seen as a means of communication in the Bible (Jacobs 2012) and is a commonly used literary device. Freud proposed that dreams are a form of wish fulfilment (Isbister 1985). The process and meaning of dreaming are beyond the scope of this chapter; for more information on dreaming see, for example, Carhart-Harris and Friston 2010 or Hobson 2002.

3.7 Sleep cycles, sleep architecture and changes in sleep architecture during life

When the repeating stages of sleep are mapped overnight, a chart known as a hypnogram is produced. The pattern, which resembles a city skyline, is known as sleep architecture. Figure 3.6 illustrates how in normal sleep we move between the stages, in sequence, throughout the night in a series of cycles. The first cycle averages between 70 and 100 minutes while later cycles are 90–120 minutes in length (Carskadon and Dement 2011); we might have four or five cycles during a night. It is in the first two cycles of adult sleep that most stage N3 sleep is taken and there may be little or none by the third or fourth cycles. Sleep therefore becomes lighter as the night goes on. As the amount of N3 decreases, the length of N2 and REM sleep periods increases (see Figures 3.6a and 3.6b).

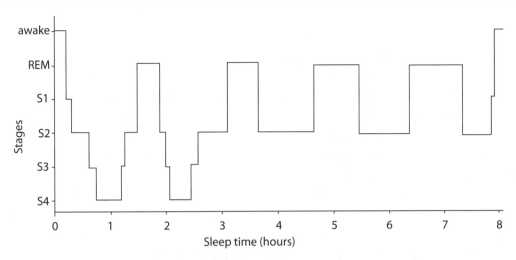

FIGURE 3.6A AN IDEALIZED HYPNOGRAM SHOWING THE STAGES OF
SLEEP AND THEIR DISTRIBUTION OVER THE COURSE OF A NIGHT

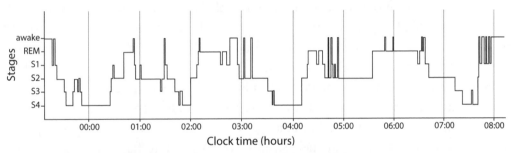

FIGURE 3.6B THE ACTUAL HYPNOGRAM OF A HEALTHY 25-YEAR-OLD MALE SHOWS
THE STAGES OF SLEEP AND THEIR DISTRIBUTION OVER THE COURSE OF A NIGHT
*Note that the individual had several very short wakenings (which he would not remember)
and one longer wakening. Although most of his deep sleep (here labelled S3 and S4) was
in the first half of the night, he also had some deep sleep just before waking up.*

Waking between cycles (and during cycles) is the norm, especially as we age. A child
or adolescent is likely to sleep 'solidly', but in adulthood it is typical to wake several
times during the night. However, it is important to realize that such waking is entirely
natural and that for the most part we are unaware of waking at all. If nothing occurs
to attract our attention, we are likely to return to sleep within moments and know
nothing more about it. Of course, if an individual wakes, hears a noise and begins
to worry about it (or has to act on it), then wakening will be prolonged and recalled
in the morning. This tendency to wake could have been selected by evolution as a
safety mechanism: without it, our ancestors would seem likely to have been eaten by

predators. In any case, it can be very reassuring to understand that short periods of time awake at night are not only natural but harmless.

Changes in sleep duration throughout life have been noted already, but there are also changes in the nature of sleep – or the amount of time spent in different stages, or in wakefulness after sleep onset. The eyes of a newborn baby do not move in REM sleep (although jerky body movements are common); this type of sleep is known as *active sleep*. It occurs soon after sleep onset and dominates sleep cycles of newborn infants: see Jones and Ball (2012). REM sleep diminishes during the first 2–3 years of life, and in the 4.5–7-year age group the first period of REM sleep does not occur until 3 or 4 hours into sleep (i.e. a young child might not have a period of REM sleep in the first sleep cycle). In mid-adolescence the adult pattern emerges where REM sleep occurs 50–70 minutes after sleep onset. During adulthood the amount of REM sleep diminishes slightly with age, but as a proportion of total sleep it continues well into old age.

Slow-wave sleep is at a peak in young children and decreases across the lifespan. A 5-year-old child might have about 3 hours of SWS and, as noted by Carskadon and Dement (2011), 'it is nearly impossible to wake youngsters in the SWS of the night's first sleep cycle' (p.22). In the second decade SWS diminishes substantially, despite total sleep time remaining the same. By the age of 60 years a man might have no SWS, while in women it remains later in life. With the slight decline in REM sleep and the more substantial decline in SWS, the sleep of older people tends to be lighter – consisting of more N2 sleep. As noted earlier, older people do not necessarily sleep less – or need less sleep – but their sleep tends to be more fragmented and lighter (Figure 3.7). It is also possible that if an older person sleeps more in the day, perhaps as a result of inactivity, less night-time sleep is needed.

In clinical practice, and for practical purposes, it may not be necessary to dwell on the details of these changes during the lifespan; however, the differences highlight two points. First, sleep in the various periods of life is qualitatively and quantitatively different, and we should not assume that what is good for one age group is good for another. For example, Jones and Ball (2012) suggest that it is unwise to try to entrain infants into a sleep pattern more convenient for parents by early weaning, which can lead to negative health consequences both in infancy and later life (see Smith and Harvey 2010). Second, the variation in stages of sleep suggests that each stage serves its own purpose and increases or decreases according to need at the particular time of life.

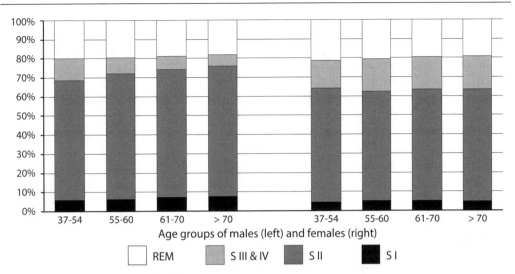

<figure>FIGURE 3.7 PROPORTION OF TIME SPENT IN DIFFERENT
STAGES OF SLEEP IN LATER ADULTHOOD AND OLD AGE</figure>

The figure shows that men of all ages tend to have less SWS (and correspondingly more stage I and stage II sleep) than women, and that the amount of SWS declines with age. The proportion of REM sleep remains fairly stable. Sleep efficiency* (not shown) decreases from 86% for the under-54-year-olds to 80% for the over-70-year-olds. Based on data summarized by Bliwise (2011) from Redline et al. (2004).

3.8 Conclusion

The exact purpose of sleep remains unclear, but its importance for health and performance is undoubted. It is not a single continuous state and comprises several stages that occur in cycles; also, waking briefly during sleep is entirely natural. The need for sleep varies between individuals, even in neonates, although we still do not know whether studies of sleep duration reflect a sleep need or whether laboratory studies simply measure what we have, whereas surveys ask what we think we have. The timing of sleep also varies between individuals and the structure of sleep changes naturally during the course of life. There is some scope for choice in when and how long we sleep, and a key message is that we must not assume that everyone's needs are the same.

Notes

1 Rechtshaffen (1971) continued: 'Sleep precludes hunting for and consuming food. It is incompatible with procreation. It produces vulnerability to attack from enemies. Sleep interferes with every voluntary, adaptive motor act in the repertoire of coping mechanisms. How could natural selection with its irrevocable logic have "permitted" the animal kingdom to pay the price of sleep for no good reason? In fact, the behavior of sleep is so apparently maladaptive that one can wonder why some other condition did not evolve to satisfy whatever need it is that sleep satisfies' (p.88).

2 For example, in an informal exercise, the majority of participants attending lectures and seminars on sleep produce a chart similar to Figure 3.5.

References

Aeschbach, D., Sher, L., Postolache, T.T., Matthews, J.R., Jackson, M.A. and Wehr, T.A. (2003) 'A longer biological night in long sleepers than in short sleepers.' *Journal of Clinical Endocrinology & Metabolism 88*, 1, 26–30.

Aristotle (2011) *On Sleep and Sleeplessness* [Illustrated]. Kindle Edition.

Aserinsky, E. and Kleitman, N. (1953) 'Regularly occurring periods of eye motility, and concomitant phenomena, during sleep'. *Science 118*, 3062, 273–274.

Ballard, J.G. (2006) *The Complete Short Stories: Vol 1.* London: Harper Perennial.

Blair, P.S., Humphreys, J.S., Gringras, P., Taheri, S. *et al.* (2012) 'Childhood sleep duration and associated demographic characteristics in an English cohort.' *Sleep 35*, 3, 353–360.

Bliwise, D.L. (2011) 'Normal Aging.' In M.H. Kryger, T. Roth and W.C. Dement (eds) *Principles and Practice of Sleep Medicine*, 5th edn. St Louis, MO: Elsevier Saunders.

Bonnet, M.H. and Arand, D.L. (1995) 'We are chronically sleep deprived.' *Sleep 18*, 10, 908–911.

Borbély, A.A. (1982) 'A two process model of sleep regulation.' *Human Neurobiology 1*, 3, 195–204.

Bruce, H.A. (n.d.) *Sleep and Sleeplessness.* Kila, MT: Kessinger Publishing. (Original work published in 1915.)

Cappuccio, F.P., Cooper, D., D'Elia, L., Strazzullo, P. and Miller, M.A. (2011) 'Sleep duration predicts cardiovascular outcomes: a systematic review and meta-analysis of prospective studies.' *European Heart Journal 32*, 12, 1484–1492.

Cappuccio, F.P., D'Elia, L., Strazzullo, P. and Miller, M.A. (2010) 'Sleep duration and all-cause mortality: a systematic review and meta-analysis of prospective studies.' *Sleep 33*, 5, 585–592.

Carhart-Harris, R.L. and Friston, K.J. (2010) 'The default-mode, ego-functions and free-energy: a neurobiological account of Freudian ideas.' *Brain 133*, 4, 1265–1283.

Carskadon, M.A. and Dement, W.C. (2011) 'Normal Human Sleep.' In M.H. Kryger, T. Roth and W.C. Dement (eds) *Principles and Practice of Sleep Medicine*, 5th edn. St Louis, MO: Elsevier Saunders.

Chien, K., Chen, P., Hsu, C., Su, T. *et al.* (2010) 'Habitual sleep duration and insomnia and the risk of cardiovascular events and all-cause death: report from a community-based cohort.' *Sleep 33*, 2, 177–184.

Cirelli, C. and Tononi, G. (2008) 'Is sleep essential?' *PLoS Biol 6*, 8, e216.

Czeisler, C.A., Duffy, J.F., Shanahan, T.L., Brown, E.M. et al. (1999) 'Stability, precision, and near-24-hour period of the human circadian pacemaker.' *Science 284*, 5423, 2177–2181.

De Gennaro, L. and Ferrara, M. (2003) 'Sleep spindles: an overview.' *Sleep Medicine Reviews 7*, 5, 423–440.

Eastman, C.I., Molina, T.A., Dziepak, M.E. and Smith, M.R. (2012) 'Blacks (African Americans) have shorter free-running circadian periods than whites (Caucasian Americans).' *Chronobiology International 29*, 8, 1072–1077.

Ferrara, M. and De Gennaro, L. (2001) 'How much sleep do we need?' *Sleep 5*, 2, 155–179.

Foster, R.G. and Kreitzman, L. (2005) *Rhythms of Life: The Biological Clocks that Control the Daily Lives of Every Living Thing.* London: Profile Books.

Frank, M.G. (2012) 'Erasing Synapses in Sleep: Is It Time to Be SHY?' *Neural Plasticity*. doi: 10.1155/2012/264378.

Gale, C. and Martin, C. (1998) 'Larks and owls and health, wealth, and wisdom.' *British Medical Journal 317*, 1675–1677.

Green, A. (2012a) 'Sleeping on It.' In A. Green and A. Westcombe (eds) *Sleep: Multiprofessional Perspectives.* London: Jessica Kingsley Publishers.

Green, A. (2012b) 'A Question of Balance: The Relationship Between Daily Occupation and Sleep.' In A. Green and A. Westcombe (eds) *Sleep: Multiprofessional Perspectives.* London: Jessica Kingsley Publishers.

Hobson, J.A. (2002) *Dreaming: An Introduction to the Science of Sleep.* Oxford: Oxford University Press.

Horne, J. (2010) 'Sleepiness as a need for sleep: When is enough, enough?' *Neuroscience and Biobehavioral Reviews 34*, 1, 108–118.

Horne, J.A. and Minard, A. (1985) 'Sleep and sleepiness following a behaviourally "active" day.' *Ergonomics 28*, 3, 567–575.

Huber, R., Tononi, G. and Cirelli, C. (2006) 'Exploratory behavior, cortical BDNF expression, and sleep homeostasis.' *Sleep 30*, 2, 129–139.

Hudson, N. (2012) 'Recording and Quantifying Sleep.' In A. Green and A. Westcombe (eds) *Sleep: Multiprofessional Perspectives.* London: Jessica Kingsley Publishers.

Iber, C., Ancoli-Israel, S., Chesson, A. and Quan, S.F. (2007) *The AASM Manual for the Scoring of Sleep and Associated Events: Rules, Terminology and Technical Specifications.* Westchester, IL: American Academy of Sleep Medicine.

Isbister, J.N. (1985) *Freud: An Introduction to his Life and Work.* Cambridge: Polity Press.

Jacobs, S. (2012) 'Ambivalent Attitudes Towards Sleep in World Religions.' In A. Green and A. Westcombe (eds) *Sleep: Multiprofessional Perspectives.* London: Jessica Kingsley Publishers.

Jones, C.H.D. and Ball, H.L. (2012) 'Medical Anthropology and Children's Sleep.' In A. Green and A. Westcombe (eds) *Sleep: Multiprofessional Perspectives.* London: Jessica Kingsley Publishers.

Knutson, K.L. (2010) 'Sleep duration and cardiometabolic risk: a review of the epidemiologic evidence.' *Best Practice & Research: Clinical Endocrinology & Metabolism 24*, 5, 731–743.

Kripke, D.F., Garfinkel, L., Wingard, D.L., Klauber, M.R. and Marler, M.R. (2002) 'Mortality associated with sleep duration and insomnia.' *Archives of General Psychiatry 59*, 2, 131–136.

Kripke, D.F., Simons, R.N., Garfinkel, L. and Hammond, E.C. (1979) 'Short and long sleep and sleeping pills.' *Archives of General Psychiatry 36*, 1, 103–116.

Kroker, K. (2007) *The Sleep of Others and the Transformations of Sleep Research.* Toronto: Toronto University Press.

Lacrampe, C. (2003) *Sleep and Rest in Animals.* Richmond Hill, Ontario: Firefly Books.

Landolt, H.-P. and Dijk, D.-J. (2011) 'Genetic Basis of Sleep in Healthy Humans.' In M.H. Kryger, T. Roth and W.C. Dement (eds) *Principles and Practice of Sleep Medicine,* 5th edn. St Louis, MO: Elsevier Saunders.

Lesku, J.A., Roth, T.C. 2nd, Rattenborg, N.C., Amlaner, C.J. and Lima, S.L. (2008) 'Phylogenetics and the correlates of mammalian sleep: a reappraisal.' *Sleep Medicine Reviews 12,* 3, 229–244.

Maas, J.B. (1998) *Miracle Sleep Cure.* London: Thorsons.

Maquet, P., Laureys, S., Peigneux, P., Fuchs, S. *et al.* (2000) 'Experience-dependent changes in cerebral activation during human REM sleep.' *Nature Neuroscience 3,* 8, 831–836.

Martin, P. (2003) *Counting Sheep.* London: Flamingo.

Meddis, R. (1977) *The Sleep Instinct.* London: Routledge & Kegan Paul.

Mednick, S.C., McDevitt, E.A., Walsh, J.K., Wamsley, E. *et al.* (2013) 'The critical role of sleep spindles in hippocampal-dependent memory: a pharmacology study.' *Journal of Neuroscience 13,* 10, 4494–4504.

National Institutes of Health (2003) *Sleep, Sleep Disorders, and Biological Rhythms.* Colorado Springs, CO: BSCS. Available at http://science.education.nih.gov/supplements/nih3/sleep/guide/nih_sleep_curr-supp.pdf, accessed on 2 November 2012.

National Sleep Foundation (2002) '2002 "Sleep in America" Poll.' Available at www.sleepfoundation.org/sites/default/files/2002SleepInAmericaPoll.pdf, accessed on 25 October 2013.

Nielsen, L.S., Danielsen, K.V. and Sørensen, T.I.A. (2011) 'Short sleep duration as a possible cause of obesity: critical analysis of the epidemiological evidence.' *Obesity Reviews 12,* 2, 78–92.

Ohayon, M.M. (2005) 'Insomnia: a dangerous condition but not a killer?' *Sleep 28,* 9, 1043–1044.

Paterson, L. (2012) 'The Science of Sleep: What is it, What Makes it Happen and Why Do We Do it?' In A. Green and A. Westcombe (eds) *Sleep: Multiprofessional Perspectives.* London: Jessica Kingsley Publishers.

Phillips, B. and Mannino, D.M. (2005) 'Does insomnia kill?' *Sleep 28,* 8, 965–971.

Rattenborg, N.C., Lesku, J.A., Martinez-Gonzalez, D. and Lima, S.L. (2007) 'The non-trivial functions of sleep.' *Sleep Medicine Reviews 11,* 5, 405–409.

Rechtschaffen, A. (1971) 'The Control of Sleep.' In W.A. Hunt (ed) *Human Behavior and Its Control.* Cambridge, MA: Shenkman Publishing Company.

Rechtschaffen, A. and Kales, A. (1968) *A Manual of Standardised Terminology, Techniques and Scoring System for Sleep Stages in Normal Subjects.* Washington, DC: United States Department of Health and Welfare.

Redline, S., Kirchner, H.L., Quan, S.F., Gottlieb, D.J., Kapur, V. and Newman, A. (2004) 'The effects of age, ethnicity and sleep-disordered breathing on sleep architecture.' *Archives of Internal Medicine 164,* 4, 406–418.

Rial, R.V., Nicolau, M.C., Gamundi, A., Akaâris, M. *et al.* (2007) 'The trivial function of sleep.' *Sleep Medicine Reviews 11,* 4, 311–325.

Roenneberg, T. (2012) *Internal Time: Chronotypes, Social Jet Lag, and Why You're So Tired.* Cambridge, MA: Harvard University Press.

Roth, T.C. 2nd, Lesku, J.A., Amlaner, C.J. and Lima, S.L. (2006) 'A phylogenetic analysis of the correlates of sleep in birds.' *Journal of Sleep Research 15*, 4, 359–402.

Shapiro, C.M., Bortz, R., Mitchell, D., Bartel, P. and Jooste, P. (1981) 'Slow-wave sleep: a recovery period after exercise.' *Science 214*, 4526, 1253–1254.

Siegel, J.M. (2005) 'Clues to the functions of mammalian sleep.' *Nature 437*, 7063, 1264–1271.

Smith, J.P. and Harvey, P.J. (2010) 'Chronic disease and infant nutrition: Is it significant to public health?' *Public Health Nutrition 14*, 2, 279–289.

Sofi, F., Cesari, F., Cassini, A., Macchi, C., Abbate, R. and Gensini, G.F. (2014) 'Insomnia and risk of cardiovascular disease: a meta-analysis.' *European Journal of Preventive Cardiology 21*, 1, 57–64.

Swanson, L.E., Arnedt, J.T., Rosekind, M.R., Belenky, G., Balkin, T.J. and Drake, C. (2011) 'Sleep disorders and work performance: findings from the 2008 National Sleep Foundation "Sleep in America" poll.' *Journal of Sleep Research 20*, 3, 487–494.

Taheri, S. (2006) 'The link between short sleep duration and obesity: we should recommend more sleep to prevent obesity.' *Archives of Disease in Childhood 91*, 11, 881–884.

Tononi, G. and Cirelli, C. (2006) 'Sleep function and synaptic homeostasis.' *Sleep Medicine Reviews 10*, 1, 49–62.

Tononi, G. and Cirelli, C. (2012) 'Time to Be SHY? Some comments on sleep and synaptic homeostasis.' *Neural Plasticity.* doi: 10.1155/2012/415250. Available at www.hindawi.com/journals/np/2012/415250, accessed on 1 October 2013.

US National Institutes of Health (2003) *Sleep, Sleep Disorders, and Biological Rhythms.* Colorado Springs, CO: BSCS. Available at http://science.education.nih.gov/supplements/nih3/sleep/guide/nih_sleep_curr-supp.pdf, accessed on 25 October 2013.

Van Dongen, H.P.A., Maislin, G., Mullington, J.M. and Dinges, D.F. (2003) 'The cumulative cost of additional wakefulness: dose-response effects on neurobehavioral functions and sleep physiology from chronic sleep restriction and total sleep deprivation.' *Sleep 26*, 2, 117–126.

Van Someren, E.J.W. (2010) 'Doing with less sleep remains a dream.' *Proceedings of the National Academy of Science 107*, 37, 16003–16004.

Van Someren, E.J.W. and Riemersma-van der Lek, R.F. (2007) 'Live to the rhythm, slave to the rhythm.' *Sleep Medicine Reviews 11*, 6, 465–484.

Wallander, M.-A., Johansson, S., Ruigómez, A., Rodríguez, L.A. and Jones, R. (2007) 'Morbidity associated with sleep disorders in primary care: a longitudinal cohort study.' *Primary Care Companion to the Journal of Clinical Psychiatry 9*, 5, 338–345.

Wehr, T.A., Moul, D.E., Barbato, G., Giesen, H.A. *et al.* (1993) 'Conservation of photoperiod-responsive mechanisms in humans.' *American Journal of Physiology 265*, 4, R846–R857.

Worthman, C.M. and Melby, M.K. (2002) 'Toward a Comparative Developmental Ecology of Human Sleep.' In M.A. Carskadon (ed) *Adolescent Sleep Patterns: Biological, Social, and Psychological Influences.* Cambridge: Cambridge University Press.

Wulff, K. (2012) 'Chronobiology: Biological Rhythms that Influence Sleep.' In A. Green and A. Westcombe (eds) *Sleep: Multiprofessional Perspectives.* London: Jessica Kingsley Publishers.

Zimmer, C. (2005) *The Soul Made Flesh.* London: Arrow Books.

4

TIME FOR BED

Historical and Cultural Factors, and Time Use

Andrew Green and Claire Durant

4.1 Introduction

In Chapter 3 sleep is considered from the scientific perspective and it is noted that there is some flexibility and choice about when and how long we sleep. Figure 4.1 shows that the majority (about 80%) of a sample of people in the UK take their sleep between the hours of 10 p.m. and 8 a.m., and it seems reasonable to conclude that the expectation or hope of most people is to have a single unbroken period of sleep, roughly between 11 p.m. and 7 a.m. This period can vary by an hour or two at either end of the night – unless there is something else to do, such as working shifts, staying up partying or making an early start on a journey.

The idea that a single night-time period of sleep is the norm is reinforced by numerous medical and scientific texts, as well as self-help books for managing insomnia. This sleep pattern is described as *monophasic* (see Steger 2012) in contrast to *biphasic* and *polyphasic* patterns. Furthermore, a pattern of *segmented* sleep has been noted through examination of historical literature (see Box 4.1; Ekirch 2001, 2006). This chapter explores these different sleep patterns, demonstrating that 'normal' sleep is not as straightforward as might be thought. In addition to looking at differences over time and between cultures, it examines differences *within* cultures (chiefly between males and females, since age-related differences are discussed elsewhere). Lastly, it considers implications for therapy.

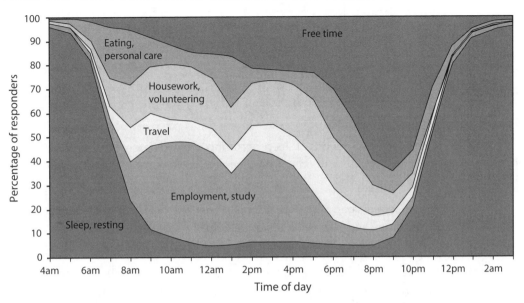

FIGURE 4.1A The distribution of activities on weekdays
Data from Lader, Short and Gershuny (2006).

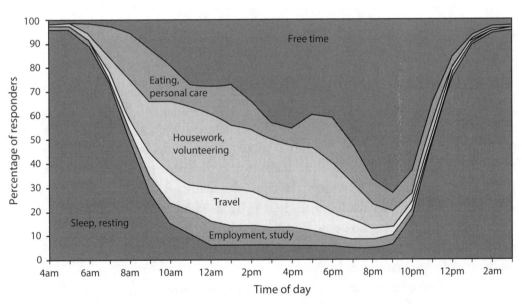

FIGURE 4.1B The distribution of activities on weekends
Data from Lader et al. (2006).

BOX 4.1 Terminology of sleep patterns

- *Monophasic sleep*: a single night-time period of sleep.

- *Segmented sleep*: two periods of sleep, occurring at night, and separated by a period of wakefulness.

- *Biphasic sleep*: two periods of sleep, occurring at two different times, separated by daytime activity, with one of the sleeps taking place during the day, such as a siesta.

- *Polyphasic sleep*: sleep periods that are short and irregular, taken at individually selected times, and taken in addition to night-time sleep.

Steger (2012) also distinguishes between the contexts in which a nap occurs: a *monochronic* nap takes place in private and the person is unavailable to social life, whereas in a *polychronic* nap the individual dozes in the presence of others who are awake and remains – 'at least in part – socially aware of what is going on and always prepared to engage…if necessary' (p.74).[1]

4.2 Monophasic sleep and time use

An idea of how people fit sleep into their 24-hour routines can be gained from time-use surveys and polls. The main pitfalls of such surveys are that they depend on self-report and produce only average figures. There are also difficulties with categorization of activities as there is often no clear distinction between *sleep* and *rest*, or between *rest* and *passive activity* such as watching television; this is further complicated, for example, when someone dozes off while watching television. These issues are discussed in more detail by Green (2012a); however, time-use studies do give a good impression of how people use their time, and when large numbers are involved, they can give insight into the habits of a population as a whole.

The findings of one study with a sample of nearly 5000 people (Lader, Short and Gershuny 2006) are summarized in Figures 4.1a and 4.1b. They indicate that within the UK population:

- 90% of people are asleep between the hours of about 1:00 and 5:30 a.m.

- 90% take their sleep in the period between the hours of 9 p.m. and 9 a.m.

- 75% are asleep or resting by 11:30 p.m. and 75% are out of bed by 8 a.m.

- 50% are in bed by 11 p.m. and 50% are up by 7 a.m.

- People tend to sleep later at weekends.

It should not be inferred from these examples that 75% of people were in bed for a whole 10 hours, or that 50% sleep for 8.5 hours; however, the average total sleep time for men was just over 8 hours (484 minutes) per day, and for women, about 8.25 hours (498 minutes). These averages compare with figures in a survey in the US involving over 47,000 respondents (Basner *et al.* 2007), which found that the average sleep time on a weekday was just less than 8 hours (472 minutes) for the 45–54-year age group (and 539 minutes for the over-75-years age group). These figures for sleep time are slightly higher than those shown in Chapter 3 (which relate to a survey specifically about sleep), perhaps because they include daytime rest and, in the case of the US study, time spent in bed in the hope of sleep.

In the next section of this chapter it is noted that, overall, the monophasic sleep pattern is associated with greater productivity. Indeed, Basner *et al.* (2007) found that work was the activity most commonly exchanged for sleep: as work time increases, the time for sleep decreases. This was also noted by Swanson *et al.* (2011) reporting on a poll of 1000 workers in the US. They observed that the 'poll…found that employed Americans get less sleep than they need to function well at work' (p.491). Respondents who slept for less than 6 hours a night were more likely to have a work schedule that did not allow sufficient sleep. Reviewing data from studies in 12 countries (in western Europe, in the former Eastern Bloc, the US and Peru) Biddle and Hamermesh (1990) calculated that an extra 1 hour of work cost about 10 minutes of sleep and found that people who were not working slept about an hour more than people in employment. As economists, Biddle and Hamermesh (1990) concluded that sleep 'is affected by the same economic variables that affect choices about other uses of time' (p.941) and that, in effect, part of our sleep time is optional – 'a reserve on which people can draw when economic circumstances make other uses of time more attractive' (p.941). This anticipated the proposal of Horne (2006) that we need 'core sleep' (between 6 and 7 hours) and can also have 'optional sleep' (pp.204–205) in the same way that we can continue eating once hunger is satisfied. (For more on the economics involved in the personal choices about sleep time see Biddle and Hamermesh 1990, Green 2012a, 2012b and Yaniv 2004.) It remains controversial as to whether, or how much, we can have 'optional' sleep, but there clearly are choices that we can make over and above our individual tendencies for sleep duration and timing.

4.3 Segmented sleep

Of all animals, only humans have a monophasic sleep pattern, and it was thought that in this respect humans were fundamentally different (Wehr 1992). Wehr (1992) cites research showing that whereas the average chimpanzee is awake for 17% of its main sleep period, a young adult human's total wakefulness amounts to only 0.86% of their main sleep time. However, when people have a longer sleep period in laboratory conditions (e.g. 14 hours) they typically have a waking interval in line with other primates. Wehr (1992) suggests that 'consolidated sleep in human beings may be an artifact of modern lighting technology' (p.103). Indeed, widespread monophasic sleep is probably a by-product of industrialization: the invention of effective and affordable artificial lighting allowed the majority to extend daytime activity well into the hours of darkness, and workers increasingly had to adapt to the long factory hours in order to maximize production (see also Scrivner 2012). In contrast, in an agrarian economy in mid-latitude temperate regions individuals could adjust more easily to the seasons and environmental changes. For example, in the summertime in the UK it was (and is) possible to start work at first light in the cooler morning hours, sleep in the heat of the early afternoon (a custom that persisted in Mediterranean countries and elsewhere) and return to work later in the day. Although in winter there is less outdoor work, afternoon sleep would have been a waste of the daylight hours. In this case, it was passing the long cold nights that presented the challenge.

Maintaining a segmented sleep pattern was such a way to spend the hours of darkness. As shown below, there is ample evidence that in preindustrial society, and perhaps still in some traditional cultures in Africa and elsewhere, people would take two periods of sleep during the night – the first sleep and the second sleep. These periods would be separated by a period of 'quiet wakefulness' in which people would typically talk with their bedfellows or roommates. They would thereby remain warm in bed (or in their sleeping quarters in the absence of beds) as well as be more alert to the dangers of the night outside. Wehr (1996) has also suggested that this allowed people to access the 'wellspring of myths and fantasies' (p.341) since people would wake from rapid eye movement (REM) sleep* and recount their dreams to their companions.

The evidence for segmented sleep has been well documented by Ekirch (2001) and widely described and discussed (e.g. Green 2012b). Briefly, Ekirch notes that he found references to the term 'first sleep' in 58 sources in English literature of the period from the fourteenth century to the seventeenth century, as well as similar references in French and Italian literature of the same era. To cite just one example from Ekirch (2001), during the reign of Queen Mary the following advice for better digestion and more tranquil repose was offered by Andrew Borde:

> Whan you be in your bedde, lye a lyttle whyle on your lefte syde, and slepe on your ryght syde. And when you do wake of your fyrste slepe, make water yf you feel your bladder charged, & then slepe on your lefte syde. (Borde 1867, p.129, first published circa 1557)

Like his contemporaries, Borde refers to waking from the first sleep in a way that indicates that it was the routine and completely normal; however, Ekirch (2001) notes that references to segmented sleep among the upper classes are less commonly found, reflecting the trend towards keeping late hours, using artificial light that only they could afford. Going to bed later engendered monophasic sleep for the wealthy centuries ahead of the masses.

Evidence of the survival of the segmented sleep pattern in traditional cultures is harder to trace. Ekirch (2001) cites anthropology texts indicating that, for example, the Tiv of central Nigeria use the terms 'first sleep' and 'second sleep' as intervals of time. Worthman and Melby (2002) explain how in traditional societies the degree of separation between sleep and wake states may vary. The !Kung of Botswana and the Efe (previously Zaire) of the Democratic Republic of the Congo, for example, do not have bedtimes. People may therefore stay up while there is something interesting happening, but after going to sleep, they might get up again if they hear something going on. This is not the more 'organized' segmented sleep of cold preindustrial Europe, but it illustrates the flexibility of sleep patterns that is possible. Worthman and Melby (2002) also mention a useful facility among the Gabra of northern Kenya where 'sleep offers one way to "check out" of interminable, slow-moving circular, or frustrating debates' (p.85). For the Gabra sleeping and waking are both social behaviours, and withdrawal to sleep in public is quite acceptable.

When the BBC referred recently to the work of Ekirch on its website (Hegarty 2012a) a range of responses was received from individuals who related their own experience of segmented sleep in the modern day (Hegarty 2012b). One correspondent recalled growing up in Papua (Indonesia) where his parents were working among the Yali people. He wrote about spending time camping with his young Yali friends:

> We would go to bed more or less after sunset and people would always wake up during the night. I would hear them talking and someone would start a fire. Sometimes we would eat some sweet potato before going back to sleep until 05:30 or 06:00. (Iain Wilson quoted by Hegarty 2012b)

Segmented sleep could be considered a waste of time in the West if it involves going to bed earlier and spending longer in bed; however, the total time asleep is not increased. The correspondents to the BBC certainly did not seem to regard it as time wasted (although the sample was self-selecting). For example, one person practised yoga while another did artwork – drawing upon material from dreams. In these instances, the individuals were possibly waking later in the night than was traditionally the case, but one woman described having 4 hours of sleep and then waking to prepare a meal for her husband who returned from work at about midnight. After eating and spending some time together, they would go to bed at 3 a.m.

Arguably, for some people this kind of segmented sleep is an adaptation to insomnia (although, on the other hand, it could be suggested that middle insomnia is merely a return to 'default mode'). One correspondent described waking at an unspecified time and, originally, being anxious:

> When I was a full-time teacher and had a busy workload in the morning, I used to get anxious that I wouldn't fall back to sleep. Now I have the luxury of knowing that I have at least two hours of wonderful sleep to come with brilliant dreaming. It is like having your very own home cinema to look forward to every night: the sheer expectation sends me to sleep again. (Bernie O'Leary quoted by Hegarty 2012b)

It appears therefore that the key is to be relaxed and not to think of the period of wakefulness as a time that one *should* be asleep: that would be a sure recipe for anxiety and insomnia. While segmented sleep may not be a practical option for the majority of people in modern life, it *is* an option.

Ekirch (2001) noted that the Christian church 'colonized' (p.367) the period of night-time wakefulness. He suggests that monks were not forced from their slumber to go and pray during the night: they were awake anyway, between their first and second sleeps. Another correspondent to the BBC observed that, as a Muslim, he would rise for voluntary night-time prayer. He continued:

> We also have a dawn prayer, which is obligatory, so sometimes I stay up until dawn and then go back to sleep. According to the Koran, Muhammad slept in this way. So segmented sleep is quite normal in the Muslim tradition. (Reham Samir quoted by Hegarty 2012b)

To sum up, segmented sleep was probably the norm for a large part of human history, but we have adapted to modern life and most of us expect unbroken night-time sleep. In some traditional cultures segmented sleep probably continues and there are also people in industrial societies who for a variety of reasons either choose or accept a segmented sleep pattern. While it was industrialization that brought about the decline of segmented sleep, it is arguable that computers and the Internet, which now make it so easy to remain active, or to spend time during the night communicating with other people around the world, could have unexpectedly encouraged a return of the ancient sleep pattern for some. Our sleep patterns appear to be capable of changing, and changing back, in response to different lifestyles.

4.4 Biphasic sleep and polyphasic sleep (napping)

Steger (2012) distinguishes segmented sleep from biphasic sleep. Although segmented sleep involves two bouts of sleep, they traditionally occur at night within a single sleeping period during the hours of darkness, and generally without leaving the sleeping space. In contrast to this, biphasic sleep involves sleeping at two different times separated by daytime activity, and one of the sleeps occurs during the daylight hours. This is the siesta – from the Latin *sexta hora*: the sixth hour. (The sixth hour is in the middle of the day in cultures where the hours of the day are counted from dawn – a potential source of confusion for travellers in Africa, for example.) As noted in Chapter 3, the siesta is a means of slowing down in the heat of the day and conserving resources, and not a direct result of eating a meal. However, Steger (2012) suggests that the siesta is not just a consequence of midday heat, or of a heavy meal, but that the *idea* of a good meal with a rest at midday relates to a perception of how a proper life should be led.

We are still 'programmed' by the circadian drive to sleep in the early afternoon, although the drive is not strong and it is usually possible to resist it, especially if sufficient sleep has been taken the previous night. In Protestant Christian cultures in particular, and in industrial society in general, afternoon sleep is often considered to be only for the very young, the very old or the infirm. As Jacobs (2012) notes, according to the Protestant ethic 'every waking hour engaged in work is regarded as spiritually valuable [implying that sleep is] inherently spiritually worthless' (p.249). However, the siesta is under threat in non-Protestant European countries, especially in urban areas. Air conditioning makes indoor work more comfortable and there is pressure through globalization to continue communicating with other countries at all available opportunities. If people commute further to work, taking time out for a long break is not practical and would diminish time at home in the evening. Mednick (2006) reports that only 7% of Spaniards in big cities now have a daytime sleep.

According to *The Daily Telegraph*, the European financial crisis has further threatened the siesta in Spain (Roberts 2012). The report notes that although many people had been taking a short lunch break for some time, the Spanish government was relaxing rules and allowing large shops to remain open through the afternoon in the hope of boosting trade. Similarly, in China an afternoon sleep persisted and, as Steger (2012) shows, there was also a political element to this. The traditional custom was officially sanctioned by the Communist government in 1950, establishing the right of workers to rest. In the 1980s, in response to the suggestion that the midday sleep was associated with communism and economic backwardness, the break was reduced to 1 hour. Although there was some ideological pressure to resist Western work practices, the short break has continued; 'people now nap at any time when they find an opportunity' (Steger 2012, p.79) and there is, at least in cities, no common break. In neighbouring Taiwan, according to Steger (2012), a short (quarter-hour) nap is common not only in the classroom, but also in the office, where lights are switched off and 'employees lay their heads on their desks and take a short nap' (p.79). This does not amount to a siesta but, equally, it is a collective sleep and thereby can be distinguished from an individual's nap.

Napping represents polyphasic sleep, in which naps are often irregular, at individually selected times and taken in addition to night-time sleep. As noted above, napping has a negative connotation in the West but is much more acceptable in some other cultures. Retreating into sleep in social gatherings among the Gabra people of Kenya has already been noted above, but in one industrial country at least, Japan, people may take a nap in a lecture or in a meeting. Steger (2012) notes that a sleeping student might be assumed to have been working hard the previous night, and that established employees might doze in a meeting as it is their *presence* that is important, while more eager, young employees take a more active part in the proceedings. In other parts of the world, the traveller might observe people napping in public, using time waiting for trade, work or other business to catch up with sleep. Such public napping might seem outlandish to British sensibilities. In the UK the only place where people are usually found sleeping in public are places like airports, trains and coaches or buses, and (unwisely) while sunbathing in a park or on a beach. Someone sleeping on the street is probably assumed to be homeless, but anyone who enjoys the guilty pleasure of a nap is likely to welcome the concept of the 'power nap' – a term coined by James Maas (Maas 1998, p.136). Maas argues that the nap is more effective at getting to the root of sleepiness (which is insufficient sleep) than consumption of caffeine, which might bring a transitory feeling of alertness. He encourages an early-afternoon 15–30-minute nap and claims that employees in companies that allow naps are more alert and productive, and less accident-prone. (See Mednick 2006 for further argument in favour of the nap.)

More recently, Ficca *et al.* (2010) carried out a detailed review of research into napping. They concluded that 'napping is an effective important countermeasure to maintain adequate performance levels during extended work shifts' and that even a 10-minute nap 'can improve alertness and performance for about 2.5 hours if prior sleep loss exists, and for almost 4 hours if preceded by normal sleep' (p.256). Furthermore, they note that naps appear to be beneficial for memory consolidation, although longer naps might be necessary for that. They add the usual caution that unplanned and longer naps might interfere with night-time sleep and be associated with negative health consequences (see Box 4.2).

BOX 4.2 Taking a nap

When having a nap it is important to restrict the time to 20–30 minutes at most. If a nap is longer, there is a strong likelihood of going into deeper sleep: resulting in an extended sleep period with unhelpful consequences. First, the extended nap may itself disrupt the afternoon schedule, making the individual late for appointments. Second, the nap could reduce the main drive to sleep, delaying the subsequent bedtime. Furthermore, if the individual is roused when in deep sleep, they are likely to wake up feeling groggy – and potentially feeling worse, since we feel better when waking naturally from lighter sleep stages. If oversleeping is a concern, it might help to set an alarm, and remaining seated might prevent the napper becoming too comfortable and drifting into deep sleep.

It remains unclear whether total sleep time in 24 hours in the case of napping is increased or whether it is just catching up on lost night-time sleep. (See Green 2012b and Horne 2010 for further discussion of napping.) A nap is not necessarily a sign of laziness, although it remains the responsibility of employees to ensure that they are fit for work by having sufficient sleep before work. On the other hand, when an employee is expected to work shifts (especially at night, or in changing time zones in the airline industry, for example) it becomes the responsibility of an employer to ensure that the worker has sufficient time for sleep – and that might be much longer than the bare hours needed for sleep, since time is needed to adjust.

4.5 Cultural factors

The different sleep patterns described above reflect varying cultural attitudes about sleep and about how life is lived. One influence on cultural values is religious belief. Jacobs (2012) notes that 'in world religions sleep usually only merits passing comments' (p.247), although, as he shows, religious beliefs do influence understanding and beliefs about sleep. Ancoli-Israel (2001) points out that in the Hebrew tradition sleep was well understood for thousands of years[2] and suggests that 'sleep is a result of divine intervention, with ordinary sleep seen as a gift from God' (p.779). Similarly, in Islam, according to BaHammam (2011), sleep is considered to be a sign of the greatness of Allāh and is mentioned frequently in the Quran. Islamic teaching clearly recognizes the importance of sleep and it also seems probable that the daily prayer rituals of devout Muslims will serve to reinforce good sleep habits. The same might be said of Eastern religions where there are requirements for routines of prayer and meditation.

There is some ambivalence towards sleep in the Christian tradition where, as Jacobs (2012) notes, the apostles are chided for sleeping while Jesus prayed in the garden at Gethsemane, whereas they were criticized for their lack of faith in failing to sleep during a storm on Galilee. However, perhaps the most influential effect of Christianity on sleep has been the Protestant ethic, mentioned above. A prominent exponent of the 'danger' of sleep was the New England Puritan minister Cotton Mather who held that the Devil laid snares 'on the *Bed*, where it is *Lawful* for us to Sleep' (Mather 1862, p.179, first published 1693). Wolf-Meyer (2012) traces ideas about sleep in the US from Mather, via Benjamin Franklin, to the pioneers of sleep medicine, Nathaniel Kleitman and William Dement. He reaches the conclusion that 'if sleep disrupts daily life, then it must be controlled' (p.78). He continues: 'The flexibility of sleep must be aligned with the variations allowed in spatiotemporal rhythms of everyday life rather than everyday life being rendered more flexible for the sake of sleep' (p.78). The Puritan legacy is strong in the West. Although few would now curtail sleep to minimize the influence of the Devil, there is still a tendency to devalue sleep and to give priority to other things.[3]

Sleep science, as well as the study of sleep in general, has emerged in the West, and Worthman and Melby (2002) observe how much of the sleep research carried out in laboratories reflects the cultural ecology of Western sleep. In the West solitary sleep – or sleep with a single co-sleeper – is the norm. Clear bedtimes are imposed in childhood and continued throughout life, and housing provides a quiet, dark and controlled environment for a consolidated sleep period. However, in non-Western and traditional societies people are much more likely to sleep in groups where conditions are less controlled, and where there is far more background noise. In traditional cultures there may be an open fire, and while the sleeping place might be less physically secure, there may be security in numbers. People in traditional societies may not use soft bedding, pillows or covers but might sleep on the ground – on a mat, skins or leaves – or on a wooden platform. As Worthman and Melby (2002) put it, 'non-Western sleep settings tend to be sensorily dynamic' (p.107). Worthman and Melby expand on some of the detailed practices of traditional societies and highlight differences between them, but such groups now represent a tiny proportion of the world's population. It seems reasonable to conclude that in most parts of the world the use of beds or mattresses, for example, has become the norm.

Although with growing prosperity and urbanization people around the world are increasingly likely to use beds and other ways to enhance comfort at night, sharing rooms remains common in much of the world. Steger (2012) observes that American students sharing a room at university often experience a degree of sleep disruption if they are used to their own bedrooms. In contrast, students from African or south Asian backgrounds thought nothing of sharing and seemed comfortable with the arrangement.

Perhaps the greatest diversity in sleeping habits around the world relates to the sleep of children. This diversity is exemplified in a review by Giannotti and Cortesi (2009) which examines sleep patterns, arrangements, settings and bedtime routines. Although a bewildering array of information is presented, their findings are worth exploring in some detail. For example, they cite research suggesting that working parents in the US, who have limited time in the evening, might prioritize spending time with their children over getting them to bed early. Similarly, Italian children usually go to bed later, as the evening 'has also become an integral part of the "quality time" that many middle-class parents devote to their children' (Giannotti and Cortesi 2009, p.856). In China, however, later bedtimes may often reflect burning the midnight oil with a strong emphasis on academic achievement (Liu *et al.* 2005) and may conversely affect daytime performance and lead to daytime sleepiness.

Daytime sleep habits in preschool children also show wide variation. Giannotti and Cortesi (2009) cite studies finding that fewer than 10% of Italian children of 4–5 years of age still nap regularly compared with over half of children of the same age in the US. Crosby, LeBourgeois and Harsh (2005) found further differences between racial groups in the US. Working in an area of Mississippi, they compared two groups of children (aged 2–8 years) which they categorized as black and white – excluding children of other races or mixed racial background. The black children continued napping at later ages than the white children, reflecting shorter nocturnal sleep, but total sleep time over 24 hours was very similar in both groups. The timing of children's sleep in traditional societies will reflect more fluid sleep-wake patterns, and in tropical climates 'an afternoon nap during the heat of the day is almost mandatory' (Giannotti and Cortesi 2009, p.857) with shorter night-time sleep.

It has been noted that the sleep environment can vary, with differences in bedding and attitudes towards sharing, and there is similar variation in co-sleeping arrangements. Giannotti and Cortesi (2009) state that it is 'only in industrialized Western societies, such as those in North America and some parts of Europe, that sleep has become a "private" affair' (p.854); however, they also note that there is variation within the US where co-sleeping varies with ethnicity and geographic area: they cite evidence that 'up to 70% of African American children, 21% of Latino children, and less than 10% of middle-class Caucasian [children] share their parents' beds' (p.854). Additionally, they suggest that 'Asian mothers believe that children are too young to sleep alone' (p.854) and report co-sleeping rates of over 90% in India and 80% in Japan. Rates of co-sleeping vary in Europe, but a figure of 10–14% of toddlers in Italy is cited, although co-sleeping is 'almost absent during the first year of life' (Giannotti and Cortesi 2009, p.855).

Although co-sleeping around the world is common, sharing with a baby carries risks and in many countries the advice is not to share a bed with a baby in any circumstances because of the increased incidence of sudden infant death syndrome (SIDS). Carpenter *et al.* (2013) examined a number of studies on SIDS and concluded:

Our findings suggest that professionals and the literature should take a more definite stand against bed sharing, especially for babies under 3 months. If parents were made aware of the risks of sleeping with their baby, and room sharing were promoted, as 'Back to Sleep' was promoted 20 years ago, a substantial further reduction in SIDS rates could be achieved. (Carpenter *et al.* 2013, p.10)[4]

The other main variable in children's sleep noted by Giannotti and Cortesi (2009) is in bedtime routines. For example, they cite an (unpublished) research finding that over 40% of a sample of Portuguese parents remained with their children until they fall asleep, as well as a study in Rome that found a high degree of parental involvement at bedtime in 50% of a sample of 3000 children. They note how an Indian study found that only 42% of a sample of 103 children (aged 3–10 years) had a bedtime routine, that two thirds refused to sleep in the absence of a parent and that television viewing delayed the bedtime of 39%; no child slept in a separate room (Bharti, Malhi and Kashyap 2006). According to other studies cited by Giannotti and Cortesi (2009) growing numbers of children around the world have television sets in their rooms or use them as part of a pre-bedtime routine or sleep aid, despite evidence of an association between television viewing and sleep disturbances in 5–6-year-olds (Paavonen *et al.* 2006).

4.6 Sociological factors

It is noted in Chapter 3 that there are few recorded objective differences between the sleep of men and women, except that, as they age, men tend to have less deep (slow-wave) sleep. The sleep of women is more prone to disturbance in later life because of the menopause, where there may be hot flushes and night sweats as well as changes in stress reactivity, for example (Lee and Moe 2011). Baker, O'Brien and Armitage (2011) also note that women have shorter sleep latency★, better sleep efficiency★ and more sleep than men.[5] Other differences between the sleep of men and women would appear to result from factors determined by culture and society. However, a study reported by Kloesch and Dittami (2008) suggests the possibility of a further biological difference or a combination of biology and culturally determined gender roles.

Kloesch and Dittami (2008) contend that the sharing of a bed by couples is a relatively recent phenomenon.[6] They state that 'pair-sleep with common bedding and close tactile and olfactory contact is primarily found in mother-infant interactions and not among siblings or in sexual pairs' (p.96). They report on their study where the sleep of unmarried heterosexual couples was assessed using subjective self-report measures and actigraphy★ both when they slept together and when sleeping apart. The results clearly showed that pair-sleep is more disturbing for females, whereas the sleep of the male is no different from his sleep if he were alone. Kloesch and Dittami (2008) speculate that one explanation could relate to upbringing and culturally determined gender roles, whereas the biological explanation would be that women need to be more reactive to the presence of others in order to fulfil a maternal role.

There are suggestions that the more socially determined sleep habits of women and men have been different for generations. Referring to German medieval literature Klug (2008) explains how it was the role of the 'brave knight' to look after his lady by day; her role was to watch over him at night while he slept. The gender differences in sleeping arrangements of the lower orders at that time are not known, but as Meadows (2012) notes, 'nowadays, women need to be alert at night because of their caring roles for children and other family members' (p.109). We could rephrase that to say that the sleep of carers, male or female, tends to be compromised – and it is not only during the period of actual care, but also long after care is over (Bianchera and Arber 2007). In reality, of course, the majority of informal care at home is provided by women. Meadows (2012) comments that the research suggests that there is actually little discussion about who undertakes physical and emotional care and that 'women's compromised access to sleep quality is, therefore, often the result of "unspoken", implicit decision-making and non-negotiation' (p.110).

In a qualitative study involving 26 couples Venn *et al.* (2008) found that mothers took on the role of responding to children at night. Only two of the fathers in the study (8%) were actively involved, but in both cases the child – or twins in one case – had a significant health problem. It appears therefore that these fathers shared care where there was an additional burden beyond the usual disturbance to sleep that children can cause (which otherwise was deemed the responsibility of the mothers). However, it was noted that the father of the twins was responding to their physical needs 'rather than anticipating or worrying about their children's needs' (Venn *et al.* 2008, p.89) in the way that, the authors contend, mothers do. The mothers simply carried on being attuned to the children's needs and continued the physical caring of the day into the night. The mothers may well have understandably prioritized the sleep of their working partner while not in employment themselves, but it was observed that when mothers returned to work there was rarely a renegotiation of care responsibilities at night. It was at a much later stage that fathers were more usually involved, when older children were out late at night; they would comment that they could not sleep until the teenagers were safely home – a common concern being who was driving them home. There appears therefore to have been some reflection of traditional stereotypes whereby mothers were nurturing and fathers were protecting the family. (It is not known how same-sex couples allocate or share care responsibilities at night.)

These findings reflect the earlier observations of Hislop and Arber (2003) in a focus group study. They argue that the sleep of 'mid-life' women (aged 40–59 years) is 'structured by the multiplicity of roles and responsibilities they carry out as part of their daily lives: as partners and/or mothers, as working women or as daughters of aging parents' (p.709). Sleep is likely to be disrupted and the authors suggest that 'being female within a family structure can thus be synonymous with a loss of sleeping rights' (p.709), which they go on to argue could be construed as compromising their basic human rights.

A quantitative perspective of sleep differences is provided by the Understanding Society project, a longitudinal survey involving 14,000 households in the UK (McFall and Garrington 2011). The first round of the survey asked seven questions on sleep, about duration and quality, problems with sleep and responses to problems. Results showed that women at all ages are more likely than men to report problems getting to sleep and remaining asleep, and to report poor sleep quality. The use of sleeping tablets was similar in men and women until about the age of 65 years after which use by women was greater (Arber and Meadows 2011). A further finding of the survey was that sleep could vary according to marital status or socio-economic class. Broadly, married people reported the best sleep followed by those who never married; divorced people reported the worst sleep, and for those who had been widowed it was not much better. It is not certain how these findings accord with those above of Kloesch and Dittami (2008). See also Meadows and Arber (2012) and Troxel (2010) on couples' sleep, and for further discussion on the effect on sleep of gender and socioeconomic status see Arber, Bote and Meadows (2009).

The relationship found in the Understanding Society survey between sleep and social class (determined by current or last occupation) and educational status seemed clear: those with the highest educational qualifications reported the fewest sleep problems, as did those with higher professional jobs, while those with no qualifications or in routine occupations reported the worst sleep. People in employment had the best sleep, followed by the retired; unemployed people reported more problems, but by far the worst sleep on all measures was reported by the disabled or sick. Similarly, there was a clear relationship between good sleep and perceived health, with those reporting poor health having much worse sleep. The findings of the survey are summed up as follows:

> Women consistently are more likely to have sleep problems than men. Several sleep problems increase with age, particularly short duration, taking sleeping medication and waking up in the night. When adjusting for age and gender, married people have better sleep patterns than divorced and separated persons and the widowed. For each sleep measure, those in more disadvantageous socio-economic circumstances are more likely to report problematic sleep. There are also very strong associations between poor sleep and negative health perceptions and having health conditions that have limiting effects. (Arber and Meadows 2011, p.96)

4.7 Implications for therapy

While Chapter 3 shows that our sleep pattern is regulated by a combination of the circadian and homeostatic drives, and that there is great natural variation in timing, duration and structure of sleep which are dependent on age and genetic make-up, this chapter shows that there is yet further variation determined by who we are and the way that we live. For most of us, our sleep mechanisms are sufficiently flexible to allow us to adopt different patterns; this might be as a society, with sleep habits reflecting cultural norms or the climate of the region, or more individual choices perhaps in response to economic demands (as in shift work) or care demands. In the last three centuries we have increasingly adopted a (monophasic) sleep pattern that departs from the pattern that evolved over millennia, and it should perhaps therefore be no surprise that sleep disturbances are as common as they are. The management of sleep disorders is discussed in Chapter 8, but some general observations are made here.

A reassuring observation from Chapter 3 was that it is quite normal (and therefore generally harmless) to wake frequently at night. To this can be added the suggestion that a lengthy period of wakefulness at night is also 'normal'. This will not be quite as reassuring to a busy person in the modern age who has only an 8-hour window, or less, in which to sleep, but it does allow the possibility of other options. For example, as seen in the examples of night-time activity (Hegarty 2012b), an option is to cease worrying about monophasic sleep and adopt a segmented sleep pattern, using the period of wakefulness for some useful or enjoyable purpose.

The natural tendency for segmented sleep also offers support for the rationale behind sleep restriction therapy (see Chapter 8) for insomnia. It is suggested that people with insomnia often extend their time in bed in the hope of getting more sleep. In fact, by doing that a person could simply be inviting a longer period of night-time wakefulness. Sleep became consolidated as people began to spend less time in bed (as lighting became more widely available and kept them up later) and this is what is recommended in sleep restriction therapy in order to achieve the same result.

Similarly, taking a nap is a natural act and people in much of the world do not give it a second thought. While daytime sleep is discouraged for people with insomnia (who, as seen in Chapter 8, find it difficult to nap anyway), a strategic nap is beneficial for many people; the key is to keep it short and not to go into deep sleep. If someone chooses to have a longer daytime sleep, or a siesta, they are also performing an entirely natural act which still occurs in many areas of the world and until relatively recently in the summer in temperate latitudes. There is nothing wrong with this as long as it fits the person's lifestyle (which may not then synchronize easily with society) and the person does not still expect a full night's sleep. There are also times when a nap is to be actively recommended, for example, if someone feels drowsy when driving (see Box 4.3).

BOX 4.3 Avoiding sleeping at the wheel

Feeling sleepy while driving should alert the driver to the danger of falling asleep, and measures such as opening windows or turning up the radio will not cure sleepiness. In the UK driving while sleepy is categorized as dangerous driving and it is no defence in law to deny feeling sleepy before dozing off, because we do not doze off without warning (Dyfed-Powys Police 2011). If a driver is sleepy, the usual advice is to stop where it is safe, have a caffeinated drink, such as two cups of coffee (Dyfed-Powys Police 2011), and then sleep for 15 minutes – the time that it takes for the caffeine to begin to take effect. Even if the nap were likely to affect night-time sleep, or if the caffeine were taken later in the day than usually recommended, the need for safety takes priority over the other considerations in this instance.

While understanding the interplay between biological factors and social and cultural factors helps to inform therapeutic intervention to improve sleep, it can also suggest alternatives for people whose health conditions do not easily permit monophasic sleep. For example, as discussed in Chapter 16, chronic pain poses a threat to consolidated sleep and, theoretically, adopting a biphasic (or segmented) sleep pattern offers a perfectly reasonable alternative for some individuals, especially given the usual advice of pacing activity and not spending too long at once in any position. Plainly, this would not work for anyone hoping to remain in traditional, regular paid employment, but some occupations and employment practices do lend themselves to fitting around different sleep patterns, where flexible working hours can be an option and where it does not matter exactly when the work involved has to be done. These are very personal, individual choices, but for some people there can be real advantages which outweigh the inconvenience of being partly out of step with society.

4.8 Conclusion

In conclusion, there is no right or wrong about sleeping patterns, although the monophasic pattern dominates in industrialized society and is probably most efficient and convenient. However, different cultural norms and historical variations indicate that other options exist and that it may be possible in managing sleep, in the context of some medical conditions, to adopt different patterns. There are also sociological and cultural aspects to consider, and it is important to take account of caring roles and differences in child-rearing practices. In summary, we must not assume that people's sleep needs or habits are consistent, any more than we would expect their dietary requirements or practices to be the same.

Notes

1   In Japan such naps are known as *inemuri*: 'literally "the sleep taken whilst present in a situation that is not oriented around sleep", such as naps during a train ride or in a business meeting' (Steger 2012, p.74).

2   Ancoli-Israel (2001) expands on the knowledge in biblical times: 'Our ancestors were aware that sleep was not one continuous stage. They referred to the function of sleep as being restorative. They deplored sleep deprivation, believing that it impaired life. They felt that excessive sleepiness was harmful. They understood that insomnia could be caused by stress and anxiety and by excessive alcohol, and that physical activity (exercise) and drinking milk could improve sleep. They suggested cures for insomnia, including some of the ideas included in today's sleep hygiene* rules. They understood that there was a rhythm or timing to sleep. They even understood that it was easier to delay the circadian rhythm than to advance it. They often took naps in the afternoon, but suggested just how long that nap should last – about one half hour. And they knew that with age, sleep is advanced, but that the elderly who were healthy did not have difficulty sleeping' (p.786).

3   It is not only people with a Protestant Christian background who might devalue sleep. The following is widely attributed to the science fiction writer Isaac Asimov: 'I never use an alarm clock. I can hardly wait until five a.m. In the army I always woke before reveille. I hate sleeping. It wastes time.' See, for example, Kendrick (2004).

4   The Back to Sleep campaign has now become the Safe to Sleep® campaign (see www.nichd. nih.gov/sts/Pages/default.aspx, accessed on 20 October 2013).

5   There is also evidence that women and men have different temperature rhythms (see, for example, Baker *et al.* 2001) and that men have a greater temperature drop at night. The latter phenomenon is reflected in the availability of 'His and Hers', or split tog, duvets with different levels of insulation in the two halves.

6   Although it is a fairly recent phenomenon, bed sharing is on the decline according to reports on the Internet and in the popular press. For example, see (all accessed on 20 October 2013):

- http://news.bbc.co.uk/1/hi/8245578.stm
- www.dailymail.co.uk/femail/article-2360193/One-couples-sleep-separate-beds.html
- www.telegraph.co.uk/news/uknews/9359342/One-in-10-British-couples-sleep-in-separate-beds.html
- www.cbc.ca/news/health/more-couples-opting-to-sleep-in-separate-beds-study-suggests-1.1316019

As found in clinical experience and, as reported by Robert Meadows of the University of Surrey (personal communication), couples may be reluctant to disclose that they sleep separately; it is therefore difficult to estimate accurately how many couples do.

References

Ancoli-Israel, S. (2001) '"Sleep is not tangible" or what the Hebrew Tradition has to say about sleep.' *Psychosomatic Medicine 63*, 6, 778–787.

Arber, S., Bote, M. and Meadows, R. (2009) 'Gender and socio-economic patterning of self-reported sleep problems in Britain.' *Social Science & Medicine 68*, 2, 281–289.

Arber, S. and Meadows, R. (2011) 'Social and Health Patterning of Sleep Quality and Duration.' In S.L. McFall and C. Garrington (eds) *Early Findings from the First Wave of the UK's Household Longitudinal Study*. Colchester: Institute for Social and Economic Research, University of Essex.

BaHammam, A.S. (2011) 'Sleep from an Islamic perspective.' *Annals of Thoracic Medicine 6*, 4, 187–192.

Baker, F.C., O'Brien, L.M. and Armitage, R. (2011) 'Sex Differences and Menstrual-Related Changes in Sleep and Circadian Rhythms.' In M.H. Kryger, T. Roth and W.C. Dement (eds) *Principles and Practice of Sleep Medicine*, 5th edn. St Louis, MO: Elsevier Saunders.

Baker, F.C., Waner, J.I., Viera, E.F., Taylor, S.R., Driver, H.S. and Mitchell, D. (2001) 'Sleep and 24 hour body temperatures: a comparison in young men, naturally cycling women and women taking hormonal contraceptives.' *Journal of Physiology 530*, 3, 565–574.

Basner, M., Fomberstein, K.M., Razavi, F.M., Banks, S. *et al.* (2007) 'American time use survey: sleep time and its relationship to waking activities.' *Sleep 30*, 9, 1085–1095.

Bharti, B., Malhi, B. and Kashyap, S. (2006) 'Patterns and problems of sleep in school going children.' *Indian Pediatrics 43*, 1, 35–38.

Bianchera, E. and Arber, S. (2007) 'Caring and Sleep Disruption Among Women in Italy.' *Sociological Research Online 12*, 5, 4. Available at www.socresonline.org.uk/12/5/4.html, accessed on 20 September 2013.

Biddle, J.E. and Hamermesh, D.S. (1990) 'Sleep and the allocation of time.' *Journal of Political Economy 98*, 5, Pt 1, 922–943.

Borde, A. (1867) 'Sleep, Rising and Dress.' In F. Furnival (ed) *John Russell's Boke of Nurture*. Bungay: John Childs and Son. (Original work published circa 1557.) Available at www.gutenberg.org/files/24790/24790-h/nurture.html#borde, accessed on 20 September 2013.

Carpenter, R., McGarvey, C., Mitchell, E.A., Tappin, D.M. *et al.* (2013) 'Bed sharing when parents do not smoke: Is there a risk of SIDS? An individual level analysis of five major case-control studies.' *BMJ Open*. doi: 10.1136/bmjopen-2012-002299.

Crosby, B., LeBourgeois, M.K. and Harsh, J. (2005) 'Racial differences in reported napping and nocturnal sleep in 2- to 8-year-old children.' *Pediatrics 115*, 1, 225–232.

Dyfed-Powys Police (2011) 'Tiredness and Driving.' Available at www.dyfed-powys.police.uk/en/advice-and-support/road-safety/driving-safely/tiredness, accessed on 20 October 2013.

Ekirch, A.R. (2001) 'Sleep we have lost: pre-industrial slumber in the British Isles.' *The American Historical Review 106*, 2, 343–386.

Ekirch, A.R. (2006) *At Day's Close: A History of Nighttime*. London: Phoenix.

Ficca, G., Axelsson, J., Mollicone, D.J., Muto, V. and Vitiello, M.V. (2010) 'Naps, cognition and performance.' *Sleep Medicine Reviews 14*, 4, 249–258.

Gianotti, F. and Cortesi, F. (2009) 'Family and cultural influences on sleep development.' *Child & Adolescent Psychiatric Clinics of North America 18*, 4, 849–861.

Green, A. (2012a) 'A Question of Balance: The Relationship Between Daily Occupation and Sleep.' In A. Green and A. Westcombe (eds) *Sleep: Multiprofessional Perspectives*. London: Jessica Kingsley Publishers.

Green, A. (2012b) 'Sleeping on It.' In A. Green and A. Westcombe (eds) *Sleep: Multiprofessional Perspectives*. London: Jessica Kingsley Publishers.

Hegarty, S. (2012a) 'The myth of the eight-hour sleep.' Available at www.bbc.co.uk/news/magazine-16964783, accessed on 20 September 2013.

Hegarty, S. (2012b) 'Segmented sleep: ten strange things people do at night.' Available at www.bbc.co.uk/news/magazine-17193783, accessed on 20 September 2013.

Hislop, J. and Arber, S. (2003) 'Sleepers Wake! The gendered nature of sleep disruption among mid-life women.' *Sociology 37*, 4, 695–711.

Horne, J. (2006) *Sleepfaring*. Oxford: Oxford University Press.

Horne, J. (2010) 'Sleepiness as a need for sleep: when is enough, enough?' *Neuroscience and Biobehavioral Reviews 34*, 1, 108–118.

Jacobs, S. (2012) 'Ambivalent Attitudes Towards Sleep in World Religions.' In A. Green and A. Westcombe (eds) *Sleep: Multiprofessional Perspectives*. London: Jessica Kingsley Publishers.

Kendrick, K. (2004) *To Sleep, Perchance to Dream: Why do We and Other Animals Sleep?* Lecture presented at Barnard's Inn Hall, Gresham College, London, 29 January. Available at www.gresham.ac.uk/lectures-and-events/to-sleep-perchance-to-dream-why-do-we-and-other-animals-sleep, accessed on 17 October 2014.

Kloesch, G. and Dittami, J.P. (2008) 'A Bed for Two? Gender Differences in the Reactions to Pair-sleep.' In L. Brunt and B. Steger (eds) *Worlds of Sleep*. Berlin: Frank and Timme.

Klug, G. (2008) 'Dangerous Doze: Sleep and Vulnerability in Medieval German Literature.' In L. Brunt and B. Steger (eds) *Worlds of Sleep*. Berlin: Frank and Timme.

Lader, D., Short, S. and Gershuny, J. (2006) *The Time Use Survey, 2005. How We Spend Our Time*. London: Office for National Statistics.

Lee, K.A. and Moe, K.E. (2011) 'Menopause.' In M.H. Kryger, T. Roth and W.C. Dement (eds) *Principles and Practice of Sleep Medicine*, 5th edn. St Louis, MO: Elsevier Saunders.

Liu, X., Liu, L., Owens, J.A. and Kaplan, D.L. (2005) 'Sleep patterns and sleep problems among schoolchildren in the United States and China.' *Pediatrics 115*, Suppl. 1, 241–249.

Maas, J.B. (1998) *Miracle Sleep Cure*. London: Thorsons.

Mather, C. (1862) *The Wonders of the Invisible World: Being and Account of the Tryals of Several Witches Lately Executed in New-England*. London: John Russell Smith. (Original work published in 1693.) Available at https://archive.org/details/wondersinvisibl00mathgoog, accessed on 20 September 2013.

McFall, S.L. and Garrington, C. (eds) (2011) *Early Findings from the First Wave of the UK's Household Longitudinal Study*. Colchester: Institute for Social and Economic Research, University of Essex.

Meadows, R. (2012) 'Beyond "Death's Counterfeit": The Sociological Aspects of Sleep.' In A. Green and A. Westcombe (eds) *Sleep: Multiprofessional Perspectives*. London: Jessica Kingsley Publishers.

Meadows, R. and Arber, S. (2012) 'Understanding sleep among couples: gender and the social patterning of sleep maintenance among younger and older couples.' *Longitudinal and Lifecourse Studies 3*, 1, 66–79.

Mednick, S.C. (2006) *Take a Nap! Change Your Life*. New York, NY: Workman Publishing.

Paavonen, E.J., Pennonen, M., Roine, M., Valkonen, S. and Lahikainen, A.R. (2006) 'TV exposure associated with sleep disturbances in 5- to 6-year-old children.' *Journal of Sleep Research 15*, 2, 154–161.

Roberts, M. (2012) 'Spanish siesta falls victim to Europe's debt crisis.' *Daily Telegraph*, 23 July 2012. Available at www.telegraph.co.uk/finance/financialcrisis/9421162/Spanish-siesta-falls-victim-to-Europes-debt-crisis.html, accessed on 20 September 2013.

Scrivner, L. (2012) 'That Sweet Secession: Sleep and Sleeplessness in Western Literature.' In A. Green and A. Westcombe (eds) *Sleep: Multiprofessional Perspectives*. London: Jessica Kingsley Publishers.

Steger, B. (2012) 'Cultures of Sleep.' In A. Green and A. Westcombe (eds) *Sleep: Multiprofessional Perspectives*. London: Jessica Kingsley Publishers.

Swanson, L.M., Arendt, J.T., Rosekind, M.R., Belenky, G., Balkin, T.J. and Drake, C. (2011) 'Sleep disorders and work performance: findings from the 2008 National Sleep Foundation "Sleep in America" poll.' *Journal of Sleep Research 20*, 3, 487–494.

Troxel, W.M. (2010) 'It's more than sex: exploring the dyadic nature of sleep and implications for health.' *Psychosomatic Medicine 72*, 6, 578–586.

Venn, S., Arber, S., Meadows, R. and Hislop, J. (2008) 'The fourth shift: exploring the gendered nature of sleep disruption in couples with children.' *British Journal of Sociology 59*, 1, 79–97.

Wehr, T. (1992) 'In short photoperiods, human sleep is biphasic.' *Journal of Sleep Research 1*, 2, 103–107.

Wehr, T. (1996) 'A "Clock for All Seasons" in the human brain.' *Progress in Brain Research 111*, 321–342.

Wolf-Meyer, M.J. (2012) *The Slumbering Masses: Sleep, Medicine and Modern American Life*. Minneapolis, MN: University of Minnesota Press.

Worthman, C.M. and Melby, M.K. (2002) 'Toward a Comparative Developmental Ecology of Human Sleep.' In M.A. Carskadon (ed) *Adolescent Sleep Patterns: Biological, Social, and Psychological Influences*. Cambridge: Cambridge University Press.

Yaniv, G. (2004) 'Insomnia, biological clock, and the bedtime decision: an economic perspective.' *Health Economics 13*, 1, 1–8.

5

THE EFFECTS OF SLEEP AND SLEEP LOSS ON PERFORMANCE

Andrew Green and Chris Alford

5.1 Introduction

The associations between sleep loss and poor health are mentioned in Chapter 3 (see also Möller-Levet *et al.* 2013); these are long-term consequences, but sleep loss has consequences in the very short term. Although most people will have noticed a difficulty in concentrating, or just staying awake after a bad night, or when experiencing jet lag, we might not always be so aware of how much our performance is impaired by as little as one night's poor sleep. This chapter therefore emphasizes the importance of sleep by focusing on the psychological and performance deficits that result from sleep deprivation. It shows why it is important to take patients' sleep problems seriously and provides the evidence for advising caution when sleep is impaired – even if an individual does not complain of poor sleep.

The mechanisms by which sleep deficit affects cognitive function are complex, but Alhola and Polo-Kantola (2007) suggest a broad two-way classification of theories whereby there are 'general effects on alertness and attention or selective effects on certain brain structures and function' (p.554). These theories are explored briefly before a more detailed look at some of the key performance areas that are affected by sleep loss: alertness in driving and similar tasks, and cognitive performance in memory and learning. Lastly, implications for clinical practice are considered.

5.2 Mechanisms

According to the wake-state instability hypothesis, lapses of attention result from the homeostatic pressure to sleep causing microsleeps* which have the characteristic electroencephalogram (EEG)* activity of sleep. This is in line with the synaptic homeostasis hypothesis (see Chapters 3 and 6), which suggests that if the brain is deprived of the chance to go offline in an orderly fashion in night-time sleep, certain parts will go offline in a more haphazard manner as wakefulness persists (Lucassen *et al.* 2010; Tononi and Cirelli 2006). The continued instability of the wake state and fluctuations in alertness leads to the variability of performance.

Doran, Van Dongen and Dinges (2001) trace the history of research on performance in the context of sleep deprivation from early experiments by Patrick and Gilbert in the 1890s where 90 hours without sleep resulted in motor and cognitive deficits in three participants. Research in the following decades showed that people could often perform at baseline levels after extended periods of wakefulness, but that in longer tasks performance was affected. By the 1930s evidence suggested that 'sleep deprivation affected neurobehavioural functions by initially destabilizing performance rather than by eliminating capacity to perform' (p.253). Subsequently, it was found in the 1950s that lapses in performance were most likely when the EEG showed evidence of transition to sleep onset, leading to development of 'the "lapse hypothesis", which posited that performance during sleep deprivation was punctuated by brief moments of low arousal during which subjects appeared to be unable to respond to the task at hand' (Doran *et al.* 2001, p.254).

According to Doran *et al.* (2001) when the drive to sleep is overpowering, lapses and slower responses occur, whereas if there is compensatory effort, performance may appear relatively normal for a short time at least. Their experiment, in which participants repeated reaction time tests over a period of 88 hours of wakefulness, showed increasing variability in performance as time went on (with normal responses even after 80 hours awake). They conclude that their findings provide support for the state-instability hypothesis which creates 'an unstable state which fluctuates within seconds and cannot be characterized as either fully awake or asleep' (p.265). It could be argued that it is adaptive to be able to function at baseline after no sleep, but in the modern world that can present a hazard, where it is possible for someone to believe that their ability to drive, for example, remains satisfactory, but where it is in fact impaired because of the variability of performance. As a parallel to this, analysis of lapses has been examined in on-the-road tests of driving as a result of drug-induced impairment (Verster *et al.* 2014).

The major alternative mechanism that has been suggested is the 'sleep-based neuropsychological perspective' (Babkoff *et al.* 2005, p.8) where sleep loss is said to have a variable effect in different parts of the brain. According to one theory – the prefrontal vulnerability hypothesis (Horne 1993) – sleep loss principally affects functions that are associated with the prefrontal cortex. Reviewing evidence of blood flow and EEG activity during sleep, Harrison and Horne (2000) suggest that the prefrontal cortex could be among the first regions of the brain to be affected by sleep deprivation. They go on to note that it is the area that deals with novelty and the unexpected (and therefore routine tasks are less dependent on it) and is responsible for divergent thinking and for memory for contextual detail. Not surprisingly, sufferers of disturbed sleep may put off difficult tasks including planning and problem solving which are key aspects of frontal lobe function (Tucker *et al.* 2010; Ward *et al.* 2013). Similarly, their emotional control may be affected (Killgore 2013).

5.3 Staying alert, reactions and driving

Driving is an activity that many adults do as part of their daily routine without much thought and which others do for their living. It is important for all, but especially the latter, to be alert and able to concentrate on the task, but sleepiness is a significant cause of road traffic collisions, injuries and deaths: it accounts for around 20% of traffic accidents in industrialized countries (Alford 2009; Philip and Åkerstedt 2006). Sleepiness can lead to anything from a driver having a fright on being alerted harmlessly when passing over a rumble strip (or sleeper line) to leaving the road and causing a major incident (see, for example, MacKinnon 1994 or Oliver 2002).

The scale of the problem was assessed in a study in New Zealand by Connor *et al.* (2002). They interviewed 571 drivers who had been involved in a road crash where at least one person had been admitted to hospital or died from their injuries (or interviewed a proxy, if the driver had been killed or seriously injured); they also interviewed 588 randomly selected drivers in a control group designed to represent the population of road users in the Auckland area. Respondents were asked about levels of alertness before the crash (or at the time of the survey for the control group), their sleep times in the preceding 24 hours and the number of nights in the preceding week when less than 7 hours of sleep had been taken. They also completed the Epworth Sleepiness Scale* to measure usual levels of sleepiness. Controlling for other factors, such as alcohol consumption, the researchers found an eightfold increased risk if drivers reported sleepiness and a threefold increase if driving after 5 hours of sleep or less. They summarized their findings as follows:

> Driving while feeling sleepy, driving after five hours or less of sleep, and driving between 2 a.m. and 5 a.m. were associated with a substantial increase in the risk of a car crash resulting in serious injury or death. Reduction in the prevalence of these three behaviours may reduce the incidence of injury crashes by up to 19%.
> (Connor *et al.* 2002, p.5)

It would be easy to dismiss the idea that driving on insufficient sleep is something that responsible people would do; however, it is common to get up early ahead of a long journey, or to get to work early, but it is unlikely that anyone rising at 4 a.m. for an early start would have gone to sleep at 8 p.m. the previous evening. Furthermore, it is a common experience to have a disturbed night's sleep anticipating a 'big day' or through worrying about waking up in time, but few of us are likely to cancel a trip because of a poor night's sleep and will push on regardless. Evidence for this is provided by Philip and Åkerstedt (2006) who cite their own work showing that there is an association between long-distance driving and curtailing sleep. They had found in a study in 1993 at a motorway rest area in France during the summer holiday period that as many as 50% of drivers had reduced sleep in the preceding 24 hours and that 10% had taken no sleep in that time. In a subsequent study, with a larger and more varied sample of car drivers ($n = 2196$) carried out at toll booths (avoiding the selection bias towards fatigued drivers at a rest area), they found that 50% of the drivers had slept less in the previous 24 hours than their usual sleep time; 10% of the sample had slept for less than 5 hours (Philip *et al.* 1999). Philip and Åkerstedt (2006) report that in tests comparing the sleep-deprived drivers with controls there was a reduced level of vigilance and shorter sleep latency* among the drivers.

If it is a matter of concern that vacation drivers and more regular car drivers are sleep deprived and showing signs of reduced performance, it would be yet more worrying if professional drivers' performance were impaired by lack of sleep. Mitler *et al.* (1997) investigated the sleep of 80 male truck drivers in the US and Canada working on different routes and schedules. They found that during the study period the drivers spent an average of 5.18 hours in bed per day and slept for 4.78 hours per day. It was recorded that two of the drivers had stage 1 sleep* while they were driving and also picked up that two others had undiagnosed sleep apnoea. More recently, Sharwood *et al.* (2011) reviewed the literature on sleep problems and the risk of commercial vehicle crashes. It was found that the evidence was somewhat inconclusive because of small sample sizes, for example, but it was concluded that there is an association between crashes and both daytime sleepiness (as measured on the Epworth Sleepiness Scale) and sleep debt.

The association between sleep loss and vigilance has been examined in controlled laboratory conditions by Van Dongen *et al.* (2003) where the neurobehavioural performance of 48 adults (aged 21–38 years) was monitored every 2 hours during wakefulness. Participants were randomly assigned to one of four groups in which different sleep durations were imposed: 8, 6 or 4 hours of sleep for 2 weeks or no sleep at all for 3 days. It was found that restriction to 6 and 4 hours of sleep progressively eroded performance in a battery of tests measuring vigilance, working memory and cognitive throughput (using a serial addition/subtraction task). The researchers conclude that there is no evidence therefore that humans can adapt to chronic sleep restriction; the performance after 14 days of 4 or 6 hours of sleep per night was comparable to that after 1 or 2 days of total sleep deprivation.

A further finding by Van Dongen *et al.* (2003) was that sleep restriction led to increased subjective sleepiness in the first days but increased only slightly as time went on (never approaching levels equivalent to those after two nights of complete sleep deprivation). At the end of the 14 days, participants in the 4- and 6-hour sleep groups performed at their worst in the tests but reported feeling only slightly sleepy. It is suggested that, after chronic sleep restriction, if people are having at least 4 hours of sleep, they do not experience sleepiness as they would after total deprivation; they therefore have a subjective impression that they have adapted to short sleep because they do not feel sleepy. The meaning of this is worth reflecting on: people with chronic partial sleep loss might be less aware of the need for sleep and believe that they can manage with less sleep than others, whereas their performance is on a par with someone who is totally sleep deprived. This gives further reason for concern with the 2005 'Sleep in America' poll reporting a rise to 16% in those sleeping less than 6 hours on weeknights (Banks and Dinges 2007).

Cohen *et al.* (2010) provide more evidence that individuals are not the best judge of their need for sleep and challenge the belief of many that they adapt to chronic sleep loss or that only a single extended period of sleep is necessary for recovery. In a study that manipulated sleep schedules to include extended periods of wakefulness over 3 weeks, they found that a chronic sleep debt can develop despite apparent full recovery from acute sleep loss. The relatively common practice of having short sleep on work or school days and longer sleep at weekends could lead someone with chronic sleep restriction to have a false sense of recovery from sleep debt because of performing well in the early part of their usual waking day. The authors point to the vulnerability of shift workers to accidents and errors after extended wakefulness, combined with the tendency towards worse functioning when operating at times when one would usually be asleep (at the circadian performance nadir).

A further observation by Cohen *et al.* (2010) is that acute sleep loss alone is hazardous, reminding us that 19 hours of continued wakefulness from 8 a.m. to 3 a.m. is linked with deficits in performance that are equivalent to a blood alcohol concentration (BAC) that would be illegal in most European countries (0.05%): after 24 hours awake, the deficit is equivalent to a level (0.10%) that exceeds the legal limit in the UK and the US. A study reported by Verster *et al.* (2011) provides support for such observations. Drivers were allowed to sleep between the hours of 11 p.m. and 7 a.m. on the night before driving the following night. Accompanied by professional driving instructors in dual-control vehicles, they drove on a two-lane highway for different lengths of time finishing at 5 a.m. and their performance was monitored by use of a video camera that measured deviation from the lane markings. It was found that the impairment observed in 2 hours of continuous driving at night was comparable to that seen with a BAC of 0.05%, and after 3 hours it was equivalent to a BAC of 0.08% (which is the UK 'drink-drive' limit). As Verster *et al.* (2011) conclude, it is important that drivers take sleepiness at the wheel seriously. Furthermore, our own data reveal that combining extended waking with driving in the early morning between 2 and 5 a.m. (the peak time for sleep-related accidents) can show impairment equivalent to 0.1% BAC, well over the legal driving limit (Alford 2009).

Although the discussion here focuses mainly on driving, a great deal of research has been done in other areas where vigilance is essential (for example, for guidelines on sleep to promote safety in aviation maintenance see Hobbs *et al.* 2011, and for a military perspective see Lindsay and Dyche 2011). However, there are two particular circumstances in which sleep and performance are compromised: shift working and obstructive sleep apnoea.

Shift working is a significant problem because of the interaction between circadian and diurnal rhythms of alertness with sleep duration and extended waking. Daytime sleep is shorter and more disturbed than night-time sleep, resulting in poorer performance and the need for recovery sleep (Gillberg 1995; Häkkänen *et al.* 1999; Kecklund and Åkerstedt 1995; Mawdsley, Grasby and Talk 2014). Those people who are adapted to day working feel more sleepy during night shifts, and rotating shifts result in extended waking, with more than 16 hours of work being associated with performance impairment (Rosa 1995; Van Dongen *et al.* 2003). The overall risk of traffic accidents may be doubled by shift working and extended waking (Barger *et al.* 2005; Ftouni *et al.* 2013; Mets *et al.* 2009).

Sleep apnoea is a clinical condition that results in chronic sleep disturbance affecting over 2–4% of the population, although other estimates are higher (Bearpark *et al.* 1995; Young *et al.* 1993). The condition is defined by the cessation of breathing during sleep and consequent arousals when breathing is restored, resulting in chronic sleep disruption (Chugh, Weaver and Dinges 1996). There are currently no drug treatments available with the standard treatment being continuous positive airway pressure (CPAP) delivered through a mask, although these are often only worn for about 5 hours per night, again resulting in reduced sleep (Gay *et al.* 2006). Worse still, untreated apnoea patients may turn to sedative drugs, such as alcohol, in an attempt to sleep, but this further exacerbates their condition through respiratory depression (Scrima *et al.* 1982). Marked daytime sleepiness is a major consequence and can be picked up by diagnostic tools such as the Epworth Sleepiness Scale (Johns 1991). Whilst it is not surprising that diagnosis may result in withdrawal of the driver's licence until effective treatment has been established and performance restored (Krieger *et al.* 1997; Turkington *et al.* 2004), this may make suffering drivers less likely to come forward, just as they may be reluctant to admit the offence of falling asleep at the wheel. Apnoea represents a particular example of the adverse consequences of chronic sleep disturbance on waking performance (Adams *et al.* 2001; Dinges *et al.* 1998). Consequently, an increased risk of driving accidents has been reported (Howard, Jackson and Baulk 2009).

5.4 Learning and memory

To make sense of the research on sleep and memory, it is necessary to appreciate the different types of memory. A declarative memory is something that can be called to mind and may be a *semantic* memory, such as the name of the capital of France, or an *episodic* memory of a particular event, such as last night's dinner. Non-declarative memory, which includes *conditioning* and *procedural skills*, involves memory of how to do things without conscious recollection, such as riding a bicycle (Stickgold 2005).

Wamsley and Stickgold (2011) suggest that one of sleep's functions is to consolidate new memory traces – conceptualized previously as a process of 'strengthening' a fragile trace and making it resistant to interference. They go on to point out that recent research has shown that, in sleep, new information is integrated into established memory networks, meaning is extracted and insight is developed. It is beyond the scope of this chapter to explore in any detail the mechanisms by which memories are retained, and readers are referred elsewhere; for example, Mednick *et al.* (2011) provide a review of theories to explain the role of slow-wave sleep (SWS) in the consolidation of declarative memory. They note that non-declarative memory is thought to be enhanced by rapid eye movement (REM) sleep*, whereas the facilitation of declarative memories is related to the period of non-REM sleep* consisting of both stage 2 sleep* and SWS; they point to a long history of research that shows that a period of SWS is more beneficial for memory than a similar period of REM sleep or waking activity. Mednick *et al.* (2011) outline hypotheses to explain the role of SWS in memory consolidation; the unique-to-sleep hypothesis suggests that memory consolidation depends on mechanisms that exist only in SWS, whereas other theories suggest that SWS eliminates interference that might disturb the process, whether or not SWS is the *only* means by which interference is reduced. Recent research suggests that SWS may also help prepare the brain to encode or form new memories following sleep (Antonenko *et al.* 2013; Wamsley 2013).

Research on sleep and memory can be traced back to the 1880s (Payne *et al.* 2012), but Wamsley and Stickgold (2011) note that it is 'well established that post-learning sleep is beneficial for human memory performance' (p.97). A suggestion by Vertes (2004) that there was insufficient evidence that a function of sleep is memory consolidation brought a response from Stickgold and Walker (2005) who noted that 83% of published articles on the subject in the previous 3 years supported a role for sleep. In a more detailed review Stickgold (2005) concludes that 'each stage of sleep seems to contribute differently…and we have proposed that the multiplicity of sleep stages has evolved, in part, to provide optimal brain states for a range of distinct memory consolidation processes' (p.1273; see also Walker and Stickgold 2006).

Stickgold and his colleagues at Harvard University, and elsewhere, have continued to provide further evidence of the role of sleep, typically in experiments involving learning of information which has to be recalled after a period of sleep or a similar period of wakefulness. Box 5.1 provides an illustration of the range of work that has been done.

BOX 5.1 Examples of sleep and memory research

- Ellenbogen *et al.* (2006): participants learned word pairs at either 9 a.m. or 9 p.m and half of each group (wake and sleep) were given a further set of words (an 'interfering list') to learn just before testing on the first list. The better performance of the group that slept led the researchers to conclude that 'sleep protects declarative memories from associative interference in the subsequent day' (p.1292) and that sleep has an active role in the consolidation of declarative memory.

- Tamminen *et al.* (2010): participants learned novel (made-up) words, such as 'cathedruke', and were tested for recall after 9–10 hours. The performance of the group that learned the words in the evening and slept before the first test was superior to those who learned the words in the morning and remained awake before testing. Because the study involved use of polysomnography*, the researchers were able to identify an involvement of sleep spindles (see Chapter 3) in the integration of new information into the existing framework of knowledge.

- Payne *et al.* (2012): tested for learning of sets of related and unrelated word pairs, where participants underwent training periods at different times of day and were tested after a variety of intervals. Retention after 12 hours was enhanced if there was a period of sleep, although a period of wakefulness had no impact on retention of related word pairs. Where there was a longer delay before retesting (24 hours) sleep had a beneficial effect if it came soon after learning (and not after 16 hours awake). Finally, 'when sleep shortly follows declarative task learning, it actually slows the subsequent rate of deterioration during the post-sleep wake period, suggesting that an important function of sleep is to stabilize newly learned declarative memories' (p.6).

- Wamsley *et al.* (2010) explored the role of dreaming in memory consolidation. Participants took part in an exercise involving navigating a virtual maze before taking a daytime nap or having a period of wakefulness. Sleep during the nap period was monitored with polysomnography and participants were woken on entering REM sleep. Participants in both the sleep and wake groups were asked to record what was going through their mind during the interval – including the dreams of the sleepers. It was found that dreaming of the maze task predicted better performance on subsequent testing, whereas thinking about the task while awake did not help. The researchers do not suggest that the experience of dreams cause memory consolidation, rather that dreaming might reflect the brain processes that support memory processing.

There is some evidence that memories that are likely to be of future relevance are selectively processed in sleep. Wilhelm *et al.* (2011) demonstrated this in a simple experiment where participants learned three tasks involving both declarative and non-declarative memory that have been found to be sensitive to sleep-dependent memory consolidation: learning of word pairs, object location and tapping a sequence on a keyboard. Groups performed each task and memory consolidation was tested after a period of wakefulness or after a similar period of sleep. A further distinction was that one subgroup of sleepers was told that there would be an additional test, whereas the others did not expect the retesting. It was found that when participants were informed of retesting, consolidation during sleep was enhanced in both declarative memory and procedural memory tasks. Furthermore, the researchers observed that there was also enhancement of sleep-related consolidation among participants who *suspected* there would be a further test. The inference is that 'sleep preferentially consolidates memories to be retrieved in the future' (Wilhelm *et al.* 2011, p.1569).

Although the focus here has been on the effect of sleep on the memory process, there is also some evidence of an effect on other cognitive processes, such as insight, as well as decision-making and judgement of risk. For example, a study by Wagner *et al.* (2004) suggests that sleep is involved in the process of developing insight, or the 'mental restructuring that leads to a sudden gain of explicit knowledge allowing qualitatively changed behaviour' (p.352). Volunteers (aged 18–31 years) took part in an experiment involving a mathematical puzzle where they had to convert a sequence of eight numbers into another sequence according to two simple rules. Unknown to the participants, there was a third hidden rule, which, once they had discovered it, meant that the puzzle could be solved more quickly. This enabled the researchers to identify the point at which the participants gained insight. After a training period, three groups of participants had an 8-hour interval in which they slept at night, remained awake at night, or remained awake during the day. The period of sleep was found to double the probability of spotting the hidden rule. Wagner *et al.* (2004) concluded that sleep 'not only strengthens memory traces quantitatively, but can also "catalyse" mental restructuring' (p.354).

It is noted in Chapter 1 that many major incidents have occurred when people are sleep deprived; this is likely to reflect impaired judgement. As in the case of memory and learning, there is a great deal of research on decision-making (see Harrison and Horne 2000 for an early review). For example, Drummond, Paulus and Tapert (2006) found that after two nights of total sleep deprivation, people were able to respond normally in a task when it was appropriate, but they had difficulty withholding inappropriate responses. In a gambling task, Killgore, Balkin and Wesensten (2006) observed that after 49.5 hours of sleep deprivation, participants made riskier decisions than they had done at baseline: they noted that the pattern of decisions reflected a pattern seen where there is damage to parts of the prefrontal cortex. In a subsequent study, Killgore, Kamimori and Balkin (2011) found that after three nights of total sleep deprivation, research participants showed an increase in risk-taking behaviour (in a laboratory exercise) but without a corresponding change in self-reported risk-taking propensity. (See Venkatraman *et al.* 2007 for a study using brain imaging that provides further evidence that sleep deprivation threatens decision-making ability in gambling tasks.)

Venkatraman *et al.* (2007) note that one reason why it is important to understand why we make poor decisions when sleep deprived is that 'there are now unprecedented opportunities to incur damaging losses by means such as online gambling' (p.603). However, while many people might gamble online or on interactive television programmes late at night and threaten their own financial stability, others are involved in work that affects the safety of themselves and others. These few examples from the research suggest that without sufficient sleep people might be able to take routine decisions but are less quick to react when a different response is necessary. They are also more likely to take risks but without the awareness of the increased likelihood of danger. When impaired judgement is coupled with decreased vigilance and increased reaction times, as described in the previous section, the potential for harm is increased greatly.

5.5 Conclusions and implications for practice

To summarize, deficits in performance as a result of sleep deprivation can be as dangerous as those caused by alcohol consumption. Accordingly, sleep loss is associated with increased risk of road traffic crashes (as is driving at night), but people often sleep less before a long journey, and many professional drivers may also be sleep deprived. Continuing sleep restriction has been shown to erode performance, but there is no evidence that humans can adapt to chronic sleep restriction although, as it goes on, people are less aware of being sleepy and may therefore believe that their performance is unimpaired. Sleep is necessary for learning and memory but also appears to have an important role in decision-making, risk-taking and insight.

Research into the effects of sleep loss continues, but there is sufficient existing evidence to conclude that sleep contributes to a range of cognitive functions that we depend on for the performance of daily activity. The evidence supports our everyday experience (that is, what we know without being told by scientists): we need sleep in order to be alert to carry out tasks such as driving, and sleep is necessary to facilitate learning and other cognitive processes. However, the evidence also suggests that we might underestimate the importance of sleep and, for example, forgo sleep before driving in order to get ahead of the traffic. Occupational therapists involved in driving assessments might routinely include screening questions for sleep problems.

If a patient is sleeping badly, it is our duty to warn them of the risk (and document it) that they pose to themselves or others; a therapist may have to decide at which point safety concerns outweigh the imperative of confidentiality (see Chapter 7). We cannot assume that a patient experiencing poor sleep will concentrate fully in any kind of assessment or, for example, that they will be able to fully comprehend instructions. Furthermore, they will not consolidate learning without sleep. Lastly, while the evidence presented in this chapter emphasizes the need for sleep, it cannot be assumed that patients will be able to make effective plans to improve their sleep without being given explicit instructions and guidance.

References

Adams, N., Strauss, M., Schluchter, M. and Redline, S. (2001) 'Relation of measures of sleep-disordered breathing to neuropsychological functioning.' *American Journal of Respiratory and Critical Care Medicine 163*, 7, 1626–1631.

Alford, C. (2009) 'Sleepiness, Countermeasures and the Risk of Motor Vehicle Accidents.' In J.C. Verster, S.R. Pandi-Perumal, J.G. Rameakers and J.J. De Gier (eds) *Drugs, Driving and Traffic Safety*. Boston, MA: Birkhäuser.

Alhola, P. and Polo-Kantola, P. (2007) 'Sleep deprivation: impact on cognitive performance.' *Neuropsychiatric Disease and Treatment 3*, 5, 553–567.

Antonenko, D., Diekelmann, S., Olsen, C., Born, J. and Mölle, M. (2013) 'Napping to renew learning capacity: enhanced encoding after stimulation of slow wave oscillations.' *European Journal of Neuroscience 37*, 7, 1142–1151.

Babkoff, H., Zukerman, G., Fostick, L. and Ben-Artzi, E. (2005) 'Effect of the diurnal rhythm and 24 h of sleep deprivation on dichotic temporal order judgement.' *Journal of Sleep Research 14*, 1, 7–15.

Banks, S. and Dinges, D.F. (2007) 'Behavioral and physiological consequences of sleep restriction.' *Journal of Clinical Sleep Medicine 3*, 5, 519–528.

Barger, L.K., Cade, B.E., Ayas, N.T., Cronin, J.W. *et al.* (2005) 'Extended work shifts and the risk of motor vehicle crashes among interns.' *New England Journal of Medicine 352*, 2, 125–134.

Bearpark, H., Elliott, L., Grunstein, R., Cullen, S. *et al.* (1995) 'Snoring and sleep apnea. A population study in Australian men.' *American Journal of Respiratory and Critical Care Medicine 151*, 5, 1459–1465.

Chugh, D.K., Weaver, T.E. and Dinges, D.F. (1996) 'Neurobehavioral consequences of arousals.' *Sleep 19*, Suppl. 10, S198–S201.

Cohen, D.A., Wang, W., Wyatt, J.K., Kronauer, R.E. *et al.* (2010) 'Uncovering residual effects of chronic sleep loss on human performance.' *Science Translational Medicine 2*, 14, 14ra3.

Connor, J., Norton, R., Ameratunga, S., Robinson, E. *et al.* (2002) 'Driver sleepiness and risk of serious injury to car occupants: population based case control study.' *British Medical Journal 324*, 7346, 1125. Available at www.ncbi.nlm.nih.gov/pmc/articles/PMC107904/pdf/1125.pdf, accessed on 11 October 2013.

Dinges, D., Maislin, G., Staley, B., Pack, F., Woodle, C. and Pack, A. (1998) 'Sleepiness and neurobehavioral functioning in relation to apnoea severity in a cohort of commercial motor vehicle operators.' *Sleep 21*, Suppl., 83.

Doran, S.M., Van Dongen, H.P.A. and Dinges, D.F. (2001) 'Sustained attention performance during sleep deprivation: evidence of state instability.' *Archives Italiennes de Biologie 139*, 3, 253–267.

Drummond, S.P.A., Paulus, M.P. and Tapert, S.F. (2006) 'Effects of two nights sleep deprivation and two nights recovery sleep on response inhibition.' *Journal of Sleep Research 15*, 3, 261–265.

Ellenbogen, J.M., Hulbert, J.C., Stickgold, R., Dinges, D.F. and Thompson-Schill, S.L. (2006) 'Interfering with theories of sleep and memory: sleep, declarative memory, and associative interference.' *Current Biology 16*, 13, 1290–1294.

Ftouni, S., Sletten, T.L., Howard, M., Anderson, C. *et al.* (2013) 'Objective and subjective measures of sleepiness, and their associations with on-road driving events in shift workers.' *Journal of Sleep Research 22*, 1, 58–69.

Gay, P., Weaver, G.P.T., Loube, D. and Iber, C. (2006) 'Evaluation of positive airway pressure treatment for sleep related breathing disorders in adults: a review by the Positive Airway Pressure Task Force of the Standards of Practice Committee of the American Academy of Sleep Medicine.' *Sleep 29*, 3, 381–401.

Gillberg, M. (1995) 'Sleepiness and its relation to the length, content, and continuity of sleep.' *Journal of Sleep Research 4*, Suppl. 2, 37–40.

Häkkänen, H., Summala, H., Partinen, M., Tiihonen, M. and Silvo, J. (1999) 'Blink duration as an indicator of driver sleepiness in professional bus drivers.' *Sleep 22*, 6, 798–802.

Harrison, Y. and Horne, J.A. (2000) 'The impact of sleep deprivation on decision making: a review.' *Journal of Experimental Psychology: Applied 6*, 3, 236–249.

Hobbs, A., Bedell Avers, K. and Hiles, J.J. (2011) 'Fatigue risk management in aviation maintenance: current best practices and potential future countermeasures.' Washington, DC: Office of Aerospace Medicine, Federal Aviation Administration. Available at https://primis.phmsa.dot.gov/crm/docs/FRMS_in_MX_OAM_TR_HobbsAversHiles.pdf, accessed on 14 October 2013.

Horne, J.A. (1993) 'Human sleep, sleep loss and behaviour: implications for the prefrontal cortex and psychiatric disorder.' *British Journal of Psychiatry 162*, 413–419.

Howard, M.E., Jackson, M.L. and Baulk, S. (2009) 'Drugs, Driving and Traffic Safety in Sleep Apnea.' In J.C. Verster, S.R. Pandi-Perumal, J.G. Rameakers and J.J. De Gier (eds) *Drugs, Driving and Traffic Safety*. Boston, MA: Birkhäuser.

Johns, M.W. (1991) 'A new method for measuring daytime sleepiness: the Epworth sleepiness scale.' *Sleep 14*, 6, 540–545. Kecklund, G. and Åkerstedt, T. (1995) 'Effects of timing of shifts on sleepiness and sleep duration.' *Journal of Sleep Research 4*, Suppl. 2, 47–50.

Killgore, W.D.S. (2013) 'Self-reported sleep correlates with prefrontal-amygdala functional connectivity and emotional functioning.' *Sleep 36*, 11, 1597–1608.

Killgore, W.D.S., Balkin, T.J. and Wesensten, N.J. (2006) 'Impaired decision making following 49 h of sleep deprivation.' *Journal of Sleep Research 15*, 1, 7–13.

Killgore, W.D.S., Kamimori, G.H. and Balkin, T.J. (2011) 'Caffeine protects against risk-taking propensity during severe sleep deprivation.' *Journal of Sleep Research 20*, 3, 395–403.

Krieger, J., Meslier, N., Lebrun, T., Levy, P. *et al.* (1997) 'Accidents in obstructive sleep apnea patients treated with nasal continuous positive airway pressure: a prospective study.' *Chest 112*, 6, 1561–1566.

Lindsay, D.R. and Dyche, J. (2011) 'Sleep disturbance implications for modern military operations.' *Journal of Human Performance in Extreme Environments 10*, 1, Article 2. Available at: http://docs.lib.purdue.edu/jhpee/vol10/iss1/2, accessed on 28 October 2013.

Lucassen, P.J., Meerlo, P., Naylor, A.S., Van Dam, A.M. *et al.* (2010) 'Regulation of adult neurogenesis by stress, sleep disruption, exercise and inflammation: implications for depression and antidepressant action.' *European Neuropsychopharmacology 20*, 1, 1–17.

MacKinnon, I. (1994) 'M40 crash driver "probably fell asleep".' *Independent*, 30 June. Available at www.independent.co.uk/news/uk/m40-crash-driver-probably-fell-asleep-1425967.html, accessed on 11 October 2013.

Mawdsley, M., Grasby, K. and Talk, A. (2014) 'The effect of sleep on item recognition and source memory recollection among shift-workers and permanent day-workers.' *Journal of Sleep Research.* doi: 10.1111 jsr.12149.

Mednick, S.C., Cai, D.J., Shuman, T., Anagnostaras, S. and Wixted, J.T. (2011) 'An opportunistic theory of cellular and systems consolidation.' *Trends in Neurosciences 34*, 10, 504–514.

Mets, M.A.J, van Deventer, K.R, Olivier, B., Volkerts, E.R. and Verster, J.C. (2009) 'Drugs, Driving and Traffic Safety in Shift Workers.' In J.C. Verster, S.R. Pandi-Perumal, J.G. Rameakers and J.J. De Gier (eds) *Drugs, Driving and Traffic Safety*. Boston, MA: Birkhäuser.

Mitler, M.M., Miller, J.C., Lipsitz, J.J., Walsh, J.K. and Wylie, C.D. (1997) 'The sleep of long-haul truck drivers.' *New England Journal of Medicine 337*, 11, 755–761.

Möller-Levet, C.S., Archer, S.N., Bucca, G., Laing, E.E. *et al.* (2013) 'Effects of insufficient sleep on circadian rhythmicity and expression amplitude of the human blood transcriptome.' *PNAS 110*, 12, E1132–E1141.

Oliver, M. (2002) 'Selby crash motorist receives five year sentence.' *Guardian*, 11 January. Available at www.guardian.co.uk/uk/2002/jan/11/selby.railtravel, accessed on 11 October 2013.

Payne, J.D., Tucker, M.A., Ellenbogen, J.M., Wamsley, E.J. *et al.* (2012) 'Memory for semantically related and unrelated declarative information: the benefit of sleep, the cost of wake.' *PLoS ONE 7*, 3, e33079.

Philip, P. and Åkerstedt, T. (2006) 'Transport and industry safety: How are they affected by sleepiness and sleep restriction?' *Sleep Medicine Reviews 10*, 5, 347–356.

Philip, P., Taillard, J., Guilleminault, C., Quera Salva, M.A., Bioulac, B. and Ohayon, M. (1999) 'Long distance driving and self-induced sleep deprivation among automobile drivers.' *Sleep 22*, 4, 474–480.

Rosa, R.R. (1995) 'Extended workshifts and excessive fatigue.' *Journal of Sleep Research 4*, Suppl. 2, 51–56.

Scrima, L., Broudy, M., Nay, K.N. and Cohn, M.A. (1982) 'Increased severity of obstructive sleep apnea after bedtime alcohol ingestion: diagnostic potential and proposed mechanism of action.' *Sleep 5*, 4, 318–328.

Sharwood, L.N., Elkington, J., Stevenson, M. and Wong, K.K. (2011) 'Investigating the role of fatigue, sleep and sleep disorders in commercial vehicle crashes: a systematic review.' *Journal of the Australasian College of Road Safety 22*, 3, 24–30.

Stickgold, R. (2005) 'Sleep-dependent memory consolidation.' *Nature 437*, 7063, 1272–1278.

Stickgold, R. and Walker, M.P. (2005) 'Sleep and memory: the ongoing debate.' *Sleep 28*, 10, 1225–1227.

Tamminen, J., Payne, J.D., Stickgold, R., Wamsley, E.J. and Gaskell, M.G. (2010) 'Sleep spindle activity is associated with the integration of new memories and existing knowledge.' *Journal of Neuroscience 30*, 43, 14356–14360.

Tononi, G. and Cirelli, C. (2006) 'Sleep function and synaptic homeostasis.' *Sleep Medicine Reviews 10*, 1, 49–62.

Tucker, A.M., Whitney, P., Belenky, G., Hinson, J.M. and Van Dongen, H.P. (2010) 'Effects of sleep deprivation on dissociated components of executive functioning.' *Sleep 33*, 1, 47–57.

Turkington, P.M., Sircar, M., Saralaya, D., Elliott, M.W. (2004) 'Time course of changes in driving simulator performance with and without treatment in patients with sleep apnoea hypopnoea syndrome.' *Thorax 59*, 1, 56–59.

Van Dongen, H.P.A., Maislin, G., Mullington, J.M. and Dinges, D.F. (2003) 'The cumulative cost of additional wakefulness: dose-response effects on neurobehavioral functions and sleep physiology from chronic sleep restriction and total sleep deprivation.' *Sleep 26*, 2, 117–126.

Venkatraman, V., Chuah, Y.M.L., Huettel, S.A. and Chee, M.W.L. (2007) 'Sleep deprivation elevates expectation of gains and attenuates response to losses following risky decisions.' *Sleep 30*, 5, 603–609.

Verster, J.C., Bervoets, A.C., de Klerk, S. and Roth, T. (2014) 'Lapses of attention as outcome measure of the on-the-road driving test.' *Psychopharmacology 231*, 1, 283–292.

Verster, J.C., Taillard, J., Sagaspe, P., Olivier, B. and Philip, P. (2011) 'Prolonged nocturnal driving can be as dangerous as severe alcohol-impaired driving.' *Journal of Sleep Research 20*, 4, 585–588.

Vertes, R.P. (2004) 'Memory consolidation in sleep: dream or reality.' *Neuron 44*, 1, 135–148.

Wagner, U., Gais, S., Haider, H., Verlager, R. and Born, J. (2004) 'Sleep inspires insight.' *Nature 427*, 6972, 352–355.

Walker, M.P. and Stickgold, R. (2006) 'Sleep, memory and plasticity.' *Annual Review of Psychology 57*, 139–166.

Wamsley, E.J. (2013) 'Engineering sleep to discover the function of slow wave activity (Commentary on Antonenko *et al.*).' *European Journal of Neuroscience 37*, 7, 1140–1141.

Wamsley, E.J. and Stickgold, R. (2011) 'Memory, sleep and dreaming: experiencing consolidation.' *Sleep Medicine Clinics 6*, 1, 97–108.

Wamsley, E.J., Tucker, M., Payne, J.D., Benavides, J.A. and Stickgold, R. (2010) 'Dreaming of a learning task is associated with enhanced sleep-dependent memory consolidation.' *Current Biology 20*, 9, 850–855.

Ward, A.M., McLaren, D.G., Schultz, A.P., Chhatwal, J. *et al.* (2013) 'Daytime sleepiness is associated with decreased default mode network connectivity in both young and cognitively intact elderly subjects.' *Sleep 36*, 11, 1609–1615.

Wilhelm, I., Diekelmann, S., Molzow, I., Ayoub, A., Mölle, M. and Born, J. (2011) 'Sleep selectively enhances memory expected to be of future relevance.' *Journal of Neuroscience 31*, 5, 1563–1569.

Young, T., Palta, M., Dempsey, J., Skatrud, J., Weber, S. and Badir, S. (1993) 'The occurrence of sleep-disordered breathing among middle-aged adults.' *New England Journal of Medicine 328*, 17, 1230–1235.

6

THE EFFECTS OF DAYTIME ACTIVITY ON SLEEP

Andrew Green

6.1 Introduction

This chapter explores the influence of daily activity on sleep; it builds on Chapter 3, which looks at some of the key factors involved in the regulation of sleep and its timing, and it complements Chapter 5, which looks at how sleep affects performance of occupations. Although this chapter does not dwell on scientific theory, it is worth recalling the synaptic homeostasis hypothesis, which is outlined in Chapter 3, as a possible explanation for some of what follows. The hypothesis suggests that the homeostatic pressure to sleep (or the pressure for deep, slow-wave sleep in particular) relates to the need for the synapses of the brain to recalibrate themselves after the day during which they have become stronger in response to environmental stimuli (see Tononi and Cirelli 2006, 2012).

The factors that are discussed here can be difficult to disentangle from each other in research studies: they are exercise, activity and social contact, and regularity or routine, which are examined in turn before exploring their overall relevance for therapy. In reviewing published work it is necessary to use the terminology of sleep research; terms are explained in the glossary, and in other chapters, and abbreviations are listed in Box 6.1.

BOX 6.1 Abbreviations used in this chapter

- EEG: electroencephalogram

- PSG: polysomnography

- PSQI: Pittsburgh Sleep Quality Index

- RCT: randomized controlled trial

- REM sleep: rapid eye movement sleep (cf. non-REM sleep)

- SOAR: Scale of Older Adults' Routine

- SOL: sleep onset latency

- SRM: Social Rhythm Metric

- SWS: slow-wave sleep

- TST: total sleep time

6.2 Exercise

It is only relatively recently that more sedentary lifestyles have become common in Western society, but there is an intuitive logic in the idea that exercise should enhance sleep if it is assumed that there are natural cycles of activity that persisted through millennia of human history. It has been noted previously that exercise is a particularly quantifiable activity (Green 2012) in that it is possible to time it, or to count the number of repetitions, to record weights lifted or to measure a distance covered. Furthermore, physiological responses to exertion can be measured and it has therefore been possible to conduct a great deal of research in relation to exercise and its effect on sleep, and also on circadian rhythms (see Atkinson *et al.* 2007), despite the problem of controlling for the effects of light and of pre-existing fitness levels of participants. Essentially, studies on the relationship between sleep and exercise can be categorized as follows: those that explore the relationship between exercise levels and a person's habitual sleep (or changes in sleep in response to exercise) and those that aim to find whether exercise as an intervention can improve poor sleep.

Investigation of the possible mechanisms of any associations is beyond the scope of this chapter, but an introduction is provided by Driver and Taylor (2000) in their review of the literature on the links between exercise and sleep. They distinguish between the thermogenic hypothesis, which builds on the evidence that a trigger for sleep onset is the decline in body temperature in the evening (and the effects of exercise on body temperature) and hypotheses related to energy conservation and body restoration. These theories propose that there is a need for increased sleep after exercise. In their review, Passos *et al.* (2012) suggest other possible mechanisms where the antidepressant and anxiety-reducing effects of exercise led to improved sleep.

A clear link between exercise and sleep architecture* is exemplified in an extreme case: an early study involving runners in a 92-kilometre road race (more than a double marathon) in South Africa (Shapiro *et al.* 1981). Sleep was recorded in the laboratory for a total of six nights (one each for a 'baseline' measure two weeks before the race and a post-race control measure two weeks afterwards, and for the four nights from race day). It was found that the six participants not only had more sleep than usual for two nights after the event (over 1 hour on the night after the race, and about 2 hours extra on the second night), but they also had about twice as much deep, slow-wave sleep (SWS)* and less rapid eye movement (REM) sleep*; the percentage of SWS on the third and fourth nights was not significantly raised.

Where less extreme activity is involved it can be difficult to determine which variables are significant. For example, in a study in Switzerland Brand *et al.* (2009) investigated the sleep of 36 males (aged 15 years) who were regular footballers, and 34 matched controls. Comparing sleep diaries and questionnaires, including the Pittsburgh Sleep Quality Index (PSQI)* (Buysse *et al.* 1989), they found that the footballers were getting to sleep more quickly (in less than 10 minutes – less than half the time of the control group) and sleeping for about half an hour longer with fewer awakenings; they also had higher sleep-quality scores and reported improved levels of concentration and less tiredness by day. Several factors could be involved in explaining the differences. It could be simply that regular exercise and increased fitness improve sleep, although participation in a pleasurable activity might lead to improved mood and reduced anxiety, which in turn could enhance sleep. A dedicated team member might also be more likely to keep to regular routines and to pay more attention to general health.

Youngstedt and Kline (2006) note that many studies involve good sleepers who have little room for improvement (i.e. ceiling/floor effects; see Youngstedt 2003) and also tend to involve small samples. They examined surveys and epidemiological studies and cite two surveys where, when asked an open question, respondents named exercise as the most important habit that helped sleep. Youngstedt and Kline (2006) also observed that epidemiological studies have 'consistently shown associations of exercise and better sleep' (p.217). For example, in an epidemiological study using a questionnaire sent to 722 respondents (aged 40 years or over), Sherrill, Kotchou and Quan (1998) asked about sleep problems and exercise levels (among other factors). Regular exercise (jogging or cycling at least once a week) was associated with a lower risk of any sleep disorder.

Several relatively small studies have been carried out with people with impaired sleep attempting to evaluate the effect on sleep of different types of exercise. The quality of the research is variable, but the following examples illustrate what can be achieved, as well as some of the difficulties involved in investigating the issue. A rigorously conducted randomized controlled trial (RCT) was reported by King *et al.* (1997), where 20 volunteers (aged 50–76 years) with moderate sleep problems recruited from the community underwent a 16-week exercise programme with 30–40-minute sessions held four times a week; exercise included aerobics and brisk walking. Participants' subjective sleep quality increased, as measured on the PSQI, and total sleep time (TST) increased by an average of 42 minutes, while sleep onset latency (SOL)* halved. Compared with the waiting-list control group, there was a significant difference in all these measures after 16 weeks; however, there was no significant improvement in sleep after 8 weeks, suggesting it is important not to assume that exercise is a 'quick fix' and to persist with it.

The improvement was not replicated in a subsequent RCT by King *et al.* (2008) with 36 adults (aged over 55 years) with mild to moderate non-clinical sleep complaints, which used polysomnography (PSG)* to assess the effect of a year-long exercise programme. Participants attended twice-weekly 60-minute classes of moderate-intensity exercise and were asked to exercise on their own another three times a week; members of a control group attended weekly health education classes (without exercise). Objective improvement in sleep after a year was only modest, although there was some subjective improvement with the exercisers reporting getting to sleep more quickly and feeling more refreshed in the morning. Further examination of data from the same study by Buman *et al.* (2011) indicated that the moderate-intensity exercise programme brought about a small decrease in self-rated SOL (an average of 10 minutes) and reduced fluctuations from night to night.

In another RCT, which involved sedentary adults (aged 55 years and over), 10 people recruited through advertisements took part in a carefully planned 16-week exercise and sleep hygiene* education programme, and 7 others joined in control group with a 45-minute recreation or education session three times a week (Reid *et al.* 2010). Actigraphy* was used to screen for sleep disorders, and the PSQI and other measures were used for measuring outcomes. Total sleep time for the experimental group increased by 1.25 hours – a larger increase than in other studies according to the authors, who observe that it could reflect the low baseline sleep duration (less than 6.5 hours).

The studies by King *et al.* (1997, 2008) and Reid *et al.* (2010), and three other randomized trials, are reviewed in a meta-analysis by Yang *et al.* (2012), who conclude that 'participation in exercise training has a moderately beneficial effect on sleep quality and decreases both sleep latency and use of sleep medication' (p.162). Yang *et al.* (2012) go on to recommend exercise as an additional therapy for sleep problems since it is inexpensive, widely available and generally safe; they might have added that even if it failed to help sleep, it would still be likely to be beneficial to the individual.

These studies cited so far included non-clinical samples, which lays them open to the criticism that exercise cannot be conclusively shown to help insomnia. Accordingly, an RCT by Passos *et al.* (2010) involved 48 patients (aged 30–55 years) with a clinical diagnosis of chronic primary insomnia (that is, insomnia for over 6 months that is not attributable to any other medical condition; see Chapter 7). Participants were randomly assigned to one of four groups: control, moderate-intensity aerobic exercise, high-intensity aerobic exercise and moderate-intensity resistance exercise, and all but the control group took part in a single exercise session lasting about 50 minutes. Sleep was recorded using PSG at baseline and following the exercise session. It was found that those in the moderate-intensity aerobic exercise group had significantly improved sleep in terms of reduced SOL, increased TST and increased sleep efficiency*. Improvements in the other groups (including the control) were consistent but more modest. As so often, the sample was small, and at baseline the sleep of the moderate-intensity aerobic exercise group was markedly, and inexplicably, worse on all measures when compared with the other groups. Add to this the single-exercise-session design and it makes the results very difficult to interpret, except at face value.

The last problem is addressed in a further randomized study by Passos *et al.* (2011) where exercise was continued for a period of 6 months with a similar patient group – but without a control group; instead, participants were randomly assigned to 50-minute exercise sessions three times a week in either the morning (10 a.m. $\pm$ 1 hour) or the late afternoon (6 p.m. $\pm$ 1 hour). Sleep was recorded by PSG at baseline and after 6 months and showed significant improvements in SOL and sleep efficiency. Sleep diaries showed improvements in sleep quality, and other measures recorded improvements in some aspects of quality of life and mood. Although there was no significant improvement in TST, 'anecdotal accounts indicated that the participants felt there had been a remarkable improvement in sleep' (Passos *et al.* 2011, p.1023). It is also noted that there were few differences between the effect of morning or late afternoon exercise and that either is beneficial to patients with chronic primary insomnia (see below).

Looking at less vigorous exercise Li *et al.* (2004) conducted an RCT to investigate the effect of low-to-moderate-intensity tai chi (1 hour three times a week for 24 weeks). The 62 previously inactive participants (aged 60–92 years), who were recruited through advertisement, reported significant improvements in their sleep (as measured by the PSQI) compared with members of the control group who attended low-impact exercise classes (mostly involving seated exercise, with stretching and controlled breathing). There was an average decrease in SOL of 18 minutes and average TST increased by 48 minutes. These findings compared well with those of King *et al.* (1997) where participants had engaged in moderate-intensity aerobic exercise. The authors note that the mechanism of any improvement in sleep through tai chi is not known, but they observe that movements are slow and flowing and are combined with relaxation and diaphragmatic breathing; this is 'conducive to an enhanced feeling of well-being and altered mental state, which may possibly lead to improved sleep quality' (Li *et al.* 2004, p.899). In that statement they effectively acknowledge that it may be the more meditative aspect of tai chi that is involved in improved sleep as well as – or even instead of – the effect of the exercise.

Similarly, in many other studies, the effect of exercise can be difficult to distinguish from other factors (and, conversely, exercise could be a factor in some of the studies cited in the next section on activity). For example, Gebhart, Erlacher and Schredl (2011) combined moderate physical exercise with 'sleep education' in a study in Germany. Participants with insomnia (*n* = 70; mean age 55 years) attended six sessions of Nordic walking (1 hour, weekly) and talks on sleep science, sleep hygiene *and* cognitive behavioural strategies for managing insomnia (known as CBT-I; see Chapter 8). Compared with the waiting-list control group, participants reported improved subjective sleep quality (measured on the PSQI) and improved daytime mood. It is not clear, however, whether sleep duration changed or whether it was the exercise or the sleep education (or the combination) that was effective in bringing about the improvements. As the sample was recruited by advertisement, it is also not clear how many would have met the diagnostic criteria for insomnia. In a similar-sized study carried out in Japan, Morita *et al.* (2011) concluded that 2 hours of forest walking can improve sleep. Participants with self-rated sleep complaints took part in either a 2.5-kilometre walk or a 900-metre walk with some light work such as felling small trees with a hand saw. This finding raises all kinds of questions about the effect of daylight, for example (see Chapter 3), or the effect of the woodland environment on mood, or the effect of engagement in activity (before even considering issues such as the problems of self-rating, lack of control group and the inaccessibility of forests to many people in urban areas around the world).

In summary, studies suggest that exercise enhances sleep, although it must be acknowledged that the reverse may still be true – that sleep quality might be a predictor of subsequent exercise behaviour – at least in sedentary older adults (Dzierzewski *et al.* 2013). There has yet to be a randomized controlled trial with a large sample of previously sedentary people (in different age groups), with diagnosed primary insomnia, who take part in a sustained exercise programme to establish whether exercise helps objectively measured sleep. In the absence of such a trial it may be reasonable to turn to what people say in surveys, and to consider the recent National Sleep Foundation 2013 poll (National Sleep Foundation 2013), which focused on exercise and sleep: 1000 people in the US (aged 23–60 years), representing the population, were polled by telephone or via the Internet. Exercise was categorized as vigorous, moderate, light and 'no activity', and the findings of the poll were summarized under the following headings:

- *Exercise is good for sleep and vigorous exercisers report best sleep.* For example, 45% of those reporting no activity complained of poor sleep – fairly bad (31%) or bad (14%) – compared with only 17% of those who did vigorous exercise (fairly bad: 14%; bad: 3%).

- *Non-exercisers report worst sleep/health.* More respondents in the no-activity group reported 'poor' (12%) or 'fair' health (30%) than the vigorous exercisers (1% and 9%, respectively) and those in the no-activity group took more and longer naps, consumed more caffeine, took more medication to help sleep and complained more of daytime sleepiness.

- *Less time sitting is associated with better sleep/health.* This appears to be another way of making the above point.

- *Exercise is good, regardless of time of day.* No significant differences were found between those who exercised within 4 hours of bedtime and those who exercised more than 4 hours before bedtime.

The last finding is at odds with much advice that is given in relation to sleep hygiene where late-evening exercise is discouraged because it increases arousal levels and raises body temperature. However, noting that there has been insufficient research on the effects of vigorous evening exercise on sleep quality, Myllymäki *et al.* (2010) used PSG, actigraphy and subjective measures with 11 physically fit young adults (aged 23–29 years), who were good sleepers, to assess the effect of an exercise session that ended 2–2.5 hours before bedtime. Their sleep was recorded after a day when they did not exercise, and on a day when they did about half an hour's vigorous exercise on an exercise bicycle, starting between 8:30 and 9:30 p.m. Comparing the two nights, the researchers found sleep was not impaired after exercise: the proportion of non-REM sleep* was greater after exercise (although the actual extra time did not reach significance); heart rate was also elevated in the first 3 hours of sleep. On this evidence Myllymäki *et al.* (2010) conclude that sleep quality was not disturbed by vigorous late-night exercise – although it is questionable whether 9:30 p.m. amounts to 'late night'. (For implications for therapy see section 6.5.)

6.3 Activity

It is not so easy to measure 'activity' as it is to measure exercise. For example, as noted by Green (2012), participation in 'church activities' (as found in some activity checklists) cannot be easily quantified: it could involve anything from quiet contemplation in a Quaker meeting to arguing in a committee, or doing physical work to help to maintain the fabric of a building. It is therefore even harder than it is with exercise to control for the multiplicity of factors that could affect sleep and, as before, it is necessary to resort to looking to small experimental studies and large epidemiological surveys in the hope of finding trends and associations.

As with exercise in the previous section, a striking case from the 1980s sets the scene. Anticipating by some years the synaptic homeostasis hypothesis (see below; also see Chapter 3), Horne and Minard (1985) observed that, even allowing for different levels of physical exertion, a day's sightseeing and travelling in a new environment could make us feel sleepy. To test this, they carried out a small innovative experiment involving a minor deception of nine female graduate students (aged 21–27 years): they believed that they would spend a day completing psychological tests as part of a trial where they also spent three uneventful days on the university campus engaged in routine study, while having their sleep monitored for five nights in a laboratory. However, the tests were 'cancelled' and, instead, the participants were taken for a surprise day out – over 12 hours – to a shopping and exhibition centre, a zoo and an amusement park, and a cinema. On the night after the trip, they slept no longer than at baseline, but they got to sleep more quickly (in about half the time, i.e. 8 minutes on average) and had significantly more deep SWS (about 25% extra). There was also increased SWS on the second night; REM sleep was unchanged.

Inevitably, on a day out it is all but impossible to control for all variables, and the most significant in this case could be exercise, but the researchers point out that the activities mostly involved sitting or walking. The conclusion therefore is that it was the novelty of the new environment that induced the deep sleep. Twenty years later, Huber, Tononi and Cirelli (2006) noted that, according to the synaptic homeostasis hypothesis, slow-wave activity in sleep should depend not only on the length of prior waking, but also on the quality of waking. In a laboratory experiment rats, whose sleep was monitored by electroencephalogram (EEG)* recordings, were allowed to have varying amounts of exploratory activity, and it was found that with greater levels of exploratory behaviour, the greater was the amount of slow-wave activity in subsequent sleep. The two experiments provide very different but consistent evidence in support of the role of daytime activity in influencing sleep.

An association between social activity and sleep in working-age people has been demonstrated in an epidemiological study by Nasermoaddeli et al. (2005) using data from 1628 Japanese civil servants (across the working-age range) and 6873 British civil servants (aged over 40 years) who had taken part in a wider study. Respondents completed measures of sleep quality (the PSQI in the Japanese sample) and were asked about their leisure activities in the previous 12 months. The options were different in each study: the Japanese questionnaire included the slot machine game, pachinko, and karaoke, whereas the UK list included items such as bingo, visiting stately homes and gardening. Leisure activities were classified in both populations according to whether they entailed engagement with others ('social') or were individual pursuits. It was found that in both countries increased participation in social leisure activities was linked with fewer sleep problems. Noting other studies involving exercise, the authors propose that 'social leisure activities, that are not necessarily associated with increased physical activity, are related to improvements in sleep quality' (Nasermoaddeli *et al.* 2005, p.388). As the authors note, in a cross-sectional study it is not possible to determine the causal direction of the relationships: poor sleep quality might cause low mood which could, in turn, influence participation in social leisure activities.

In individuals who are usually more inactive, such as older people whose circadian systems also become less well synchronized (Van Someren and Riemersma-van der Lek 2007), the clinical significance of such findings might be greater. Two large studies have explored the relationships and, in one, Morgan (2003) used data from survivors of a 1985 UK sample of 1042 elderly people, reassessed in 1989 and 1993. Although social engagement showed some association with insomnia, it appeared that lower physical activity levels were a more significant risk factor for insomnia.

Ohayon *et al.* (2001) conducted a telephone survey involving 13,057 people, aged over 15 years, in Germany, Italy and the UK using methods to ensure representation of age and gender. People aged over 65 years comprised 18.6% of the sample. Interviews used an existing standard procedure designed for epidemiological studies on sleep habits and sleep problems. Among the variables measured was social activity, which the researchers defined as activity for which a salary was received or involved the person to be outside the home. Respondents were divided into four groups depending on whether they were active or not and whether they were satisfied or not with their social life. Results showed that adjustments and changes that occur in life, rather than age, are mostly responsible for sleep problems often experienced by older people: 'activity status' and satisfaction with social life were more influential on their sleep. Ohayon *et al.* (2001) note that the prevalence of insomnia symptoms in healthy older people (without physical or mental illness) is similar to the rate found in younger people; they add that 'being active and having a satisfying social life can be protective factors against insomnia symptoms at any age' (p.365).

There is less evidence from research using PSG, but one study that did use it investigated the sleep of a group of 10 elderly nuns (aged 62–82 years) who remained active in their vocations, which was compared with the sleep of 10 healthy retired women with a similar mean age (Hoch *et al.* 1987). It was observed that the nuns spent about an hour less in bed each night but that they slept more quickly (in 15 minutes on average, compared with the control group's average SOL of 27 minutes) and for longer (400 minutes, which was 45 minutes more than the control group). Their sleep was therefore much more efficient (see Chapter 8). This study could equally be cited in the next section which considers regularity, since the nuns had a highly entrained routine with a regular rising time and regular meals; however, they also had scheduled daily activities with eight of them being actively employed. (It is not known how the retired women spent their days and it is also notable that the nuns had exemplary health behaviour, being non-smokers and only light drinkers, and they had a high degree of security in the knowledge that their future needs were provided for.) Although regularity is likely to be a key factor (see below), it would seem that regularity of significant *activity*, or having purpose, was important for the nuns.

There is also much less research on the use of activity as an intervention to improve sleep than there has been with exercise, that is, experimental research as opposed to cross-sectional studies. One example of the former is a small pilot study by Benloucif *et al.* (2004) where 12 older adults (aged 67–86 years) participated in a daily social and physical activity programme. The 90-minute activity sessions took place at either 9 a.m. or 7 p.m. every day for 2 weeks and consisted of two half-hour sessions of mild to moderate physical activity with a half hour of social activity (talking and playing cards or board games). Notably, participants were not selected for sleep quality and, perhaps unsurprisingly, there were no objective changes in sleep discernible on actigraphy or PSG. However, there was a 4–6% improvement in a battery of neuropsychological tests (the main focus of the study) and participants reported a subjective improvement in sleep quality regardless of whether the activity session was in the morning or the evening.

Of particular interest to occupational therapists should be a study by Garms-Homolovà, Flick and Röhnsch (2010) which analyzed data from a cross-sectional sample of 2577 residents (average age 80 years) in 39 nursing homes in Berlin. Cognitive ability was impaired to some extent at least in most cases. The data were collected routinely by nursing home staff as part of outcome measurement and included measures of sleep, physical ability, cognitive performance, mood, activity level, communication, conflicts with others and 'activation and mobilization' (the number of days in the previous seven in which a resident had received at least 15 minutes of occupational therapy or physiotherapy provision). The data were subjected to complex statistical analysis known as structural equation modelling, and associations between the variables were sought. The findings were notable and are summarized in the words of the researchers (Garms-Homolovà *et al.* 2010, pp.750–751) as follows:

- More than half of the participants suffered from some kind of sleep disorder.

- Activation by occupational therapy and/or physiotherapists was provided on an irregular basis or not at all to the [nursing home] residents who were affected by sleep disorders.

- Individuals with sleep disorders were overrepresented among those residents who wished for change in activities within the facility.

- With rising depression and cognitive impairment, prevalence and frequency of sleep disorders increased and ability to communicate decreased.

- Individuals with sleep disorders generally seemed to have more conflicts in the nursing home.

It was concluded 'that low levels of activities and social engagement are partially the result of sleep disorders' and that 'it seems obvious that low activity levels reinforce sleep disorders' (Garms-Homolovà *et al.* 2010, p.751). It would not be surprising if a resident who had not slept well were left to sleep in, or was a little grumpy and that, as a consequence, staff focused their attention on those more likely to participate easily in activities. However, these findings highlight the importance both of addressing sleep difficulties in order to enhance participation and of providing adequate and appropriate stimulation in daytime activity that will in turn enhance sleep.

6.4 Regularity

The two previous sections note some overlap between exercise and activity, but as some of the cited studies imply, it is not just whether you participate in either of them that is important – it is also when, or how regularly, you do it. To add a further layer of complication, there is also evidence that fitness training in the long-term can improve circadian rhythms in the elderly (Van Someren *et al.* 1997); however, the sleep-wake cycle is maintained by the interaction of endogenous circadian and homeostatic drives (see Chapter 3) as well as social and environmental factors (Reid and Zee 2011). Because, in comparison with the solar day, the circadian period is slightly longer in diurnal mammals – about 24.18 hours in humans (Czeisler *et al.* 1999) – it is necessary that it be synchronized to the natural 24-hour day by time cues known as zeitgebers★.

It is well established that the prime zeitgeber is light (see Chapter 3), but social zeitgeber theory (Ehlers, Frank and Kupfer 1988) suggested that life stress could lead to changed biological rhythms (see also Grandin, Alloy and Abramson 2006). Although social zeitgeber theory developed in connection with mood disorder, it suggests that social and behavioural factors can have a role in synchronization or timing of sleep. However, in a detailed review of available evidence at the time, Mistlberger and Skene (2004) concluded that social zeitgebers are weak compared with light (although at the same time they highlight the difficulties of conducting research in humans in controlled-light conditions). Animal studies, where more control can be achieved, suggest that it is possible to override the central pacemaker (the suprachiasmatic nucleus★) in times of stress, such as starvation. Fuller, Lu and Saper (2008) suggest that after a period of starvation, a secondary master clock is adaptive in allowing the animal to change behavioural patterns in order to increase feeding opportunities if the food is only available during the normal sleep period.

As reference to Mistlberger and Skene (2004) or other literature on chronobiology will indicate, the science is complex, but some conclusions can be drawn for the purpose of the discussion here. Although light clearly is the main regulator of circadian rhythms, it also makes sense that there are checks and balances, and that the control mechanism is tempered by other factors to allow a degree of extra flexibility. Other time cues have been shown in animals, but it is less easy to demonstrate their existence in humans in laboratory conditions. It is therefore necessary to look for evidence in other ways, where conditions cannot be easily controlled, in studies of regularity.

Regularity can be given a quantitative value by using measures that record the times at which people carry out a particular daily activity or at which events occur over the course of a week or two (such as getting up, the first interaction with other people, starting work or mealtimes) and calculating the deviation from the average. For example, the Social Rhythm Metric (SRM) (Monk *et al.* 1990) uses 17 items, although this was subsequently refined to just 5 items (Monk *et al.* 2002). A more complex measure with 42 items that distinguishes basic, instrumental, social, leisure and rest activities has been devised by Zisberg, Young and Schepp (2009) specifically for use with older adults – the Scale of Older Adults' Routine (SOAR). When such measures are used alongside measures of self-reported sleep quality, such as the PSQI, correlations can be sought.

In an early exploration of the subject Monk *et al.* (2003) looked at the relationship between regularity and sleep quality in 100 healthy adults (aged 19–49 years who had previously taken part in other studies as 'healthy controls') using the 17-item SRM and the PSQI. They found that respondents with a score on the PSQI that is associated with sleep impairment had significantly lower scores on the SRM – signifying greater regularity. Further work has shown that regularity is important for the elderly whose circadian rhythms are less robust. Monk *et al.* (2011) conducted a telephone survey of 654 retired people (aged over 65 years) using scales that assess the extent to which people were evening or morning people ('owls' or 'larks'; see Chapter 3), sleep quality (the PSQI) and time spent in bed and time asleep (and therefore, sleep efficiency). They found that, as well as morning orientation, stability of bedtime and rising times were associated with better sleep. They concluded that 'within reason, it may, perhaps, be appropriate to advise seniors to go to bed earlier than they did in their younger years (while recognizing that their nocturnal sleep is likely to be shorter than that of the young)' (Monk *et al.* 2011, p.238).

In another study involving elderly participants, Zisberg, Gur-Yaish and Shochat (2010) investigated the contribution of routine to the sleep of 96 Russian-speaking older Israeli adults (mean age 75 years): routine was assessed for the whole sample using subscales of the SOAR and, for a subsample, the SRM as well; sleep quality was measured with the PSQI, and an instrumental activity of daily living scale was used to assess functional status. The researchers found a strong association between daily routine and subjective sleep quality as measured by the instruments:

routine of both basic and instrumental daily activities based on the SOAR instrument, as well as increased stability in daily routine based on the SRM, were related to positive sleep outcomes based on subjective estimates of sleep latency, sleep efficiency and overall sleep quality. (Zisberg *et al.* 2010, p.512)

It was also found that there was a stronger association between sleep quality and basic activities of daily living than there was between sleep quality and instrumental activities of daily living. Zisberg *et al.* (2010) suggest that basic activities might be more habitual physiological activities such as bathing, dressing and eating, compared with instrumental activities which are more socially oriented and might depend more on other people's priorities and routines – perhaps less likely to be daily if including shopping or attending medical appointments. Additionally, some of the basic needs will occur in the evening as part of a winding-down routine. For further discussion of regularity and the role of loneliness see Smith, Kozak and Sullivan (2010).

It is not only the elderly that might benefit from more regularity. Carney *et al.* (2006) surveyed 243 US college students (mean age about 21 years) using the SRM, PSQI and a measure of mood. They found that the routines of students with self-reported poor sleep were more variable than those of the good sleepers, and that those with limited social activity appeared to have poorer sleep quality. Furthermore, a consistent rising time appeared to be particularly important for good sleep (and in line with advice given for managing insomnia; see Chapter 8). The link with social activity could relate to the effect of others. Carney *et al.* (2006) observed that it is unlikely that someone would select a time that differs greatly from the social conventions for meeting for a meal, whereas there can be greater variability when doing an activity alone. 'Poor sleepers with a less socially active lifestyle may be more free to violate social conventions, and they may eat, go to bed, or get out of bed at later and less conventional times, thus creating more variability' (Carney *et al.* 2006, p.635).

There is a slight inconsistency in this finding. Whereas it is suggested that younger people are influenced by others to maintain regularity, it was indicated above that older people's routines might be disrupted by others. Perhaps different factors are in play, older people being more naturally advanced and the younger being delayed. Furthermore, Van Someren and Riemersma-van der Lek (2007) suggest that there may be an implicit recognition by elderly people of a less robust circadian system with 'a compensatory adherence to a stricter 24-hour zeitgeber pattern' (p.475) than seen in younger people; maybe elderly people who keep to fixed routines are not just 'set in their ways'. Lastly, it has to be acknowledged again that in such cross-sectional studies no cause can be attributed, and it still cannot be known whether regularity of routines enhances sleep or whether people who have good sleep are better able to maintain regular activity.

6.5 Conclusions and implications for therapy

The evidence presented in this chapter points to the conclusion that sleep is enhanced by:

- vigorous exercise, and some less vigorous forms of exercise

- engagement in activity, including social activity

- regularity and routines.

If good sleep is considered to be an indicator of good health, none of that is likely to come as a surprise to an occupational therapist. Most occupational therapists will naturally promote exercise and activity and stress the importance of having some kind of structure to one's time. However, the evidence cannot be accepted at face value. Few of the studies cited here could attribute cause: epidemiological or cross-sectional studies are not able to confirm cause, and findings from small surveys and experimental studies, with variable degrees of control, cannot be generalized. A key difficulty in establishing causality is that people who sleep well are more likely to feel inclined to exercise, whereas someone experiencing severe insomnia is likely to complain that they simply do not feel like meeting friends for an evening, for example. Furthermore, if poor sleep is associated, or coincident, with any kind of health difficulty, that difficulty might lead to disruption of routines or non-participation in activity. Youngstedt and Kline (2006) note these and other confounding elements in relation to exercise research (which would also hold good in research about other activity), observing that many studies rely on self-report or measures of unknown validity; other factors that could affect sleep, such as light exposure, smoking or alcohol consumption, might not be controlled for.

Acknowledging the potential shortcomings of the research evidence, and the near impossibility of controlling the variables in a study of a size that could yield significant results, some inferences can still be made. At the very least, it appears possible to conclude that, in principle, activity and routine have no adverse effects on sleep: there is no reason for an occupational therapist *not* to recommend activity to enhance sleep. However, the combined weight of evidence from such a wide range of sources suggests a more positive conclusion: that what occupational therapists (along with most others) believe to be good for health – engagement in a range of activity meaningful to the individual – is also good for sleep. This conclusion is perhaps most important for those who might lack structure and routine, or who have difficulty engaging in exercise or activity: those with long-term medical conditions or older people, especially those in institutional care – as exemplified by Garms-Homolovà *et al.* (2010).

In giving advice about timing of exercise some caution may be needed. Traditionally, it is advised not to exercise close to bedtime, and probably few people would think it reasonable to come home from a half-hour run, shower and go straight to bed with the expectation of sleeping quickly. However, there is now some evidence from surveys and research that evening exercise is not as detrimental to sleep as has been assumed. A common-sense approach is required. If a person already exercises in the evening and gets to sleep without difficulty, they might as well continue. If another person in the same exercise group sleeps poorly on training nights, they should consider experimenting with an earlier exercise time. If encouraging someone to exercise more, either for their general health or to improve their sleep, it is probably wise to start with the standard advice to exercise earlier in the day.

In Chapter 8 it is explained that one of the recommended strategies to manage insomnia, stimulus control, depends on separating waking activity from the sleeping environment, thereby increasing the behavioural cues to sleep. However, it is possible that the opposite also applies: that in order to improve sleep, there needs to be, in waking time, a greater contrast to the behavioural inactivity of sleep. In other words, the excessive rest and inactivity of a sedentary lifestyle are insufficiently distinguishable from sleep and, on going to bed, the behavioural cues are not strong enough. Furthermore, there is evidence that the homeostatic pressure for SWS is increased in individuals who have engaged more with their environment.

There is therefore a strong *prima facie* case for people who complain of poor sleep to increase engagement in active occupation, especially if they are sedentary, and, more so, if they are living in residential care settings. Occupational therapists should advise people with poor sleep to maintain regular routines (with a set rising time), to engage in appropriate social and other activity, and to take appropriate exercise.

References

Atkinson, G., Edwards, B., Reilly, T. and Waterhouse, J. (2007) 'Exercise as a synchroniser of human circadian rhythms: an update and discussion of the methodological problems.' *European Journal of Applied Physiology 99*, 4, 331–341.

Benloucif, S., Orbeta, L., Oritz, R., Janssen, I. *et al.* (2004) 'Morning or evening activity improves neuropsychological performance and subjective sleep quality in older adults.' *Sleep 27*, 8, 1542–1551.

Brand, S., Beck, J., Gerber, M., Hatzinger, M. and Holsboer-Trachsler, E. (2009) '"Football is good for your sleep": favourable sleep patterns and psychological functioning of adolescent male intense football players compared to controls.' *Journal of Health Psychology 14*, 8, 1144–1155.

Buman, M.P., Hekler, E.B., Bliwise, D.L. and King, A.C. (2011) 'Exercise effects on night-to-night fluctuations in self-rated sleep among older adults with sleep complaints.' *Journal of Sleep Research 20*, 1, Pt 1, 28–37.

Buysse, D.J., Reynolds, C.F., Monk, T.H., Berman, S.R. and Kupfer, D.J. (1989) 'The Pittsburgh Sleep Quality Index: a new instrument for psychiatric practice and research.' *Psychiatry Research 28*, 2, 193–213.

Carney, C.E., Edinger, J.D., Meyer, B., Lindman, L. and Istre, T. (2006) 'Daily activities and sleep quality in college students.' *Chronobiology International 23*, 3, 623–637.

Czeisler, C.A., Duffy, J.H., Shanahan, T.L., Brown, E.N. *et al.* (1999) 'Stability, precision, and near-24-hour period of the human circadian pacemaker.' *Science 284*, 5423, 2177–2181.

Driver, H.S. and Taylor, S.R. (2000) 'Exercise and sleep.' *Sleep Medicine Reviews 4*, 4, 387–402.

Dzierzewski, J.M., Buman, M.P., Giacobbi, P.R., Roberts, B.L. *et al.* (2013) 'Exercise and sleep in community-dwelling older adults: evidence for a reciprocal relationship.' *Journal of Sleep Research*. doi: 10.1111/jsr.12078.

Ehlers, C.L., Frank, E. and Kupfer, D.J. (1988) 'Social zeitgebers and biological rhythms: a unified approach to understanding the etiology of depression.' *Archives of General Psychiatry 45*, 10, 948–952.

Fuller, P.M., Lu, J. and Saper, C.B. (2008) 'Differential rescue of light- and food-entrainable circadian rhythms.' *Science 320*, 5879, 1074–1077.

Garms-Homolovà, V., Flick, U. and Röhnsch, G. (2010) 'Sleep disorders and activities in long-term care facilities – a vicious cycle?' *Journal of Health Psychology 15*, 5, 744–754.

Gebhart, C., Erlacher, D. and Schredl, M. (2011) 'Moderate exercise plus sleep education improves self-reported sleep quality, daytime mood, and vitality in adults with chronic sleep complaints: a waiting list-controlled trial.' *Sleep Disorders*. doi: 10.1155/2011/809312.

Grandin, L.D., Alloy, L.B. and Abramson, L.Y. (2006) 'The social zeitgeber theory, circadian rhythms, and mood disorders: review and evaluation.' *Clinical Psychology Review 26*, 6, 679–694.

Green, A. (2012) 'A Question of Balance: The Relationship Between Daily Occupation and Sleep.' In A. Green and A. Westcombe (eds) *Sleep: Multiprofessional Perspectives.* London: Jessica Kingsley Publishers.

Hoch, C.H., Reynolds, C.F., Kupfer, D.J., Houck, P.R., Berman, S.R. and Stack, J.A. (1987) 'The superior sleep of elderly nuns.' *International Journal of Aging and Human Development 25*, 1, 1–9.

Horne, J.A. and Minard, A. (1985) 'Sleep and sleepiness following a behaviourally "active" day.' *Ergonomics 28*, 3, 567–575.

Huber, R., Tononi, G. and Cirelli, C. (2006) 'Exploratory behavior, cortical BDNF expression, and sleep homeostasis.' *Sleep 30*, 2, 129–139.

King, A.C., Orman, R.F., Brassington, G.S., Bliwise, D.L. and Haskell, W.L. (1997) 'Moderate-intensity exercise and self-rated quality of sleep in older adults: a randomized controlled trial.' *Journal of the American Medical Association 277*, 1, 32–37.

King, A.C., Pruitt, L.A., Woo, S., Castro, C.M. *et al.* (2008) 'Effects of moderate-intensity exercise on polysomnographic and subjective sleep quality in older adults with mild to moderate sleep complaints.' *Journals of Gerontology: Medical Sciences 63A*, 9, 997–1004.

Li, F., Fisher, K.J., Harmer, P., Irbe, D., Tearse, R.G. and Weimer, C. (2004) 'Tai chi and self-rated quality of sleep and daytime sleepiness in older adults: a randomized controlled trial.' *Journal of the American Geriatrics Society 52*, 6, 892–900.

Mistlberger, R.E. and Skene, D.J. (2004) 'Social influences on mammalian circadian rhythms: animal and human studies.' *Biological Reviews of the Cambridge Philosophical Society 79*, 3, 533–556.

Monk, T.H., Buysse, D.J., Billy, B.D., Fletcher, M.E. *et al.* (2011) 'Circadian type and bed-timing regularity in 654 retired seniors: correlations with subjective sleep measures.' *Sleep 34*, 2, 235–239.

Monk, T.H., Flaherty, J.P., Frank, E., Hoskinson, K. and Kupfer, D.J. (1990) 'The Social Rhythm Metric: an instrument to quantify the daily rhythms of life.' *Journal of Nervous and Mental Disease 178*, 2, 120–126.

Monk, T.H., Frank, E., Potts, J.M. and Kupfer, D.J. (2002) 'A simple way to measure daily lifestyle regularity.' *Journal of Sleep Research 11*, 3, 183–190.

Monk, T.H., Reynolds, C.F., Buysse, D.J., DeGrazia, J.M. and Kupfer, D.J. (2003) 'The relationship between lifestyle regularity and subjective sleep quality.' *Chronobiology International 20*, 1, 97–107.

Morgan, K. (2003) 'Daytime activity and risk factors for late-life insomnia.' *Journal of Sleep Research 12*, 3, 231–238.

Morita, E., Imai, M., Okawa, M., Miyaura, T. and Miyazaki, S. (2011) 'A before and after comparison of the effects of forest walking on the sleep of a community based sample of people with sleep complaints.' *BioPsychoSocial Medicine.* doi: 10.1186/1751-0759-5-13.

Myllymäki, T., Kyröläinen, H., Savollainen, K., Hokka, L. *et al.* (2010) 'Effects of vigorous late-night exercise on sleep quality and cardiac autonomic activity.' *Journal of Sleep Research 20*, 1, Pt 2, 146–153.

Nasermoaddeli, A., Sekine, M., Kumari, M., Chandola, T., Marmot, M. and Kagamimori, S. (2005) 'Association of sleep quality and free time leisure activities in Japanese and British civil servants.' *Journal of Occupational Health 47*, 5, 384–390.

National Sleep Foundation (2013) *National Sleep Foundation 2013 Poll: Exercise and Sleep.* Arlington, VA: National Sleep Foundation. Available at http://sleepfoundation.org/2013poll.

Ohayon, M.M., Zulley, J., Guilleminualt, C., Smirne, S. and Priest, R.G. (2001) 'How age and daytime activities are related to insomnia in the general population: consequences for older people.' *Journal of the American Geriatrics Society 49*, 4, 360–366.

Passos, G.S., Poyares, D., Santana, M.G., Garbuio, S.A., Tufik, M.D. and Mello, M.T. (2010) 'Effect of acute physical exercise on patients with chronic primary insomnia.' *Journal of Clinical Sleep Medicine 6*, 3, 270–275.

Passos, G.S., Poyares, D., Santana, M.G., Rodrigues, C.V. *et al.* (2011) 'Effects of moderate aerobic exercise training on chronic primary insomnia.' *Sleep Medicine 12*, 10, 1018–1027.

Passos, G.S., Poyares, D.L., Santana, M.G., Tufik, S. and Mello, M.T. (2012) 'Is exercise an alternative treatment for chronic insomnia?' *Clinics (São Paulo) 67*, 6, 653–659.

Reid, K.J., Baron, K.G., Lu, B., Naylor, E., Wolfe, L. and Zee, P.C. (2010) 'Aerobic exercise improves self-reported sleep and quality of life in older adults with insomnia.' *Sleep Medicine 11*, 9, 934–940.

Reid, K.J. and Zee, P.C. (2011) 'Circadian Disorders of the Sleep-Wake Cycle.' In M.H. Kryger, T. Roth and W.C. Dement (eds) *Principles and Practice of Sleep Medicine*, 5th edn. St Louis, MO: Elsevier Saunders.

Shapiro, C.M., Bortz, R., Mitchell, D., Bartel, P. and Jooste, P. (1981) 'Slow-wave sleep: a recovery period after exercise.' *Science 214*, 4526, 1253–1254.

Sherrill, D.L., Kotchou, K. and Quan, S.F. (1998) 'Association of physical activity and human sleep disorders.' *Archives of Internal Medicine 158*, 17, 1894–1898.

Smith, S.S., Kozak, N. and Sullivan, K.A. (2010) 'An investigation of the relationship between subjective sleep quality, loneliness and mood in an Australian sample: can daily routine explain the links?' *International Journal of Social Psychiatry 58*, 2, 166–171.

Tononi, G. and Cirelli, C. (2006) 'Sleep function and synaptic homeostasis.' *Sleep Medicine Reviews 10*, 1, 49–62.

Tononi, G. and Cirelli, C. (2012) 'Time to Be SHY? Some comments on sleep and synaptic homeostasis.' *Neural Plasticity 2012.* doi: 10.1155/2012/415250.

Van Someren, E.J.W., Lijenga, C., Mirmiran, M. and Swaab, D.F. (1997) 'Long-term fitness training improves the circadian rest-activity rhythm in healthy elderly males.' *Journal of Biological Rhythms 12*, 2, 146–156.

Van Someren, E.J.W. and Riemersma-van der Lek, R.F. (2007) 'Live to the rhythm, slave to the rhythm.' *Sleep Medicine Reviews 11*, 6, 465–484.

Yang, P.-Y., Ho, K.-H., Chen, H.-C. and Chien, M.-Y. (2012) 'Exercise training improves sleep quality in middle-aged and older adults with sleep problems: a systematic review.' *Journal of Physiotherapy 58*, 3, 157–163.

Youngstedt, S.D. (2003) 'Ceiling and floor effects in sleep research.' *Sleep Medicine Reviews 7*, 4, 351–365.

Youngstedt, S.D. and Kline, C.E. (2006) 'Epidemiology of exercise and sleep.' *Sleep and Biological Rhythms 4*, 3, 215–221.

Zisberg, A., Gur-Yaish, N. and Shochat, T. (2010) 'Contribution of routine to sleep quality in community elderly.' *Sleep 33*, 4, 509–514.

Zisberg, A., Young, H.M. and Schepp, K. (2009) 'Development and psychometric testing of the Scale of Older Adults' Routine.' *Journal of Advanced Nursing 65*, 3, 672–683.

7

SLEEP DISORDERS

Andrew Green and Dietmar Hank

7.1 Introduction

People are seldom likely to be referred to occupational therapists for sleep disorders alone, although many patients with other conditions also have sleep difficulties, and in order to help manage such difficulties, and to know when to refer, it is important to have an understanding of sleep disorders. Essentially, sleep disorders can be categorized as insufficient sleep (insomnia), too much sleep (hypersomnia or excessive daytime sleepiness), unusual behaviours in sleep (parasomnia), sleeping at the wrong time (circadian-rhythm disorders) and movement disorders in sleep. Most sleep disorders are managed by either medication or cognitive and behavioural strategies, or a combination of these approaches. For example, in the case of insomnia the more effective long-term management is cognitive behavioural therapy for insomnia, whereas in the case of narcolepsy, medication is often effective and there is less emphasis on behavioural management. This chapter explores the major sleep disorders and outlines the principles of their management, but it is not intended as a guide to treatment of sleep disorders. The next chapter focuses on the non-pharmacological management of some insomnia and excessive daytime sleepiness. (For a concise but full guide to sleep disorders see Wilson and Nutt 2013, or for more detailed information see, for example, Avidan and Zee 2011.)

7.2 Insomnia

The most common sleep problem is insomnia, which affects about 10–15% of the population (Wilson and Nutt 2013). It is defined as complaints of disturbed sleep in the presence of adequate opportunity and circumstance for sleep. The disturbance may consist of one or more of three features: (1) difficulty in initiating sleep; (2) difficulty in maintaining sleep; or (3) waking up too early. A fourth characteristic, non-restorative or poor-quality sleep, has frequently been included in the definition, although there is controversy as to whether individuals with this complaint share similar pathophysiological mechanisms with the others (NIH 2005, p.5).

A diagnosis of insomnia requires that the poor sleep have consequences for daytime performance; otherwise, a person might just be a short sleeper (and less likely to complain). It is also important to establish whether the person has had sufficient opportunity to sleep and whether or not they have been trying to sleep at the appropriate time for them.

Traditionally, a distinction has been made between primary insomnia, which is not a consequence of another medical or psychiatric condition, and secondary insomnia, which is a consequence of another disorder. Among the subtypes of primary insomnia, according to the *International Classification of Sleep Disorders* (American Academy of Sleep Medicine 2005), are psychophysiological insomnia and paradoxical insomnia (see below). Psychophysiological insomnia is typically associated with increased arousal levels and learned associations that hinder sleep; it is commonly accompanied by over-concern about the ability (or inability) to sleep. Secondary insomnia is sometimes known as co-morbid insomnia so as to imply no cause. Whether insomnia coexists with another condition, or results from it, might be an academic question, but the picture is complicated by different classification systems (see Hicks and Green 2012). However, it is important not to assume that secondary or co-morbid insomnia will take care of itself if the primary condition is treated. The 'habit' of insomnia may persist after the original condition is resolved; on the other hand, insomnia could be helped despite the continuation of the other problem (see Chapter 8). Insomnia is considered to be 'chronic' after 30 days (NIH 2005, p.5), although a figure of 6 months has also been used to define chronicity. Prevalence of insomnia can be difficult to estimate, but Wilson and Nutt (2013) suggest that 'somewhere around 10–15% of the population have persistent or chronic insomnia' (p.26).

The idea that insomnia becomes a habit underlies some models. For example, the 3P model (Spielman, Caruso and Glovinsky 1987) suggests that, first, there are *predisposing* biological, psychological or environmental factors. Second, life stresses can *precipitate* poor sleep – an understandable and commonly experienced reaction to stress. Third, the response to poor sleep may in fact *perpetuate* insomnia, for example if the individual spends longer in bed in an attempt to compensate for lost sleep or begins to engage in waking activity in the bedroom. People who sleep poorly also tend to worry about their sleep which, in turn, tends to accentuate the problem.

Another suggestion is that on being unable to sleep, the person's *attention* is drawn to the process of going to sleep – a usually automatic process that cannot be willed. This inhibits the decrease of arousal and the disengagement with the environment that are necessary for falling asleep, and the subsequent *intention* and *effort* to sleep further prevent sleep from taking over. This is the 'attention–intention–effort pathway' (see Espie *et al.* 2006). There is evidence, for example, that compared with good sleepers (and with people with a circadian rhythm disorder; see below), people with insomnia show greater levels of attention bias; for example, MacMahon, Broomfield and Espie (2006) found that poor sleepers paid greater attention to sleep-related words presented among neutral words. (For full exploration of the more influential models of insomnia see Perlis *et al.* 2011a.)

The role of arousal in insomnia has been reviewed by Bonnet and Arand (2010) and Riemann *et al.* (2010). Riemann *et al.* observe that chronic insomnia is 'a disorder of 24-hour hyperarousal' (p.29) and that chronic sleep loss may mask the hyperarousal and account for daytime fatigue. In an earlier review of the literature, Riedel and Lichstein (2000, p.279) 'safely conclude that there is no objective elevation in daytime sleepiness associated with insomnia based on the MSLT' (multiple sleep latency test, which is a standardized measure of sleepiness; see below). However, they question whether the reason that people with insomnia cannot fall asleep in the day is that they are not actually sleep deprived. Whether or not that is the case, this observation accords with clinical experience where people with insomnia typically report not being sleepy and an inability to doze off in quiet moments by day.

A bad night's sleep, whatever the cause, is something that is familiar to most people, but insomnia sufferers most commonly report fatigue, mood disturbances, memory and concentration problems, work-related mistakes and difficulties making decisions. For example, in a meta-analysis of studies, Fortier-Brochu *et al.* (2012) found statistically significant impairments in several cognitive domains, including working memory, episodic memory and problem-solving. Objective research evidence of the effects of poor sleep is discussed in Chapter 5, but the numerical data relating to concentration or reaction time tests, for example, cannot describe the individual's experience of continued poor sleep. Three small focus-group studies have attempted to understand that experience.

Carey *et al.* (2005), in a study involving 16 insomnia patients at a sleep clinic in the US, found that insomnia had a 'pervasive impact on a person's quality of life' (p.80) that was minimized by other people and led to a sense of isolation. Participants also felt that their experience was not fully understood by health care providers and, worse, they found it difficult when the effects of insomnia were diagnosed as depression. They also complained that doctors could be preoccupied with the amount of sleep they had, rather than focus on the daytime consequences of insomnia.

A UK study by Green, Hicks and Wilson (2008), also in a tertiary care centre, involved six women with insomnia. Findings were very similar in that participants felt that, as one said, insomnia 'impacts on your *whole* life' (p.199). The sense of isolation was expressed by another: 'Absolute frustration. Why me? – Why am I the only person awake in the world when everybody else is sleeping soundly?' (p.199), and they shared the feeling that others, including doctors, did not understand. There was some relief to have been seen, finally, by a sleep specialist who listened.

Also in the UK, Kyle, Espie and Morgan (2010) recruited their 11 focus-group participants through newspaper adverts and posters and subsequently verified a diagnosis of insomnia. They identified three superordinate themes in their data: 'just struggle through', 'isolated, feeling like an outsider' and 'insomnia as an obstruction to the desired self'. The last of those themes relates to the ways in which poor sleep can hold people back in their education or careers because of functional deficits, or affect social life by causing someone to be too tired to be sociable. Kyle *et al.* (2010) conclude that insomnia measurably impacts on, and reduces, the health-related quality of life for mental, social and physical functioning. (For a recent review of the literature relating to the patient experience of insomnia see Cheung *et al.* 2012.)

These qualitative studies involve small numbers in different settings, and the data are interpreted in different ways. Although the findings from such studies cannot be generalized, when the quoted words of the individuals are looked at collectively a picture does emerge, and it is recognizable in clinical experience. It is not just the night-time experience that is isolating – the daytime consequences can be very disabling, and together they make insomnia a serious problem for the individual, which is all the worse if it accompanies another illness. However, it should be noted that all the focus-group participants volunteered to take part, perhaps because they wanted to be heard. Other poor sleepers who did not volunteer could be coping differently with their sleep difficulties, and many notable figures in history achieved great things despite their insomnia. For example, Isaac Newton, Charles Dickens, Napoleon Bonaparte, Abraham Lincoln and Thomas Edison were all said to have insomnia, although it can never be known whether or not their complaint would have met modern diagnostic criteria.

Investigations are not usually necessary in making a diagnosis of insomnia. Overnight monitoring in a sleep laboratory (i.e. polysomnography) is normally only used if it is suspected that something is disturbing sleep, such as a movement or breathing disorder, for example. It would be likely just to confirm that the person does indeed not sleep well, or possibly that the person sleeps better than believed and has paradoxical insomnia (see below). Actigraphy* (see Chapter 8) might be used if it is helpful to have an understanding of a person's sleep pattern over a few weeks.

The first line of treatment for short-term insomnia is often medication, specifically, hypnotics such as the 'z-drugs' (e.g. zaleplon and zolpidem) and benzodiazepines (e.g. temazepam), or sometimes antidepressants with sedative properties (see Wilson 2012). However, family doctors are often reluctant to prescribe hypnotics even in the very short term, and in the UK it is recommended that they be prescribed for severe insomnia 'only after due consideration of the use of non-pharmacological measures' (National Institute for Clinical Excellence 2004, p.18). The difficulty with the preferred treatment, cognitive behavioural therapy for insomnia (CBT-I), is that it is not widely available, although this is gradually changing. Espie (2009) has advocated a stepped-care approach for delivery and Espie *et al.* (2012) have demonstrated that online delivery can be effective. CBT-I is considered in greater detail in Chapter 8, but although it 'is a standard, recommended treatment, and is commonly regarded as the treatment modality of choice' (Kyle *et al.* 2011, p.735), it is unhelpful in situations where there is disagreement between clinician and the person experiencing insomnia about the objective severity of sleep loss, as in paradoxical insomnia.

Paradoxical insomnia

Also known as sleep-state misperception, paradoxical insomnia sometimes becomes evident when a person has had polysomnography and subjectively reports sleeping, for example, only 1 or 2 hours despite the objective neurophysiological evidence of several hours of sleep. Alternatively, a patient might complain of persistent wakefulness at night without the significant daytime impairment that would be expected to result from such sleep loss. There has long been a debate over how insomnia is a reflection of misperception of time awake, and the extent to which insomnia can be considered to be objective or subjective (see, for example, Edinger and Krystal 2003 and Tang and Harvey 2005). More recently, Manconi *et al.* (2010) compared the objective and subjective sleep times of insomnia patients and members of a control group using a misperception index and found that insomnia patients were poor sleep perceivers who were unaware of a third of their sleep; however, they also found 'a specific group of highly misperceiver insomniacs' (*sic*) (p.484).

Further discussion about the existence of paradoxical insomnia and its management is beyond the scope of this chapter. (Interested readers are referred to Geyer *et al.* 2011 and Harvey and Tang 2012.) However, it is important to be aware that, first, overestimation of night-time wakefulness is common, both by someone who regularly has poor sleep and by a good sleeper having a bad night; it is easy to estimate sleep on a good night. Second, just because someone is underestimating sleep does not mean that they are having sufficient sleep in terms of quantity or quality. Lastly, if a person seriously misperceives or underestimates their sleep, the usual approaches to management of insomnia are unlikely to be successful.

7.3 Excessive daytime sleepiness

It might be assumed that insomnia will cause excessive daytime sleepiness (EDS) but, as noted above, people with psychophysiological insomnia tend not to be sleepy by day. Assuming that an individual is not sleep deprived for some reason, the main sleep disorders involving EDS are obstructive sleep apnoea, narcolepsy and idiopathic hypersomnia. The cause of idiopathic hypersomnia is by definition unknown, but there may be a hereditary element: it is diagnosed by exclusion and is rare.

There are two ways of measuring sleepiness. For example, the Epworth Sleepiness Scale (Johns 1991) is a widely used subject-rated tool that gives an indication of the degree of sleepiness (see Chapter 8). An objective measure of sleepiness, or propensity to sleep, is the multiple sleep latency test (MSLT)*. Using electroencephalography (EEG)* to record sleep, the individual is given timed opportunities to sleep in a darkened, comfortable room following polysomnography the night before. An average time that it takes to get to sleep (the mean sleep latency*) of 8 minutes or less over the four or five naps would, for example, suggest (but not confirm) narcolepsy; at least two sleep-onset rapid eye movement (REM) periods (see below) would add further evidence for diagnosis.

Obstructive sleep apnoea

Obstructive sleep apnoea (OSA) is a major cause of EDS and affects up to 7% of adult men and 5% of adult women (Punjabi 2008). It is a respiratory problem that occurs in sleep where the airway becomes narrowed with the consequence that breathing stops (apnoea) or is limited (hypopnoea). A reflex response wakes the person who then typically falls back to sleep, unaware of the disturbance. This may be repeated, dozens of times per hour, with the result that sleep is fragmented and diminished. The individual may perceive that sleep has been sufficient – in terms of the time in bed asleep – but will not know that the quality has been compromised and feels sleepy by day. It is a particular hazard for professional drivers, and suspension of a licence, and potential loss of livelihood, will be a great concern and a possible disincentive to seek help.

The mechanisms that maintain the airway are complex, but the cross-section of the airway tends to be smaller in OSA patients and is then reduced further by fat deposits in the neck. A larger neck size is a better predictor of OSA than body mass index alone. Snoring is commonly (but not exclusively) associated with OSA and a bed partner is also likely to notice periods of silence while breathing pauses, and a snort or a gasp when it restarts. The patient might complain of a dry mouth during the night or on waking, or of headaches in the morning; however, the chief daytime feature is sleepiness with accompanying deficits in performance.

OSA is a particular concern because the disruption of respiration can have far-reaching physiological consequences, especially on the cardiovascular system. There is, for example, an increased risk of hypertension (Phillips and Somers 2003), of atrial fibrillation (Gami *et al.* 2004) and of stroke, even with mild to moderate OSA (Redline *et al.* 2010). There is also a close association with type II diabetes, although the direction of causality is uncertain, and the close relationship of obesity with both conditions is a complicating factor. Additionally, OSA frequently has neuropsychological consequences such as diminished attention, memory and executive function, to name a few (see, for example, Alchanatis *et al.* 2005; Aloia *et al.* 2004; Antonelli Incalzi *et al.* 2004 and El-Ad and Lavie 2005). Treatment is therefore important in order to reduce such risks in the longer term, as well as to reduce the disruption to everyday life in the short term.

A study by O'Donoghue and McKay (2012) illustrates the effect of OSA on the individual. Many everyday activities become difficult, simply because the individual struggles to remain awake or because of diminished concentration and memory; relationships can change because of snoring disturbing a spouse (leading perhaps to separate sleeping arrangements) or the embarrassment of falling asleep in the company of friends. The effects of OSA can lead people to give up work; one participant in the study by O'Donoghue and McKay (2012) had to retire early because of OSA, while another (a health professional) was at some risk when she 'fell asleep one day with a drill in my hand and another day with a scalpel…I just nodded off' (p.512). Another participant reported driving when 'One time I woke on the other side of the road' (p.512). In the UK an individual is obliged by law to inform the licensing authorities of a diagnosis of OSA and not to drive until the condition is under control. However, regulations are not consistent within the European Union where 'the present system resembles chaos more than a rational plan' (Mwenga and Rodenstein 2012, p.192), and a driver from a country where untreated OSA is not a limitation on driving is free to drive in a country where there are restrictions for its own nationals with OSA. In the US regulations vary between states (see, for example, Boehlecke 2011).

Drivers and others can be reassured that OSA is treatable – principally by continuous positive airway pressure (CPAP), which requires the patient to sleep wearing a facemask through which air is blown in order to keep the airway open. Modern devices are relatively quiet and compact and, as long as the patient can tolerate the mask, CPAP can make a huge difference to sleep, daytime performance and overall quality of life. Unfortunately, many people do not easily get used to sleeping with CPAP and adherence is a great problem. (Several chapters in Perlis *et al.* 2011b outline innovative methods of enhancing management of OSA.) One possibility is a self-management programme (Stepnowsky 2011), which is an area where an occupational therapist could become involved. The intervention of occupational therapists in the management of sleep apnoea is also advocated by O'Donoghue and McKay (2012).

Narcolepsy

In comparison with OSA, narcolepsy is a relatively uncommon condition (found in about 1 in 2000 people) (Ohayon *et al.* 2002). It affects the regulatory mechanism that controls sleep and wakefulness. It is characterized by two main features: (1) daytime sleepiness with an irresistible need to sleep, resulting in the individual taking naps up to five times a day; and (2) cataplexy, which is the loss of skeletal muscle tone, as occurs in REM sleep, occurring in the context of emotion such as surprise, anger or amusement. Where loss of tone is complete, the person will fall to the floor, but in partial cataplexy there may be weakness of the knees and slumping of the head. Consciousness is not lost in cataplexy. A further feature of the dysregulation of control of REM sleep is that the patient goes rapidly into REM sleep on first falling asleep (without passing through the other stages). This is known as a sleep-onset REM period and may be detected in the MSLT. Other features of narcolepsy include hallucinations on going to sleep or on waking (known respectively as hypnagogic and hynopompic hallucinations), sleep paralysis (see section 7.4) and fragmented and unrefreshing sleep at night.

No published qualitative studies of patient experience have been identified, but clinical experience indicates how life can be severely disrupted by narcolepsy. In many respects it is similar to epilepsy in that people can experience social embarrassment, inability to drive and difficulty finding and/or retaining employment; all of these can lead to social isolation. The scale of disruption to life can perhaps be most readily appreciated by considering the difficulty that cataplexy can cause when precipitated by simply sharing a joke or having a chance encounter with a friend. The limitations that can be caused by narcolepsy are confirmed by a quantitative study using a questionnaire and depression and quality-of-life measures with a sample from a UK narcolepsy patient association (Daniels *et al.* 2001). When compared with normative data, respondents had a poorer health status on all measures with more than half of them showing signs of depression. Narcolepsy had affected schooling and caused over a third of respondents to lose a job or leave it and a similar proportion reported everyday tasks (such as cooking, ironing and childcare) to be difficult, and leisure activities were also restricted. Daniels *et al.* (2001) report avoidance of social situations where falling asleep or cataplexy could be embarrassing or harmful. However, a study by Stores, Montgomery and Wiggs (2006) indicated that it may be excessive sleepiness, rather than other factors related to narcolepsy, that causes the problems. They compared children ($n = 42$) between the ages of about 7 and 18 years with narcolepsy, children having excessive sleepiness without cataplexy and a control group; they found little difference between the narcolepsy and EDS groups on measures of depression and behavioural problems, as well as educational problems, when compared with the control group. The findings suggested that narcolepsy puts children at a higher risk of psychosocial problems and are consistent with the conclusion of Bruck (2001) that narcolepsy can have a negative impact on psychosocial adjustment.

A person with narcolepsy in the UK is legally obliged to inform the Driver and Vehicle Licensing Agency (DVLA) of the diagnosis and to stop driving (and only resume once the condition is under control). If a doctor is aware that a patient continues to drive in spite of advice not to, she or he is permitted under General Medical Council (GMC) guidelines to contact the DVLA and to inform their medical advisor (GMC 2009), preferably having advised the patient in advance.[1] Despite the difficulties presented by narcolepsy, it should be stressed that many people with the condition are still able to retain jobs and to cope with other responsibilities, as is the case for people with epilepsy, for example.

Medication is the main treatment for narcolepsy (see Mignot 2012),[2] but in terms of non-pharmacological management it is important to optimize night-time sleep, and when it is compromised, the advice that might be given for insomnia (see Chapter 8) can be just as relevant. In contrast to the usual advice in the case of insomnia, it may be helpful to take planned daytime naps in order to pre-empt uncontrolled sleep. There could be a role for an occupational therapist in helping an individual in coping with the condition – in the same way that one might work with a person with epilepsy – in developing confidence and looking at safety strategies. (For general behavioural management of EDS see Chapter 8.)

7.4 Parasomnias

Parasomnias are defined as 'undesirable nondeliberate motor or subjective phenomenon (*sic*) that arise during the transition from wakefulness into sleep or during arousals from sleep' (Avidan 2011, p.67). They amount to a failure to make a smooth or complete transition from one of the three states of being (wakefulness, REM sleep and non-REM sleep) to another, and are 'the unwanted motor, verbal, or experiential manifestations that may occur from such overlap between sleep states' (Plante and Winkelman 2006, p.969). They are classified according to the type of sleep in which, or from which, they occur: REM sleep or non-REM sleep.

REM sleep parasomnias

The most serious REM sleep parasomnia is REM sleep behaviour disorder (RBD) which amounts to a failure of the safety mechanism that prevents us acting out dreams. It is therefore a potentially dangerous condition – leading to sleep disturbance of, and injury to, sleeping partners – and to the death of a sleeping partner in one notable case in the UK (Morris 2009). RBD occurs almost exclusively in men over 50 years of age and is strongly associated with current or future neurodegenerative disorders, in particular Parkinson's disease (Wilson and Nutt 2013). Medication is the main treatment option: clonazepam or synthetic melatonin* (Aurora *et al.* 2010b). There is no specific behavioural management, although it is appropriate to look at safety measures.

Nightmares are a commonly experienced REM sleep parasomnia. Quoting DSM-IV-TR (APA 2000), Spoormaker, Schredl and van den Bout (2006) define them as 'an "extremely frightening dream" from which a person wakes up directly. After a nightmare, orientation is fast and the nightmare leaves a detailed memory "usually involving threats to survival, security or self-esteem"' (Spoormaker *et al.* 2006, pp. 19–20). Spoormaker *et al.* (2006) also observe that nightmares are highly visual and have a complex plot; in relation to cause they distinguish between post-traumatic and idiopathic nightmares – the latter being unrelated to a particular traumatic experience. As in the case of other parasomnias, fear of nightmares can be a serious disincentive to sleep and lead to insomnia. Various cognitive behavioural interventions are available and, of these, imagery rehearsal therapy is recommended (Aurora *et al.* 2010a); this involves recalling and writing down the nightmare and rehearsing a more positive conclusion. Such methods are the treatment of choice, and it has been shown that self-help interventions can be effective (Lancee, Spoormaker and van den Bout 2011).

The other commonly experienced REM sleep parasomnia is *sleep paralysis* where the muscle atonia of REM sleep persists for a short time after waking. It can be a frightening experience, especially where there is a feeling of the chest being crushed, perhaps accompanied by a sense of an ominous (usually) female presence sitting on the chest (known as 'the old hag'). Wilson and Nutt (2013) suggest that this crushing feeling could be experienced because the intercostal muscles 'needed to take a terrified gasp, are paralysed during REM' (p. 52). (For more on this curious phenomenon – the original meaning of 'nightmare' – see Green 2012 and Ness 1978.) Sleep paralysis can often occur in daytime recovery sleep and is made more likely by the consumption of alcohol; however, if occurring in isolation, sleep paralysis is a harmless experience, despite the potential for distress, and no particular treatment is usually necessary. Maintaining regular hours of sleep and moderating alcohol intake will help to prevent it, and vigorous eye movements, or a light touch by another person, might help to abort an episode. (For a self-help guide see Hurd 2011.)

Non-REM parasomnias

Non-REM parasomnias are characterized by sudden arousal from deep, slow-wave sleep*. The arousal is related to a dissociated reaction between cortical activity and motor activity or autonomic arousal (Espa *et al.* 2002). Among non-REM sleep parasomnias, *sleep terrors* (also known as night terrors) should be distinguished from nightmares which, being dreams, occur almost exclusively in REM sleep. There is no narrative content in sleep terrors, as there is in a dream, and the individual wakes (usually earlier in the night when there is more deep non-REM sleep) with a sense of intense fear. The individual typically screams (whereas in a nightmare they do not) and might try to escape from the room while still in a confused state before being fully awake. There is therefore potential for danger to the individual or a sleeping partner. Sleep terrors are fairly common in children, with a prevalence of 5% compared with 1–2% in adults (Plante and Winkelman 2006), and most 'grow out of it'; behavioural management is possible (see below).

Sleepwalking is also relatively common and mostly harmless, although it can disturb other members of a household, but if someone does it persistently, they can put themselves at risk and, more rarely, they can do harm to others. Schenck *et al.* (1989) reported on 100 consecutive adults attending a sleep centre with repeated nocturnal injuries and found sleep terrors and/or sleepwalking in 54% and RBD in 36%; the remainder had dissociative disorders, nocturnal seizures or sleep apnoea. (See Siclari *et al.* 2010 for a detailed review of violence in sleep.) On waking after sleepwalking, there is usually no recall of night-time episodes. In *confusional arousals*, which occur on arousal from deep sleep, the individual is unresponsive, as in sleepwalking, to environmental cues; a person might talk nonsense or might prepare and eat food (sleep-eating disorder).

A person complaining of persistent experiences of parasomnia should be properly assessed by an appropriate service, because it is necessary to rule out other causes for the night-time events and provide the optimum treatment. Medication can assist in the management of non-REM parasomnia by decreasing arousal, but also there are behavioural changes that can help (these are summarized in Box 7.1). Pilon, Montplaisir and Zadra (2008) show how sleepwalkers are vulnerable to increased homeostatic pressure to sleep after sleep deprivation and that they have an abnormal reaction to arousal which predisposes them to sleepwalk. The first steps in behavioural management involve the individual having a good sleep routine and avoiding sleep deprivation: a regular rising time is important as part of this. Although waking in the night (if recalled) can be an irritation for most people, for sleepwalkers it is particularly important to minimize disturbances. A standard treatment for sleepwalking and sleep terrors in children is scheduled wakening, where the child is woken up about half an hour before the event typically occurs, thereby disrupting the sleep stages (for example, see Frank *et al.* 1997 and Owens, France and Wiggs 1999).

Most people who sleepwalk will have already thought about safety themselves, but they might benefit from further advice. Occupational therapists should be well placed to assist in this instance and pay particular attention to security, and they might consider the possibility of additional locks or alarms if the sleepwalker attempts to leave the house, for example. A key factor is stress. Most people with non-REM parasomnia notice an increase in night-time activity when they are stressed. Methods of stress management will be familiar to most occupational therapists, especially those working in mental health.

There has been some debate over the potential association of alcohol and sleepwalking because of the effect of alcohol on slow-wave sleep being similar to the effect of sleep deprivation or fragmentation; however, Bornemann and Mahowald (2011) state that there is no evidence that alcohol will prime or trigger sleepwalking, although the best advice, as ever, remains moderation. Other misconceptions about sleepwalking (for example, that it is the enactment of dreams or that waking a sleepwalker can cause injury) are corrected by Pressman (2011), who cautions that waking a sleepwalker could still be unwise since in confusion, he or she may react defensively.

Sleep starts (also known as hypnic jerks) are a common experience occurring in light sleep early in the night. They are often associated with a falling sensation and are harmless.

BOX 7.1 Summary of behavioural management of non-REM parasomnias

- Make the sleeping environment as safe as possible (especially away from home).

- Maintain regular hours and avoid becoming sleep deprived.

- Minimize night-time disturbances.

- Use alcohol moderately (for those individuals who drink).

- Manage stress.

7.5 Circadian-rhythm disorders

Circadian-rhythm disorders affect the timing of sleep but may manifest as insomnia or EDS, or both. They occur when the internal timing mechanism is disrupted or, in the case of jet lag and shift work sleep disorder, when a person is not aligned with the 24-hour cycle.

In *advanced sleep phase syndrome* (ASPS) individuals have a need to sleep about 3 hours earlier than the norm. They will therefore appear sleepy in the evening and tend to wake early (attracting a suspicion of depression). It is rare in young people, uncommon in middle-aged and older adults, and seldom seen clinically, perhaps because people adjust their lives to their natural sleep preference. Delay of melatonin onset (see Chapter 3) by the use of bright light in the evening is a possibility for management.

Delayed sleep phase syndrome (DSPS), where sleep is typically delayed by several hours, is more common than ASPS and particularly affects young people, perhaps reflecting the natural tendency for a delay in circadian rhythm among normal-sleeping adolescents and young adults when compared with children (Wyatt and Cvengros 2011). It is also less easily accommodated in society. The individual might not sleep naturally until 2 or 3 a.m., or later, and if undisturbed wakes correspondingly later – and therefore has difficulty in getting to school or work on time, or in being alert after a relatively short sleep. It may seem like insomnia, but in contrast to insomnia, EDS will be likely. In fact, the sleep duration of a person with a circadian rhythm disorder is likely to be longer than average (Okawa and Uchiyama 2007). Things are made worse if, on not getting to sleep, the person engages in activity late at night involving computers or video games that increase exposure to light and stimulation which may further delay sleep. The challenges are described by Wilhelmsen-Langeland *et al.* (2012) in a report of their qualitative study. A particular difficulty is the suggestion of others (or the belief of a person with DSPS) that individuals might be lazy and to blame for the problem because, for example, of not going to bed 'on time'. Treatment by chronotherapy (see Box 7.2) is difficult, and maintaining conventional sleep patterns involves keeping to a strict sleep-wake schedule with close attention to light exposure. Melatonin administered in the evening can be helpful in advancing sleep onset (Sack *et al.* 2007b).

BOX 7.2 Chronotherapy

It may seem logical that to adapt to a conventional sleep pattern an individual might try to move the rising time gradually earlier in the hope of being ready to sleep earlier at the end of the day; however, in chronotherapy the rising time is set progressively *later*. It is easier to get to sleep after a longer period awake than to go to bed after a short day and expect to sleep (in the same way that it is easier to adjust to jet lag after an east-to-west flight). Protocols vary but, for example, the individual could get up 2 hours later and go to bed 2 hours later each day with the result that they go through a period of complete reversal – sleeping during the day and remaining awake all night – until the desired hours are reached. The process might be supplemented with the use of bright light and melatonin. The patient will still be likely to have difficulty maintaining the new pattern.

Free running, or non-24-hour circadian rhythm disorder, is probably caused by reduced light perception with the result that the body clock is not reset daily and runs on a longer cycle than the 24 hours 10 minutes average of the majority. The result is that sleep and wake times become later each day and, if unchecked, the individual's sleep times will continually change – cycling through the day and night. Management is difficult and involves rigorous adherence to routines and good sleep habits, including exposure to morning light. The condition is rare among sighted people but more common in totally blind people where light exposure is of no help, whereas melatonin has been used successfully to align to a 24-hour circadian rhythm (see Sack *et al.* 2007b and Hayakawa *et al.* 2005).

Jet lag is a short-term circadian rhythm disorder and is therefore unlikely to affect many patients and clients of occupational therapists. Readers interested in managing their own jet lag can find advice in Foster and Kreitzman (2005; see also Sack *et al.* 2007a).

Shift work can be severely disruptive to sleep patterns and has associated health risks (see Foster and Wulff 2005). *Shift work sleep disorder* is characterized by insomnia when trying to sleep after a night shift, or excessive sleepiness when needing to be awake and alert for work (see Roth 2012 and Sack *et al.* 2007a for a full review). Younger people are better able to cope with shift work, but it may become a problem in later life, perhaps in the context of changing family circumstances. Management is by detailed attention to sleep schedules and exposure to light, planned naps and careful use of stimulants so as not to prevent sleep when desired. For some people it becomes necessary to be redeployed from shift work or to modify their hours. (See Wilson and Nutt 2013 for advice on managing sleep when working irregular hours, or Gumenyuk and Drake 2011 for detailed analysis.)

7.6 Sleep-related movement disorders

Restless leg syndrome (RLS), also known as Willis-Ekbom disease, is commonly associated with periodic limb movement disorder and is characterized by a strong and almost irresistible urge to move the legs. This feeling is worse in inactivity and is relieved by movement; it is worse at night. Pigeon and Yurcheshen (2009) note that the feeling may be described as tingling or stinging, and that in up to 50% of cases the sensation is also in the upper limbs. Up to 50% of people with RLS also report the sensations as painful (Montplaisir *et al.* 2011). The feelings, or having to move to relieve them, can seriously interfere with sleep.

Periodic limb movement disorder involves repetitive movements of the leg several times a minute for periods up to an hour, mostly in lighter non-REM sleep (stage N2*). It may cause arousals and fragmentation of sleep (also for a partner in bed) and lead to daytime sleepiness.

Management of both conditions is principally pharmacological but, as Pigeon and Yurcheshen (2009) observe, there are also behavioural approaches, although they acknowledge that the evidence for much of it is anecdotal. Since the conditions are chronic, it is also reasonable to look at self-management approaches. Hornyak *et al.* (2008) report a trial 8-week programme which had promising outcomes: topics included medical background, stress management and aggravating factors (see URL in Appendix 7.1).

7.7 Conclusion

It is intended that information here be sufficient for therapists carrying out assessment of patients to be alert to the possibility of sleep disorders and to recommend appropriate referral. It is not expected that therapists become involved in management of sleep disorders on the strength of the information in this chapter. However, there is advice that holds good in any event – principally, managing daily activity in order to keep regular hours (specifically a consistent rising time), coping with stress and dealing with environmental factors – all of which is the familiar territory of an occupational therapist. It is also suggested that occupational therapists could be more involved in promoting the self-management of chronic conditions such as OSA and RLS, transferring the skills used in relation to managing chronic pain or chronic fatigue, for example. Dealing with the main symptoms of disordered sleep (too much or too little) that might be encountered most commonly by a therapist working with people with other health problems is the subject of the next chapter.

Lastly, it is important for a therapist, or other clinician, who is not an expert in sleep to:

- have a low threshold for – or not hold back from – asking about sleep complaints

- acknowledge that sleep complaints interfere with the patient's life and well-being (quality of life), and instil hope that improvement is possible

- encourage the patient to seek medical input and support, and to advocate on the patient's behalf if the complaints are not taken seriously

- be particularly vigilant about the risks associated with sleep disorders, such as hypersomnia/sleepiness, which can lead to accidents (particularly traffic accidents), and be aware that there tend to be regulations and possibly a responsibility to report? However, it is ultimately the patient's responsibility to keep themselves and others safe and to seek medical help.

Notes

1   Occupational therapists are advised to discuss any concerns about patient safety with the multidisciplinary team but the College of Occupational Therapists Code of Ethics and Professional Conduct (2010) is less explicit than GMC guidance. Section 2.4.3 stipulates that 'the disclosure of confidential information regarding the service user's diagnosis, treatment, prognosis or future requirements is only possible where: the service user gives consent (expressed or implied); there is legal justification (by statute or court order); or it is considered to be in the public interest in order to prevent serious harm, injury or damage to the service user or to any other person. Local procedures should be followed' (COT 2010, p.12; emphasis added).

2   There is some evidence that nicotine might have an effect on symptoms of narcolepsy with a report of a patient having cataplexy after quitting smoking and subsequently using nicotine patches as management (Ebben and Krieger 2012).

Appendix 7.1 Further resources

Driving

- *Tiredness can Kill* leaflet from UK Department for Transport (www.direct.gov.uk/prod_consum_dg/groups/dg_digitalassets/@dg/@en/@motor/documents/digitalasset/dg_065252.pdf)
- 'Obstructive sleep apnoea syndrome and driving' (www.gov.uk/sleep-apnoea-and-driving)
- North Bristol Trust leaflet: *Driving Regulations and Obstructive Sleep Apnoea Syndrome* (www.nbt.nhs.uk/sites/default/files/attachments/Driving%20Regulations%20and%20Obstructive%20Sleep%20Apnoea%20Syndrome_NBT002289.pdf)

Further information on specific conditions: management and support

- Narcolepsy UK (www.narcolepsy.org.uk)
- *A Practical Guide to the Therapy of Narcolepsy and Hypersomnia Syndromes* (Mignot 2012; focuses on medication only; http://med.stanford.edu/psychiatry/narcolepsy/articles/Neurotherapeutics20102.pdf)
- Children's sleep terrors information sheet, *Information for Parents on Sleep Terrors* (www.epic.edu.au/sites/default/files/Sleep/PDFed/Night%20terrors.pdf)
- *Restless leg syndrome*: online addendum to Hornyak *et al.* (2008) including outline of management programme for restless leg syndrome (http://jnnp.bmj.com/content/suppl/2008/05/27/79.7.823.DC1/797823webonlyapp.doc)
- Parkinson's Disease Society (www.parkinsons.org.uk)

All websites were assessed in April 2014. See also Appendix 8.1.

References

Alchanatis, M., Zias, N., Deligiorgis, N., Amfilochiou, A., Dionellis, G. and Orphanidou, D. (2005) 'Sleep apnea-related cognitive deficits and intelligence: an implication of cognitive reserve theory.' *Journal of Sleep Research 14*, 1, 69–75.

Aloia, M.S., Arnedt, J.T., Davis, J.D., Riggs, R.L. and Byrd, D. (2004) 'Neuropsychological sequelae of obstructive sleep apnea-hypopnea syndrome: a critical review.' *Journal of the International Neuropsychological Society 10*, 5, 772–785.

American Academy of Sleep Medicine (2005) *International Classification of Sleep Disorders: Diagnostic and Coding Manual*, 2nd edn. Westchester, IL: American Academy of Sleep Medicine.

American Psychiatric Association (2000) *Diagnostic and Statistical Manual of Mental Disorders*, 4th edn, revised. Washington, DC: American Psychiatric Association.

Antonelli Incalzi, R., Marra, C., Salvigni, B.L., Petrone, A. *et al.* (2004) 'Does cognitive dysfunction conform to a distinctive pattern in obstructive sleep apnea syndrome?' *Journal of Sleep Research 13*, 1, 79–86.

Aurora, R.N., Zak, R.S., Auerbach, S.H., Casey, K.R. *et al.* (2010a) 'Best practice guide for the treatment of nightmare disorder in adults.' *Journal of Clinical Sleep Medicine 6*, 4, 390–401.

Aurora, R.N., Zak, R.S., Maganti, R.K., Auerbach, S.H. *et al.* (2010b) 'Best practice guide for the treatment of REM sleep behavior disorder (RBD).' *Journal of Clinical Sleep Medicine 6*, 1, 85–95.

Avidan, A. (2011) 'Parasomnias.' In A.Y. Avidan and P.C. Zee (eds) *Handbook of Sleep Medicine*, 2nd edn. Philadelphia, PA: Lippincott Williams & Wilkins.

Avidan, A.Y. and Zee, P.C. (eds) (2011) *Handbook of Sleep Medicine*, 2nd edn. Philadelphia, PA: Lippincott Williams & Wilkins.

Boehlecke, B. (2011) 'Sleep, Driving, and the Law.' In A.Y. Avidan and P.C. Zee (eds) *Handbook of Sleep Medicine*, 2nd edn. Philadelphia, PA: Lippincott Williams & Wilkins.

Bonnet, M.H. and Arand, D.L. (2010) 'Hyperarousal and insomnia: state of the science.' *Sleep Medicine Reviews 14*, 1, 9–15.

Bornemann, M.A.C. and Mahowald, M.W. (2011) 'Sleep Forensics.' In M.H. Kryger, T. Roth and W.C. Dement (eds) *Principles and Practice of Sleep Medicine*, 5th edn. St Louis, MO: Elsevier Saunders.

Bruck, D. (2001) 'The impact of narcolepsy on psychological health and role behaviours: negative effects and comparisons with other illness groups.' *Sleep Medicine 2*, 5, 437–446.

Carey, T.J., Moul, D.E., Pilkonis, P., Germain, A. and Buysse, D.J. (2005) 'Focusing on the experience of insomnia.' *Behavioral Sleep Medicine 3*, 2, 73–86.

Cheung, J.M.Y., Bartlett, D.J., Armour, C.L. and Saini, B. (2012) 'The Insomnia Patient Perspective: a Narrative Review.' *Behavioral Sleep Medicine.* doi: 10.1080/15402002.2012.694382.

College of Occupational Therapists (2010) *Code of Ethics and Professional Conduct. London: College of Occupational Therapists.* Available at www.cot.co.uk/sites/default/files/publications/public/Code-of-Ethics2010.pdf, accessed on 9 October 2014.

Daniels, E., King, M.A., Smith, I.E. and Shneerson, J.M. (2001) 'Health-related quality of life in narcolepsy.' *Journal of Sleep Research 10*, 1, 75–81.

Ebben, M.R. and Krieger, A.C. (2012) 'Narcolepsy with cataplexy masked by the use of nicotine.' *Journal of Clinical Sleep Medicine 8*, 2, 195–196.

Edinger, J.D. and Krystal, A.D. (2003) 'Subtyping primary insomnia: Is sleep state misperception a distinct clinical entity?' *Sleep Medicine Reviews 7*, 3, 203–214.

El-Ad, B. and Lavie, P. (2005) 'Effect of sleep apnea on cognition and mood.' *International Review of Psychiatry 17*, 4, 277–282.

Espa, F., Dauvilliers, Y., Ondze, B., Billiard, M. and Besset, A. (2002) 'Arousal reactions in sleepwalking and night terrors in adults: the role of respiratory events.' *Sleep 25*, 8, 32–36.

Espie, C.A. (2009) '"Stepped care": a health technology solution for delivering cognitive behavioural therapy as a first line insomnia treatment.' *Sleep 32*, 12, 1549–1558.

Espie, C.A., Broomfield, N.M., MacMahon, K.M.A., Macphee, L.M. and Taylor, L.M. (2006) 'The attention–intention–effort pathway in the development of psychophysiologic insomnia: a theoretical review.' *Sleep Medicine Reviews 10*, 4, 215–245.

Espie, C.A., Kyle, S.D., Williams, C., Ong, J.C. *et al.* (2012) 'A randomized, placebo-controlled trial of online cognitive behavioural therapy for chronic insomnia disorder delievered via an automated media-rich web application.' *Sleep 35*, 6, 769–781.

Fortier-Brochu, É., Beaulieu-Bonneau, S., Ivers, H. and Morin, C.M. (2012) 'Insomnia and daytime cognitive performance: a meta-analysis.' *Sleep Medicine Reviews 16*, 1, 83–94.

Foster, R.G. and Kreitzman, L. (2005) *Rhythms of Life: The Biological Clocks that Control the Daily Lives of Every Living Thing.* London: Profile Books.

Foster, R.G. and Wulff, K. (2005) 'The rhythm of rest and excess.' *Nature Reviews Neuroscience 6*, 5, 407–414.

Frank, N.C., Spirito, A., Stark, L. and Owens-Stively, J. (1997) 'The use of scheduled awakenings to eliminate childhood sleepwalking.' *Journal of Pediatric Psychology 22*, 3, 345–353.

Gami, A.S., Pressman, G., Caples, S.M., Kanagala, R. *et al.* (2004) 'Association of atrial fibrillation and obstructive sleep apnea.' *Circulation 110*, 4, 364–367.

General Medical Council (2009) 'Confidentiality: reporting concerns about patients to the DVLA or the DVA.' Available at www.gmc-uk.org/Confidentiality_reporting_concerns_DVLA_2009. pdf_27494214.pdf, accessed on 20 October 2013.

Geyer, J.D., Lichstein, K.L., Ruiter, M.E., Ward, L.C., Carney, P.R. and Dillard, S.C. (2011) 'Sleep education for paradoxical insomnia.' *Behavioral Sleep Medicine 9*, 4, 266–272.

Green, A. (2012) 'Sleeping on It.' In A. Green and A. Westcombe (eds) *Sleep: Multiprofessional Perspectives*. London: Jessica Kingsley Publishers.

Green, A., Hicks, J. and Wilson, S. (2008) 'The experience of poor sleep and its consequences: a qualitative study involving people referred for cognitive-behavioural management of chronic insomnia.' *British Journal of Occupational Therapy 71*, 5, 196–204.

Gumenyuk, V. and Drake, C.L. (2011) 'Shift-Work Sleep Disorder: Sleep and Performance in Medical Training.' In A.Y. Avidan and P.C. Zee (eds) *Handbook of Sleep Medicine*, 2nd edn. Philadelphia, PA: Lippincott Williams & Wilkins.

Harvey, A.G. and Tang, N. (2012) '(Mis)Perception of sleep in insomnia: a puzzle and a resolution.' *Psychological Bulletin 138*, 1, 77–101.

Hayakawa, T., Uchiyama, M., Kamei, Y., Shibui, K. *et al.* (2005) 'Clinical analyses of sighted patients with non-24-hour sleep-wake syndrome: a study of 57 consecutively diagnosed cases.' *Sleep 28*, 8, 945–952.

Hicks, J. and Green, A. (2012) 'Broken Sleep: Sleep Disorders.' In A. Green and A. Westcombe (eds) *Sleep: Multiprofessional Perspectives*. London: Jessica Kingsley Publishers.

Hornyak, M., Grossmann, C., Kohnen, R., Schlatterer, M. *et al.* (2008) 'Cognitive behavioural group therapy to improve patients' strategies for coping with restless legs syndrome: a proof-of-concept trial.' *Journal of Neurology, Neurosurgery & Psychiatry 79*, 7, 823–825.

Hurd, R. (2011) *Sleep Paralysis: A Guide to Hypnagogic Visions & Visitors of the Night*. Los Altos, CA: Hyena Press.

Johns, M.W. (1991) 'A new method for measuring daytime sleepiness: the Epworth sleepiness scale.' *Sleep 14*, 6, 540–545.

Kyle, S.D., Espie, C.A. and Morgan, K. (2010) '"… Not just a minor thing, it is something major, which stops you from functioning daily": quality of life and daytime functioning in insomnia.' *Behavioral Sleep Medicine 8*, 3, 123–140.

Kyle, S.D., Morgan, K., Spiegelhalder, K. and Espie, C.A. (2011) 'No pain, no gain: an exploratory within-subjects mixed-methods evaluation of the patient experience of sleep restriction therapy for insomnia.' *Sleep Medicine 12*, 8, 735–747.

Lancee, J., Spoormaker, V.I. and van den Bout, J. (2011) 'Long-term effectiveness of cognitive-behavioural self-help intervention for nightmares.' *Journal of Sleep Research 20*, 3, 454–459.

MacMahon, K.M.A., Broomfield, N.M. and Espie, C.A. (2006) 'Attention bias for sleep-related stimuli in primary insomnia and delayed sleep phase syndrome using the dot-probe task.' *Sleep 29*, 11, 1420–1427.

Manconi, M., Ferri, F., Sagrada, C., Punjabi, N.M. *et al.* (2010) 'Measuring the error in sleep estimation in normal subjects and in patients with insomnia.' *Journal of Sleep Research 19*, 3, 478–486.

Mignot, E.J.M. (2012) 'A practical guide to the therapy of narcolepsy and hypersomnia syndromes.' *Neurotherapeutics.* doi: 10.1007/s13311-012-0150-9.

Montplaisir, J., Allen, R.P., Walters, A. and Ferini-Strambi, L. (2011) 'Restless Legs Syndrome and Periodic Limb Movements During Sleep.' In M.H. Kryger, T. Roth and W.C. Dement (eds) *Principles and Practice of Sleep Medicine*, 5th edn. St Louis, MO: Elsevier Saunders.

Morris, S. (2009) 'Devoted husband who strangled wife in his sleep walks free from court.' *Guardian*, 20 November. Available at www.guardian.co.uk/uk/2009/nov/20/brian-thomas-dream-strangler-tragedy, accessed on 28 May 2013.

Mwenga, G.B. and Rodenstein, D. (2012) 'Medicolegal and Economic Aspects of Sleep Disorders.' In A.K. Simonds and W. de Backer (eds) *ERS Handbook of Respiratory Sleep Medicine*. Sheffield: European Respiratory Society.

National Institute for Clinical Excellence (2004) *Guidance on the Use of Zaleplon, Zolpidem and Zopiclone for the Short-term Management of Insomnia.* London: NICE.

National Institutes of Health (2005) 'NIH State-of-the-Science Conference Statement on Manifestations and Management of Chronic Insomnia in Adults.' *NIH Consensus and State of the Science Statements 22*, 2, 1–30. Available at http://consensus.nih.gov/2005/insomniastatement.pdf, accessed on 1 August 2013.

Ness, R.C. (1978) 'The Old Hag phenomenon as sleep paralysis: a biocultural interpretation.' *Culture, Medicine and Psychiatry 2*, 1, 15–39.

O'Donoghue, N. and McKay, E.A. (2012) 'Exploring the impact of sleep apnoea on daily life and occupational engagement.' *British Journal of Occupational Therapy 75*, 11, 509–516.

Ohayon, M.M., Priest, R.G., Zulley. J., Smirne, S. and Paiva, T. (2002) 'Prevalence of narcolepsy symptomatology and diagnosis in the European general population.' *Neurology 58*, 12, 1826–1833.

Okawa, M. and Uchiyama, M. (2007) 'Circadian rhythm sleep disorders: characteristics and entrainment pathology in delayed sleep phase and non-24 sleep-wake syndrome.' *Sleep Medicine Reviews 11*, 6, 485–496.

Owens, J.L., France, K.G. and Wiggs, L. (1999) 'Behavioural and cognitive-behavioural interventions for sleep disorders in infants and children: a review.' *Sleep Medicine Reviews 3*, 4, 281–302.

Perlis, M., Aloia, M. and Kuhn, B. (eds) (2011a) *Behavioral Treatments for Sleep Disorders: A Comprehensive Primer of Behavioral Sleep Medicine Interventions.* London: Elsevier.

Perlis, M., Shaw, P.J., Cano, G. and Espie, C.A. (2011b) 'Models of Insomnia.' In M.H. Kryger, T. Roth and W.C. Dement (eds) *Principles and Practice of Sleep Medicine*, 5th edn. St Louis, MO: Elsevier Saunders.

Phillips, B.G. and Somers, V.K. (2003) 'Hypertension and obstructive sleep apnea.' *Current Hypertension Reports 5*, 5, 380–385.

Pigeon, W.R. and Yurcheshen, M. (2009) 'Behavioral sleep medicine interventions for restless legs syndrome and periodic limb movement disorder.' *Sleep Medicine Clinics 4*, 4, 487–494.

Pilon, M., Montplaisir, J. and Zadra, A. (2008) 'Precipitating factors of somnambulism: impact of sleep deprivation and forced arousals.' *Neurology 70*, 24, 2284–2290.

Plante, D.T. and Winkelman, J.W. (2006) 'Parasomnias.' *Psychiatric Clinics of North America 29*, 4, 969–987.

Pressman, P.R. (2011) 'Common misconceptions about sleepwalking and other parasomnias.' *Sleep Medicine Clinics 6*, 4, xiii–xvii.

Punjabi, N.M. (2008) 'The epidemiology of adult obstructive sleep apnea.' *Proceedings of the American Thoracic Society 5*, 2, 136–143.

Redline, S., Yenokyan, G., Gottlieb, D.J., Shahar, E. *et al.* (2010) 'Obstructive sleep apnea-hypopnea and incident stroke: the sleep heart health study.' *American Journal of Respiratory and Critical Care Medicine 182*, 2, 269–277.

Riedel, B.W. and Lichstein, K.L (2000) 'Insomnia and daytime functioning.' *Sleep Medicine Reviews 4*, 3, 277–298.

Riemann, D., Spiegelhalder, K., Feige, B., Voderholzer, U. *et al.* (2010) 'The hyperarousal model of insomnia: a review of the concept and its evidence. *Sleep Medicine Reviews 14*, 1, 19–31.

Roth, T. (2012) 'Shift work disorder: overview and diagnosis.' *Journal of Clinical Psychiatry 73*, 3. doi: 10.4088/JCP.11073br2.

Sack, R.L., Auckley, D., Auger, R.R., Carskadon, M.A. *et al.* (2007a) 'Circadian rhythm sleep disorders. Part I: Basic principles, shift work and jet lag disorders – an American Academy of Sleep Medicine review.' *Sleep 30*, 11, 1460–1483.

Sack, R.L., Auckley, D., Auger, R.R., Carskadon, M.A. *et al.* (2007b) 'Circadian rhythm sleep disorders. Part II: Advanced sleep phase disorder, delayed sleep phase disorder, free-running disorder, and irregular sleep-wake rhythm – an American Academy of Sleep Medicine review.' *Sleep 30*, 11, 1494–1501.

Schenck, C.H., Milner, D.M., Hurwitz, T.D., Bundlie, S.R. and Mahowald, M.W. (1989) 'A polysomnographic and clinical report on sleep-related injury in 100 adult patients.' *American Journal of Psychiatry 146*, 9, 1166–1173.

Siclari, F., Khatami, R., Urbaniok, F., Nobili, L. *et al.* (2010) 'Violence in sleep.' *Brain 33*, 12, 3494–3509.

Spielman, A.J., Caruso, L.S. and Glovinsky, P.B. (1987) 'A behavioral perspective on insomnia treatment.' *Psychiatric Clinics of North America 10*, 4, 541–553.

Spoormaker, V.I., Schredl, M. and van den Bout, J. (2006) 'Nightmares: from anxiety symptom to sleep disorder.' *Sleep Medicine Reviews 10*, 1, 195–131.

Stepnowsky, C. (2011) 'Sleep Apnea Self-Management Program.' In M. Perlis, M. Aloia and B. Kuhn (eds) *Behavioral Treatments for Sleep Disorders: A Comprehensive Primer of Behavioral Sleep Medicine Interventions.* London: Elsevier.

Stores, G., Montgomery, P. and Wiggs, L. (2006) 'The psychosocial problems of children with narcolepsy and those with excessive daytime sleepiness of uncertain origin.' *Paediatrics 118*, 4, e1116–e1123.

Tang, N.Y. and Harvey, A.G. (2005) 'Time estimation ability and distorted perception of sleep in insomnia.' *Behavioral Sleep Medicine 3*, 3, 134–150.

Wilhelmsen-Langeland, A., Dundas, I., West Saxvig, I., Pallesen, S., Nordhus, I.-H. and Bjorvatn, B. (2012) 'Psychosocial challenges related to delayed sleep phase disorder.' *Open Sleep Journal 2012*, 5, 51–58.

Wilson, S. (2012) 'Medication and Sleep.' In A. Green and A. Westcombe (eds) *Sleep: Multiprofessional Perspectives*. London: Jessica Kingsley Publishers.

Wilson, S. and Nutt, D. (2013) *Sleep Disorders*, 2nd edn. Oxford: Oxford University Press.

Wyatt, J.K. and Cvengros, J.A. (2011) 'Delayed and Advanced Sleep Phase Disorders.' In M.H. Kryger, T. Roth and W.C. Dement (eds) *Principles and Practice of Sleep Medicine*, 5th edn. St Louis, MO: Elsevier Saunders.

8

ASSESSMENT AND NON-PHARMACOLOGICAL MANAGEMENT OF INSUFFICIENT AND EXCESSIVE SLEEP

Andrew Green and Jane Hicks

8.1 Introduction

Most occupational therapists reading this are likely to be working in a Western industrial culture where monophasic sleep is the desired norm, although, as discussed in Chapter 4, other sleeping patterns and practices are normal in other cultures and in different parts of the world. The monophasic sleep pattern is easily disrupted by illness, whether physical or psychiatric, or by one of the sleep disorders described in Chapter 7. As noted in that chapter, there are pharmacological options in the management of most sleep disorders, although medication would seldom be recommended without accompanying advice on behavioural management. Medication in the treatment of insomnia is intended to be short term, and non-pharmacological management is preferable: studies have shown it to be effective (see below). Furthermore, many people would rather not take medication unless absolutely necessary. This chapter therefore looks at the range of non-pharmacological methods of managing the sleep problems most commonly encountered in clinical practice: not sleeping enough, or disturbed sleep, or to a lesser extent, sleeping too much.

It is not appropriate for this chapter to deal with the non-pharmacological management of other sleep disorders, such as parasomnias or circadian-rhythm disorders, since they should be managed by specialist sleep services. Furthermore, they are less often seen, and management protocols are much less developed. However, caution is still necessary in approaching the management of insomnia or hypersomnia. First, if there is any doubt about diagnosis, it is essential that proper investigation be carried out by those qualified to do it. Second, a therapist should be careful in giving advice that could have an impact on a patient's capacity to carry out their responsibilities.

This chapter is not intended as a substitute for proper training or supervised experience, which it is the responsibility of therapists to access. Instead, it outlines the current advice and management strategies for insomnia, and more tentative management possibilities for hypersomnia. It is not expected that a therapist will adopt strategies such as sleep restriction therapy on the strength of what is described here, but it is reasonable that, on the basis of an enhanced understanding of the science of sleep, an occupational therapist might take the principles into account in giving advice. Occupational therapists have a further advantage in that they are well equipped to look at their clients' daytime activities that might affect sleep. This is especially important when working with an elderly or disabled client group who are less likely than people in work or education to have the same structure around which to create well-established daily routines. The role of daytime activity is discussed in Chapter 6; the greater focus here is on what happens at night. But before any treatment is undertaken, assessment is necessary, and this is explored next.

8.2 Assessment

Assessment of sleep and difficulties in sleep can serve two general purposes that are considered here. First, it can be part of a diagnostic process when a sleep problem is initially reported or disclosed and, second, it is an essential part of the process of management of a known problem: gathering the detailed information necessary before implementing changes.

Assessment in identifying sleep problems

It may be that the occupational therapist working with, say, an elderly client living in the community is the first health professional to whom the client mentions the problem. The client might complain of sleep difficulty at some stage in assessment, or during the course of intervention as trust is established. As explained in Chapter 10, an older person might share a widely held belief that poor sleep is simply a consequence of old age and not think it is worth mentioning. If the client does not mention a sleep problem spontaneously, it is still worth asking simply, 'How is your sleep?' and, depending on the response, the therapist can ask some further screening questions. Alternatively, a full set of screening questions could be incorporated into the first assessment of someone in a vulnerable client group. In these circumstances the main purpose of assessment is to establish whether the client should be referred to another service for investigation. It is also helpful to gather information to evaluate the urgency of a referral and any other information that will inform the process.

An example of a set of screening questions, designed for elderly patients, is suggested by Bloom *et al.* (2009; see also Chapter 10). Their 12 questions will highlight any common sleep difficulty and should suggest when further questions are necessary. For example, if the answers to *'Does your bed partner say (or are you aware) that you frequently snore, gasp for air or stop breathing?'* and *'Do you usually doze off without planning to during the day?'* are positive, it should suggest the possibility of obstructive sleep apnoea for which referral for assessment would be necessary. Other questions will alert the assessor to the possibility of movement disorders or parasomnia for which investigation by polysomnography* (overnight monitoring) might be the way forward: *'Does your bed partner say (or are you aware) that you kick or thrash about while asleep?'* or *'Are you aware that you ever walk, eat, punch, kick or scream during sleep?'* (For further information on polysomnography see Hudson 2012.) Another example of screening questions is the Bristol Sleep Profile (see Appendix 8.2), and Stores (2007) lists questions that neurologists are advised to ask about sleep. Different emphasis in screening questions may be necessary depending on the client group. For example, with children the influence of others (parents) is particularly important, whereas screening for undiagnosed narcolepsy is less relevant for older people. It is important in using any screening questions that the questioner know how to respond to particular answers.

Assessment in managing sleep problems

When a client is referred with an established diagnosis of a sleep problem, or a client complains of poor sleep when the therapist is confident that no referral for specialist investigation is necessary, assessment focuses on the detail of the client's sleep pattern, their behaviour associated with sleep and the environment in which it takes place. As ever, it is useful to gain an understanding of the client's perception of the problem by asking for their story of how the problem started (for example, *'When did you first notice that your sleep was a problem?'* or *'How long was it before you realized that your sleep had not gone back to normal?'* if it was disrupted by an event that would obviously affect it in the short term). It is helpful to know what their normal sleep was like before the problem. For example, many people with insomnia will preface their description of a current difficulty by saying, 'I was always a light sleeper...' Was the client a morning or evening person – a 'lark' or an 'owl' (see Chapter 3)? Did they work shifts? How much sleep did they expect before? In other words, were they a long or short sleeper?

It is likely that an occupational therapist will have made a full assessment of, or asked about, an existing client's home circumstances, but in assessing the 'sleep environment' the therapist may want to ask about the sleep habits of others in the household that may impact on the client. Are there young children who wake at night and disturb sleep, or older children who come in late? Is there anyone in the home with care needs at night? Does a bed partner have any sleep problems (such as snoring or restlessness)? Does a partner, or anyone in the household, work shifts that involve early rising or late bedtimes? Are there pets in the house and where do they sleep (or spend the night)?

Looking at the bedroom, the therapist might ask whether it is only for sleep or does the client make other use of it? Is there a television or computer in there? Is it free of unnecessary clutter? What are the heating and lighting conditions? Is there noise from elsewhere in the house, or outside, that can be heard in the bedroom? It is likely that the client will have considered most of these things and worked out solutions – whether sleeping at the back of the house to avoid traffic noise or adjusting the heating to a comfortable level – but it is always possible that some factors have been overlooked or that a client is unaware how changed circumstances could affect sleep; therefore, a thorough assessment is always advisable.

A client may also be unaware how their actions might affect their sleep, and assessment of their routines and behaviours is essential. A good place to start is to ask what time the client typically goes to bed, a question that may not be as simple to answer as it is to ask. The response may reflect the time they 'go upstairs', the time they actually get into bed or the time at which they put out the light and settle down. The desired answer is the 'lights-out' time, but other responses will give clues to the winding-down process, which may need further investigation. A key question then is whether the client is usually sleepy at that point. They might respond that, yes, they are exhausted, but it is then important to establish whether they were really *sleepy* as opposed to feeling physically tired or fatigued (for example, '*Are you close to dozing off in the chair before you go to bed?*').

Having established the winding-down routine and time of settling, the client can be asked to estimate what time they tend to get off to sleep – or how long it takes; time taken to get to sleep is known as sleep onset latency* and up to 20 minutes is considered normal. Most people will have an idea, although discussions can become complicated if someone has a variable routine. After that, a useful open question is '*What happens next?*' which invites answers ranging from 'I wake after x hours or minutes when...' to 'I wake to the alarm at half past seven.' If the client does wake in the night, it is helpful to know for roughly how long and what they do (go to the toilet and return to sleep? Lie awake and worry about the children?) and whether they wake again. However, after three or four wakenings, it is usually not helpful to know exactly how many times they wake, as it does not affect intervention whether someone wakes seven times as opposed to eight times. The client might say that after a certain point they only doze until the alarm goes off, for example, perhaps drifting in and out of dreams. Lastly, it is useful to confirm their usual rising time (with or without an alarm?) and check how much that (and their bedtime) varies at weekends or on days off, and to ask them to estimate their average total sleep time. Keeping a sleep diary (see below) could be helpful in many circumstances, not only where sleep patterns are variable, but also because it might highlight variation that the client had not previously noticed.

Turning to the daytime, a first question could be to ask about any daytime naps. If the client says that they do not sleep in the day, it can be useful to ask whether they could if given the opportunity. It is then appropriate to ask about any habits that could influence sleep: smoking or alcohol intake (if any), exercise (nature, amount and timing), regularity of meals and other routines. It is also worth checking what medication they are taking and, importantly, what time it is taken. Is analgesic medication or other drugs taken at the optimum time to relieve pain at bedtime? Are hypnotics taken at the appropriate time for getting to sleep? Has other medication been reviewed since sleep problems developed or does the patient need to see their family doctor or pharmacist for advice?

At the end of the sleep assessment interview, the therapist should have a detailed picture of the individual's 24-hour routines and of any habits that could inhibit sleep. Using other information about the client and their condition, it should be possible to begin to formulate a plan of action, but it might also be useful to use other methods of assessment, either to fill in details or to provide baseline data for measuring outcomes. Dozens of rating scales and questionnaires for assessing different aspects of sleep, behaviour affecting it or beliefs about it are available, although many are more appropriate for research. The therapist should try to select a standardized scale suitable for the client group and practice setting. Many measures are in the public domain and increasingly available for free download. Therapists need to balance the costs in terms of the time taken to use rating scales against the benefits of having well-defined outcome measures. This may also be important in demonstrating to professional colleagues, managers and funding bodies that sleep problems are a significant issue, and are problems that can be addressed. A small selection of measures is reviewed here and links to websites, with other examples, may be found among the resources at the end of this chapter and in other chapters dealing with specific client groups; for a review of measures see Smith and Wegener (2003) and Wells *et al.* (2009):

- *The Epworth Sleepiness Scale* (Johns 1991) is a commonly used tool for assessing daytime sleepiness. It consists of a list of eight situations where a person might fall asleep (e.g. sitting reading or in a car while stopped in traffic) and the respondent is asked to rate their chance of dozing on a scale of 0–3. Someone with a total score of 9 (e.g. a 'high' likelihood on three items) or more is considered 'very sleepy' and they would be advised to seek medical advice.

- *The Pittsburgh Sleep Quality Index* (Buysse *et al.* 1989) is widely used in research and in clinical practice and is a measure that covers seven domains (subjective sleep quality, sleep latency, sleep duration, sleep efficiency, sleep disturbances, use of sleep medication and daytime dysfunction) which the respondent rates on a scale of 0–3, reflecting experience over the previous month.

- *The Dysfunctional Beliefs and Attitudes about Sleep brief version* (DBAS-16) (Morin, Vallières and Ivers 2007), derived from a previous longer list of statements about sleep (see Appendix 8.1), asks respondents to rate their agreement on a scale of 1–10. The stronger the overall agreement (or the higher the total score), the more likely it is that the respondent will be anxious about sleep or worry about the consequences of poor sleep. Successful management of insomnia would be likely to bring about a reduction in the score (see, for example, Hicks, Green and Wilson 2008).

- *The Insomnia Severity Index* (Bastien, Vallières and Morin 2001) is a measure of perceived severity of insomnia for use as a screening tool and outcome measure. The respondent is asked to rate seven statements on a five-point scale. The statements relate to the extent to which sleep is disturbed, distress or worry is caused and daily activity is disrupted. From the total scores the respondent can be classified from 'no clinically significant insomnia' to 'severe clinical insomnia'.

- *The Occupational Impact of Sleep Questionnaire* (David and Morgan 2006) focuses on the extent to which work is affected by sleep quality. It asks how difficult in the past week it has been to meet work demands such as keeping to a schedule, concentrating or controlling temper. Items are scored on a five-point scale.

- *Morningness–Eveningness Questionnaire* (Horne and Östberg 1976) measures the individual preference for the morning or evening (tendency to be a 'lark' or an 'owl'). It includes 19 questions that ask, for example, about preferred times to do particular tasks in order to maximize performance and preferred sleep-wake times.

- *Glasgow Sleep Effort Scale* (Broomfield and Espie 2005) assesses sleep effort on the assumption that voluntary attempts to control sleep are likely to make insomnia worse. This measure consists of seven points relating to effort and anxiety about sleep.

The other assessment tool which is readily available, but which can take many forms, is the sleep diary. Although numerous versions can be found, essentially, the individual is asked to record the time at which they went to bed, their estimated sleep onset latency (SOL), number and estimated duration of wakenings after sleep onset, and waking and rising times. Typically, they might also be asked to rate the sleep quality on a rating scale of 0–5 or 0–10. From this data the average SOL and average total sleep times and sleep efficiency (see below) can be calculated. In practice this is sufficient, but more complex diaries might ask for other inforamtion, such as daytime sleep, caffeine or alcohol intake, or use of medication. Where there is a parasomnia it may be useful to record when events occur and any possible precipitating factors, such as estimated stress levels. If timing of sleep is an issue (if there is suspected sleep phase delay, for example), or regular napping, it can be useful to represent sleep more graphically by using a chart to represent the 24 hours of the day and to colour it in to record time in bed and time asleep.

A sleep diary can also be useful in engaging a client and provide a basis for intervention. At one level, it can be a clear 'homework' task after a first meeting whereby the client has some immediate involvement in the process but, more importantly, reviewing it jointly at the next meeting can be revealing to the client and the therapist as patterns become evident and the client explains them. In the clinical setting completion of these types of sleep charts is variable. Some people's sleep patterns are so complex that they defy easy representation on paper, while some will happily produce highly detailed logs on a spreadsheet or chart; others seem to manage to leave their diaries on the bedside table, never bringing them to appointments, and have to rely on memory. It is fairly simple to draw up a diary sheet, but numerous examples are available (see Appendix 8.1).

A possible solution to some of the difficulties in recording sleep is actigraphy*, which uses a device worn on the wrist or ankle that contains an accelerometer. The device, or *actigraph*, thereby detects movement which correlates with sleep and wakefulness. When actigraphy is used in conjunction with an activity log, over the course of 1 or 2 weeks, sleep patterns can be discerned (see Hudson 2012). Actigraphy has not been widely available in the UK outside of specialist sleep disorder services, but technology is developing rapidly and becoming cheaper and more widely available. Smartphones, for example, are equipped with accelerometers for a variety of purposes, and applications that use them and which claim to monitor sleep are increasing in number and sophistication. Not intended for clinical use, most such applications are so far untested, although Natale *et al.* (2012) compared a smartphone accelerometer with actigraphy (on 13 healthy volunteers) and found 'reasonably satisfactory' (p.287) agreement between the devices. It is possible that such devices and applications will appeal to the growing number of technologically adept people and that their use will increase the accuracy of assessment. (For a review of a range of technological devices for monitoring sleep see Kelly, Strecker and Bianchi 2012, and for a review of smartphone applications see Behar *et al.* 2013.) Other applications are increasingly available for monitoring light and noise levels which can help in identifying environmental problems.

8.3 Managing insufficient sleep

As noted earlier, an occupational therapist is unlikely to be referred anyone with 'straightforward' primary or psychophysiological insomnia in the absence of other problems, but the principles of management of psychophysiological insomnia will underpin the management of the poor sleep of patients with other conditions. Managing insomnia is well covered in textbooks (Morin and Espie 2003; Perlis, Aloia and Kuhn 2011) and in self-help books (Espie 2006; Wiedman 1999). As noted in Chapter 7, cognitive behaviour therapy for insomnia (CBT-I) is the treatment of choice for people with primary insomnia and there is increasing evidence for its effectiveness with secondary or co-morbid insomnia. For example, in relation to cancer patients, Espie *et al.* (2012) demonstrated that CBT-I was effective (when compared with 'treatment as usual') with people with breast, prostate, bowel or gynaecological cancer and a diagnosis of insomnia; a mean reduction of wakefulness of 55 minutes per night was achieved with CBT-I.

This is not the place for an in-depth review of the literature on CBT-I or the detailed rationale for the different components. Essentially, they are intended to promote or reinforce the natural processes that allow and encourage sleep. It is shown in Chapter 3 how, in order to get to sleep, the body clock needs to say that it is time to sleep (the circadian drive), the time since the last sleep should be sufficient for the need to sleep to have developed (the homeostatic drive) and arousal levels should be low. Espie and Kyle (2012) note that most CBT-I outcome research focuses on multiple-component interventions but list the single components that are endorsed by the American Academy of Sleep Medicine (Morgenthaler *et al.* 2006): stimulus control therapy, sleep restriction therapy, paradoxical intention therapy, progressive muscular relaxation and biofeedback. In multiple-component programmes it is also usual to include cognitive approaches.

Different emphasis will be placed on the components here. It is assumed, for example, that the majority of occupational therapists need little advice on relaxation training, while paradoxical intention therapy is not something that can be adopted easily and is therefore not covered in detail. Various other strategies not usually included as part of CBT-I are also discussed. Sleep hygiene is examined first.

Sleep hygiene

Sleep hygiene is a widely used term in sleep medicine that often makes little sense to 'outsiders' but can be thought of as referring to all the aspects of environment and behaviour related to sleep that can be 'tidied up'. Hauri (2012), who first used the term, has suggested the alternative 'sleep/wake lifestyle modifications' (p.151) and notes that sleep hygiene is different from CBT-I. Espie (2009) argues that sleep hygiene advice should not form part of CBT-I because, as found by Morgenthaler *et al.* (2006), there is little evidence to show that it is effective either on its own or as an adjunct to other approaches; however, this could simply mean that insufficient research has been done, as opposed to there being research evidence showing that it is unhelpful. One pilot study that has shown some promising results with sleep hygiene interventions with adolescents is reported by Tan *et al.* (2012), although it is arguable whether the intervention was wholly sleep hygiene or whether it overlapped with elements of CBT-I. The key message from studies like that is that simple interventions *can* have a positive effect, although many people with established sleep problems are likely to be already aware of major pitfalls (like drinking strong coffee at bedtime).

There are several reasons why the basics of sleep hygiene cannot be ignored:

- Patients are likely to ask about them having read advice in newspapers and magazines, for example.

- Dealing with sleep hygiene is like 'picking the low-hanging ripe fruit first' or clearing up the work space before starting on a new project.

- Tackling smaller common-sense issues can get a patient engaged and feeling that they are taking control.

- It can be argued that if a patient is unable to make smaller changes in sleep hygiene, they may not be able to take on the bigger changes that might be necessary.

Sleep hygiene advice can be confusing because, as shown by Stepanski and Wyatt (2003), sleep hygiene 'rules' are not consistently given in different publications. A further caution is offered by Hauri (2012) who suggests that sleep hygiene rules are '*not a set of absolute edicts to be followed blindly, but a set of suggestions that need to be explored with each patient*' (pp.157–158; emphasis added). For example, Hauri (2012) observes that the elements of stimulus control (see below) that are often cited as sleep hygiene instructions have no supporting evidence when used in isolation: he points out that simply prohibiting reading or watching television in bed could mean that someone then spends hours in bed becoming frustrated, increasing arousal and creating a maladaptive association. Sleep hygiene measures are categorized here under environment, food and drink, and behaviours.

Sleeping environment

With regard to sleeping environment (see also Chapter 18), a bedroom should be conducive to sleep: cool (neither cold nor hot), well ventilated, quiet and dark. Hauri (2012) observes that little research has been done on the effect on sleep of temperature outside of the range 5–24°C, but to a great extent the optimum temperature will be a matter of personal choice and differs between people (which may be a source of conflict in couples). For more information on temperature see, for example, Okamoto-Mizuno and Mizuno (2012) or Van Someren (2006); see also Chapter 18.

Complete silence is not essential for sleep, but it is difficult to habituate to occasional loud noises. Sensitivity to noise varies, and Hauri (2012, p.155) cites research that found that some sleepers wakened to 15 dBA ('approximately equivalent to a mere whisper'), whereas to wake from the same stage of sleep others needed 100 dBA ('approximately equivalent to the loudness in a nightclub'). (For further information on noise see Berglund, Lindvall and Schwela 1999.) In general, there should be minimal unnecessary disturbance, and for those who are sensitive to (or exposed to) noise, sound insulation, earplugs and white noise are possibilities.

Light is not specifically mentioned in sleep hygiene rules reviewed by Hauri (2012) except in passing as part of making the bedroom comfortable. Whereas darkness is almost universally advised (except in the context of phobias, for example), absolute darkness is not necessary for sleep, although some people do become intolerant of the smallest chink of light. Because light is an important zeitgeber*, light and darkness have a significant effect on melatonin* suppression and production. For example, Gooley et al. (2011) demonstrate how room lighting can affect melatonin synthesis. Where light is a particular concern, blackout curtains and blindfolds can be used, but reducing light levels in the period before bedtime is important for everyone; this can also include computer screens.

Ordinarily, no special equipment is necessary for sleep but, plainly, a bed should be comfortable. If changing position at night is difficult, or maintaining a particular position is important, specialized advice may be needed from an appropriate source. As discussed below (under 'Stimulus control') the bedroom, wherever possible, should be reserved for sleep only and, as well as removing any electronic equipment, it is often advisable to remove clocks because 'clock watching' tends to increase anxiety and arousal. Failing that, a clock may be placed so that the time cannot be seen from the bed but an alarm can still be heard. It is usually advised that pets sleep in another room, and certainly not on the bed, where they may be a disturbance.

Food, drink and other substances

Alcohol can shorten sleep onset latency and cause more consolidated sleep (with increased deep, slow-wave sleep* and delayed rapid eye movement (REM) sleep*) in the first half of the night, but it is disruptive in the second half when sleep can be fragmented with more awakenings – perhaps also with the need to use a toilet (see URL in Appendix 8.1 and also Meoli et al. 2005). Alcohol should never be used as an aid to sleep and it may be best to cut it out during an active programme to improve sleep. On the other hand, if someone has a glass of wine with their dinner, or a small 'nightcap' as part of their winding-down routine, it might not be worth dissuading them as long as their overall intake is low (unless it is contraindicated because of medication or another condition). As ever, a therapist should take account of individual circumstances when giving advice.

Nicotine is a stimulant that affects various neurotransmitters with effects on a number of systems in the brain. Jaehne *et al.* (2009) have reviewed a wide range of studies of the effect of nicotine on sleep and report that smokers have approximately twice the risk of sleep disturbance – mainly difficulty falling asleep – compared with non-smokers. (A temporary decrease in sleep quality could be expected on stopping smoking.) Smokers should be advised not to smoke near to bedtime if they are unable or unwilling to quit.

Caffeine is another stimulant and is in more products than is sometimes realized – including cola drinks, chocolate and tea, as well as the more obvious coffee and energy drinks. (See Table 8.1 for the caffeine content of a variety of products and for recommended maximum daily intake.) Caffeine is also in some over-the-counter medications, and it is therefore always advisable to check. The usual advice is to take no caffeine after the mid-afternoon (or about 6 hours before sleep), although individuals' sensitivity to caffeine varies: in general, older people tend to be more sensitive to it than younger people. Although there is normally no need to stop caffeine altogether (and a cup of coffee in the morning can be helpful), it could be worth an experiment for some individuals, but they should be aware of temporary withdrawal effects.

It is suggested that some foodstuffs, such as turkey, milk, pumpkin and potatoes, can help sleep because they contain the naturally occurring amino acid 5-hydroxytrytophan (5HTP), which is involved in the production of the neurotransmitter serotonin, which, in turn, has a role in promoting sleep; however, it is not clear how much 5HTP in the diet can affect levels in the brain that could influence sleep (Wilson 2012), and there is no evidence of these foods being beneficial. It is likely that any benefit of a milky drink is as part of a winding-down process, perhaps with positive associations from childhood. The best advice is usually to avoid going to bed either on a full stomach or feeling hungry. A light snack in the hour before bedtime should suffice: Posner and Gehrman (2011) suggest carbohydrates (bread, cereal or fruit) as opposed to heavily sweetened food. It is important not to take too much fluid of any kind before going to bed if waking to use the toilet is likely.

Table 8.1 Caffeine content in various products

Product	Caffeine content	Caffeine in a typical serving
Brewed coffee	55–85 mg/100 ml	135 mg/240 ml (8 oz) cup
Instant coffee	35–45 mg/100 ml	85–110 mg/240 ml (8 oz) cup
Decaffeinated coffee	2 mg/100 ml	5 mg/240 ml (8 oz) cup
Tea	25–35 mg/100 ml	55–140 mg/240 ml (8 oz) cup
Cocoa	3 mg/100 ml	7 mg/240 ml (8 oz) cup
Cola drink	11 mg/100 ml	36 mg/330 ml (11.5 oz) can
Energy drink (e.g. Red Bull)	32 mg/100 ml	80 mg/250 ml (8.5 oz) can
Milk chocolate	6 mg/28 g	12 mg/56 g (2 oz) bar
Dark chocolate	20 mg/28 g	40 mg/56 g (2 oz) bar
Typical caffeine pill	200 mg	

Health Canada suggests that a moderate caffeine intake of 400 mg per day is not harmful to an average adult (300 mg/day for women planning to become pregnant, already pregnant or breast feeding). The US Food and Drugs Administration suggests that 600 mg/day (4–7 cups of coffee) is too much (see URL in Appendix 8.1). Over 1000 mg/day is toxic.

Figures are derived from various sources: Foster and Wulff (2005) citing data from the US Food and Drugs Administration, and the websites of the University of Leeds and Health Canada (see Appendix 8.1). Figures are provided as a guide only; for example, caffeine levels in a cup of coffee can vary from day to day according to brewing time and other factors, and will vary between brands of cola drinks.

Behaviours

As discussed elsewhere, daytime naps are discouraged, although a case can be made for a nap as long as night-time sleep is not compromised or the individual is prepared to accept the possibility of delayed night-time sleep. Exercise is generally considered to be good for sleep, although because of the effects on body temperature (see below), it is not usually advised late in the day (i.e. not after the early evening). There is, however, some debate over whether evening exercise is unhelpful (see Chapter 6). A winding-down routine is usually helpful, although what it includes is a very personal choice. Generally, it is wise to switch off computers and games consoles (also because they emit light) well before bedtime, and some people find it better to switch off their telephones and other devices as well. Winding down might include a hot bath. This is usually recommended to be about 90 minutes before bedtime, because although the bath will have a warming effect, it is the subsequent drop in temperature that induces drowsiness (Murphy and Campbell 1997). The wind-down could continue with a warm drink and some time spent reading or watching a quiet television programme. If no bath is taken, it is often advisable to change for bed before winding down, as some people find that the act of getting ready for bed has the effect of waking them up.

It should be stressed that with all sleep hygiene advice there is much scope for individual variation. If a person takes the dog for a brisk walk late at night, comes home and has a large whisky and a cigar before retiring to bed to watch a horror film with the dog at their feet on the bed, and then gets to sleep quickly on putting the light out – to wake feeling refreshed 7 or 8 hours later – we need not impose advice; however, if that same person sleeps poorly, many changes would be recommended.

Relaxation

Like most sleep hygiene measures, relaxation training has intuitive appeal and it should not be difficult to explain its importance to a client. It would be illogical if we could sleep when faced with any danger, whereupon the body is prepared for fight or flight, and therefore not relaxed. It is necessary to relax before sleep. Relaxation methods are helpful for anyone with heightened arousal which interferes with sleep, and various techniques are available and will be familiar to most occupational therapists (see, for example, Payne and Donaghy 2010). No particular method of relaxation is recommended over any other to aid sleep, although, as noted by Espie and Kyle (2012), most evidence exists for progressive muscular relaxation. However, the important thing is to practise and to master the skill: as Lichstein *et al.* (2011) put it, 'patients are more skilful at being anxious than at being relaxed' (p.47).

There is some debate about when and where to practise relaxation (Lichstein *et al.* 2011) and many people like to practise in bed at bedtime: if they fall asleep in the process, they will be in the right place. However, there is a case for learning the skill during the daytime so that one can relax at will and let go of tension on going to bed without the need to run through a whole relaxation exercise, especially one involving too much tensing or a lot of movement. Arguably, introducing relaxation exercises into a bedtime routine could draw attention to the problem of going to sleep. Good sleepers do not do relaxation practice in bed; they just relax naturally as they drop off to sleep. A further possibility is self-shiatsu hand massage as a means of relaxation for people with pain; it might also help people who ruminate (see Chapter 16).

Biofeedback

Biofeedback has been used for many years as an aid to relaxation training, although the expense of equipment has been a barrier to its widespread use. Most research has been done on electromyography (where the electrical activity involved in muscle movement is detected) – see Bootzin and Rider (1997) – although Forest *et al.* (2012) report on attempts to use temperature biofeedback (with limited success). In a case report, McLay and Spira (2009) demonstrated promising results using an infrared sensor to measure heart rate variability from peripheral finger pulse. Despite the limited evidence for biofeedback, technology is becoming increasingly accessible and the possibilities for its use should not be overlooked.

Stimulus control

Some people with insomnia describe their bedroom as a 'torture chamber' – the place where they go for the regular negative experience of sleep deprivation. Stimulus control, a key component of CBT-I, aims to create and reinforce a more positive association between the bedroom and sleep and to encourage falling asleep quickly. In the same way that we might try to keep a study as a place that we associate with work or reading, the principle is to keep the bedroom for sleep and sexual activity only, and to banish other waking activity. Hence, the usual advice is that there should be no television in the bedroom, nor computers or games consoles.[1] In giving this advice an assumption is made that the person *has* somewhere else to pursue other activities, although this may not be the case, for example, for a student in a bed-sitting room, or one-room apartment, or a teenager or lodger in a family home. Instead, ways need to be found to put distance (in terms of time as well as the physical distance) between waking activity and the sleeping space.

The chief way of decreasing the likelihood of lying awake for extended periods is by going to bed only when sleepy, which is what good sleepers tend to do without thinking about it. According to the principles of stimulus control, the individual should get out of bed if they have not got to sleep within 15 minutes; this is known as the 15-minute rule. They are told to go to another room (assuming they have one) and do something fairly undemanding until they feel sleepy again; looking at a magazine in subdued light or listening to the radio, or music, are commonly recommended. If after returning to bed they are not asleep in a further 15 minutes or so, they should get up again, and so forth. The same applies on waking during the night.

The first objection that people have to the 15-minute rule is that they may have just been told not to watch the clock, to which the answer is that the 15 minutes is an estimated interval. They will often observe then that it is cold at night – so it is something they would need to prepare for by having a heater or blanket at the ready – and that it will disturb other members of the household or a sleeping partner. An answer to that is that if others are in deep sleep, they will not be aware of the movement, and if they are aware it is probably because they are awake anyway (see Chapter 3). Clinical practice suggests that it can be very difficult to persuade people to try the strategy and they tend not to want to do it repeatedly, in the same night or on successive nights. Further difficulties are that for the elderly, for example, a 15-minute sleep latency is quite short, and if there is any danger of a fall, they are safer in bed.

For someone with a physical disability it might also be very difficult or painful – and therefore particularly disturbing – to leave the bed at night. *In such cases, the 15-minute rule is not appropriate.* In these circumstances the individual would still be well advised to give up 'trying' to sleep and perhaps use paradoxical intent (see below) or bend the rules and wait in bed to become sleepy again – perhaps listening to the radio (timed to switch off) or to a podcast.

Despite the difficulty of adhering to the 15-minute rule, the basic principles of stimulus control hold good and there is ample evidence of its effectiveness (Morgenthaler *et al.* 2006; Morin *et al.* 1999) although, as Hauri (2012) notes, stimulus control is only shown to be an effective strategy when all the components are applied. There is no point in remaining awake in bed if anxiety or arousal levels have reached a point at which sleep is impossible, whether after 5, 10 or 15 minutes, or longer (cf. Bootzin and Perlis 2011). Conversely, there is little to be gained by leaving the bed for the sake of it if the person is lying there completely relaxed and at ease with the idea that sleep will follow in due course ('quiet wakefulness') (see Chapter 4).

A further consideration in creating a good association, not usually a factor in managing primary insomnia, for people with chronic pain, for example, is where to rest in the daytime if there is a flare-up of pain. A person taking to their bed when pain is worse would be less likely to view the bed positively at bedtime; resting elsewhere by day might be advisable. The key elements of stimulus control are summarized in Box 8.1.

BOX 8.1 Key elements of stimulus control

- Go to bed only when sleepy.

- Use the bedroom only for sleep (and sexual activity); no television or other devices.

- If not asleep in about 15 minutes, leave the bedroom and return only when sleepy, and repeat if necessary. The same applies on waking in the night.

- Set a regular daily rising time (using an alarm) even on days off work or at weekends, and get up no matter how much sleep has been had.

- Avoid napping.

Sleep restriction therapy

For people whose sleep is already limited, sleep restriction therapy (SRT) is a daunting name for a strategy; it is sometimes known as sleep scheduling (e.g. Morin and Espie

2003) but might be more accurately termed *bed restriction.* A person who sleeps poorly and has a bad night's sleep might think of compensating for the lost sleep by going to bed early the next night. They are in fact more likely to spend longer awake in bed, thereby reinforcing the bad association with the bed that has been described in connection with stimulus control. The aim of SRT is therefore to restrict the time in bed to the amount of time that the person normally sleeps (according to a weekly average calculated using a sleep diary).

Sleep restriction therapy works not by increasing sleep time (which plainly the person has not been able to do) but by first increasing *sleep efficiency* and then, once that is achieved, by increasing the time in bed. Sleep efficiency is calculated simply by dividing the time spent asleep by the time spent in bed and expressing it as a percentage. For example, Florence might have found her average sleep time over the course of a week or 10 days to be 6 hours and 15 minutes a night. If she has been consistently going to bed at 10:30 p.m. and getting up at 7:30 a.m., she is spending an average of 9 hours in bed. Using these two figures her sleep efficiency can be worked out:

$$\frac{\text{Total time asleep} \times 100}{\text{Time in bed}} \qquad \text{i.e. } \frac{6.25 \times 100}{9} = 69\%$$

With a sleep efficiency of 69%, Florence is asleep for only just over two thirds of the time that she is in bed. This compares poorly with a good sleeper. For example, Brian goes to bed at 11:30 p.m. and falls asleep in 15–20 minutes. He wakes to his alarm at 7:15 a.m. He tends to wake in the night to go to the toilet and takes a little while to return to sleep. His total sleep time is 7.25 hours and he spends 7.75 hours in bed. His sleep efficiency is:

$$\frac{7.25 \times 100}{7.75} = 94\%.$$

Brian expects to sleep and to go back to sleep when he wakes in the night; he has a good association between his bed and sleep. Good sleepers have a sleep efficiency of over 90%, and this should be the aim in SRT. Florence can improve her sleep efficiency in only two ways. The first way is to sleep longer (which, were it possible, she would have done), and the second way is to spend less time in bed (in this case, 6.25 hours).

It might be that another person averages about 4 hours of sleep a night; however, in a sleep restriction programme, it is usual to have a minimum time in bed rather higher than that. This allows for the possibility of underestimation of sleep duration, which is typical, and also makes the strategy a little less difficult to 'sell' to the patient. Furthermore, health care professionals might be reluctant to advise a patient, who may have to get up and drive to work, to spend only 3 or 4 hours in bed. Five hours is the commonly advised minimum time in bed in published sources (Espie 2006; Morin and Espie 2003; Spielman, Yang and Glovinsky 2011), but a minimum of 6 hours is often advised more informally. The formula for time in bed is therefore the average total sleep time or 6 (or 5) hours, whichever is the *greater*.

The choice of bedtime and rising time is up to the patient and likely to reflect their natural preference for morning or evening (are they a 'lark' or an 'owl'?) and their work or domestic commitments, but the first thing to do is to set a rising time. This is the fixed point at which the body clock is reset. If, for example, Florence is happy to rise at 7:15 a.m. to get her children ready for school, she would then set her bedtime at 1:00 a.m. On the other hand, if she likes an early-morning walk with the dog, she could get up at 5:45 a.m. and set a bedtime at 11:30 p.m. However, at either (or any) bedtime she should still only go to bed if she is actually sleepy. The bedtime is what Espie (2006, p.132) calls the 'threshold time' – the time at or after which you go to bed if you are feeling sleepy.

It is important to stick to the selected hours seven nights a week, although a slight relaxation to allow an extra hour in bed in the morning on a Sunday, or other day off, might make the strategy less unattractive. It is also necessary to keep a record of the estimated sleep time so that sleep efficiency can be calculated weekly; it need not be worked out daily. When the average sleep efficiency reaches 85–90% or more for a week, the time in bed is increased – typically by 15 minutes; it is only increased further when weekly average efficiency has stabilized again at 85–90%. A point will be reached when no further increase in sleep time can be achieved. Although the individual can then start to pay less attention to their sleep, it is important to continue keeping to the hours in bed and not to revert to unhelpful habits.

The therapist and client should be aware that SRT is a very difficult strategy. It is common to warn a client that their sleep might well get worse before it gets better – almost inevitably if they are to spend in bed only the time that they normally sleep, since they will still take some time to get to sleep and therefore sleep for less time. Kyle *et al.* (2011) found that although SRT brought about improvement after 4 weeks and at 3-month follow-up, in the first week of treatment more than half of the 18 participants in their study experienced 8 out of a list of 12 side effects (such as fatigue, extreme sleepiness and reduced motivation and energy). Over a third of participants expressed some concern about their ability to drive. Such findings reinforce the need to be clear when discussing SRT that it will be hard to select a good time to try the method (when commitments are fewer) and to provide support during the process. Group treatment can be particularly helpful in that members can offer support to each other (see Green *et al.* 2005).

Spielman *et al.* (2011) show how sleep restriction, which is described in rather formulaic terms here, can be refined, for example, by allowing an extra 30 minutes 'getting to sleep time' in addition to the prescribed time in bed. Spielman *et al.* (2011) also suggest that time in bed can be reduced more gradually in a variant known as sleep compression. More usually the aim in sleep compression is to reduce wake time in bed – being mainly for people whose poor sleep is accompanied by little daytime impairment (Lichstein, Thomas and McCurry 2011) – rather than to increase sleep time. In that case, time in bed is cut incrementally by 15–30 minutes per week. For some patients, particularly those with chronic health problems, such a gradual approach might be more acceptable.

Clinical experience confirms that adherence to SRT is sometimes poor. In some cases, it is possible that the client's sleep was not as bad, or short, as they thought (as in paradoxical insomnia; see Chapter 7) and that they were therefore reducing their sleep opportunity considerably, and consequently having much less sleep. In such cases it could be helpful to use actigraphy, or perhaps a smartphone application, so that the patient might have a more objective measure. It has been observed in practice that those who pay close attention to the plan and keep good records tend to do well – that is, those who 'buy into it'. It may be that there is something about taking control of the problem that is helpful – a kind of placebo response in addition to the effect of the strategy itself.

Cognitive strategies: calming the mind

A very common complaint of people with insomnia is that of 'racing thoughts' or of their mind being 'in overdrive'. They may be preoccupied with particular worries but often will admit that the thoughts concern trivial issues. In either case, the activity in the mind increases the level of arousal which hinders sleep, and strategies for calming the mind are needed. A simple method to deal with everyday concerns is 'rehearsal and planning' or 'putting the day to rest' (Espie 2006, p.146). This involves taking time in the evening, perhaps as a start of a winding-down routine, to sit and reflect on the day, and on things in general, and to consider outstanding issues from the past day and plans for the next. The idea is not to solve any particular problems there and then, but to make an action plan which can be put aside. On thinking about the same issues in bed the individual can choose to disregard them with a reminder that there is a plan in place;[2] however, the next consideration is what to do instead, since nature does not like a vacuum and we have to think about something. Rather than try *not* to think about problems at work or how to manage a family issue – guaranteed to make anyone think about them – it is better to think deliberately about something else; something neutral.

Imagery is a commonly recommended strategy and, as Espie (2006) points out, this is something that has to be planned and practised – perhaps in conjunction with relaxation training. Trying to think of a new scenario in bed is unlikely to help and, instead, it should be prepared in advance. Espie (2006) recommends developing 'a screenplay' (p.150) which engages all the senses in a 10-minute sequence; the story should be calming and not evoke strong emotions. Some people find that they can create a personal paradise where they can escape to, but in practice, many others find it difficult to focus on visual imagery; for them it may be that the words of their anxious thoughts still trump the images. These people might find instead that they can focus better on a narrative using words, for example, by imagining that they are drafting an account of the scenario (writing a long letter about it), or perhaps rehearsing it in their mind as if they were going to tell the story to someone. The important things are that the content be just stimulating enough to maintain interest, but neither anxiety provoking nor too exciting, and that the individual does not attempt to stay awake to reach the end of the story.

A particularly troublesome set of thoughts relate to sleep itself and the effects of poor sleep – typically, 'I'll never cope tomorrow after so little sleep' inevitably leading to even less sleep. Most people will recognize this on going to bed and not getting off to sleep ahead of an early start on a big day of some kind; the difference is that for many people with insomnia it is a nightly experience that helps to perpetuate the problem. The extent to which someone believes such unhelpful thoughts regarding sleep can be measured with the Dysfunctional Beliefs about Sleep Scale (Morin, Vallières and Ivers 2007). On a scale of 0–10 respondents are asked to rate their belief in statements such as:

- 'When I sleep poorly on one night, I know that it will disturb my sleep schedule for the whole week.'

- 'When I have trouble falling asleep or getting back to sleep after night-time awakening, I should stay in bed longer and try harder.'

- 'I am concerned that chronic insomnia may have serious consequences on my physical health.'

These kinds of thoughts can be challenged in the same way as other negative thoughts in cognitive behaviour therapy through discussion and behavioural experiments. Harvey and Eidelman (2011) suggest, for example, that the belief that poor sleep is dangerous 'needs to be pulled out by the roots' (p.81) and they show how an experiment of curtailing sleep by 60–90 minutes can begin to alter the belief when the dire predictions do not come true. Many occupational therapists are used to using a cognitive behavioural approach in other contexts and might adapt easily; they also know that it is not something to attempt lightly without proper training or supervision.

Paradoxical intention therapy

This is a means of challenging beliefs about sleep in people who are preoccupied by sleep or the lack of it, and it involves giving up trying. *Trying* to sleep, as has been noted, is a sure way of not sleeping, and as Espie (2011) observes, good sleepers do not try to sleep and do not give much thought to how they do it. In paradoxical intention therapy the idea is to give up trying to sleep and to try to remain awake in bed. Espie (2011) cautions that it is not suited to anyone whose approach is concrete, and demonstrates that it is a very subtle approach. Although giving detailed advice on paradoxical intent is perhaps best left to experienced practitioners, Espie (2006) provides some self-help suggestions that individuals might follow. In any event, there could be particular situations where circumstances are such that sleep is very unlikely (e.g. when neighbours are having a noisy party), and it may be best to 'give up' and allow sleep another chance later.

Other strategies

Thought blocking

The technique of thought blocking, often included among CBT-I strategies, is likened by Morin and Espie (2003) to the opposite of remembering a telephone number, where we need to rehearse the number to the exclusion of everything else in order to keep it in the short-term memory long enough to use it. In other words, if that space in the mind is occupied by some meaningless word or sound, other thoughts cannot be a distraction to the person attempting to sleep. The process is simply to repeat the word 'the' in the head every second or so while lying with eyes closed in bed. The word, which could be mouthed but not spoken aloud, is repeated for about 5 minutes 'or until sleep ensues' (Morin and Espie 2003, p.98). It is uncertain how much evidence exists for the effectiveness of this technique, but it could be a useful addition to the armoury of someone who has difficulty calming the mind.

Mindfulness

A mindfulness-based therapy for insomnia (MBT-I) has been developed by Ong and Sholtes (2010) and aims to 'help individuals increase awareness of the mental and physical states that develop with chronic insomnia and to develop adaptive ways of working with these undesirable states' (p.1176). It combines meditation with CBT-I strategies, and one possible advantage is that practice of mindfulness meditation could increase awareness of internal cues and perhaps help to distinguish between tiredness and fatigue. Ong and Sholtes (2011) show in a case study how sleep can improve and suggest that it is a promising treatment method for insomnia; however, it is not a method that can be adopted without specialized training. (For further information see, for example, Lundh 2005.)

8.4 Managing excessive sleepiness

Managing excessive daytime sleepiness (EDS) is more complicated in many respects than managing insufficient sleep. First, EDS may result from a number of causes that should be properly investigated and which may be successfully treated. Second, it is necessary to distinguish *sleepiness* from fatigue (Pigeon, Sateia and Ferguson 2003; Shen, Barbera and Shapiro 2006; Westcombe and O'Dowd 2012; see also Chapter 17). Fatigue, as Pigeon *et al.* (2003) observe, may accompany a variety of conditions (such as cancer, depression, renal failure and multiple sclerosis) and is, of course, the major feature of chronic fatigue syndrome. A difficulty is that in everyday English we tend to use the word 'tired' to mean either 'fatigued' or 'being in need of sleep' or 'sleepy'; therefore, there are many factors to consider before attempting behavioural management of EDS, and perhaps these complications are also why there are not the same well-established protocols that exist in the case of insomnia. For that reason it is only possible to discuss general principles here.

It is assumed that any remediable causes of EDS, such as insufficient night-time sleep, mood disorder, narcolepsy, sleep apnoea or periodic limb movement disorder, have been ruled out and treated appropriately before an occupational therapist thinks about any management strategy. However, pharmacological management is rarely entirely effective and it is therefore particularly important to ensure that night-time sleep is optimized and that regular hours are maintained, as ever, with a regular rising time; this is essential in cases where an individual has previously allowed insufficient time for sleep.

Although daytime napping is discouraged, even 'prohibited' in the management of insomnia, there is a case for planned naps when dealing with EDS – since sleep remains the best cure for sleepiness, and a nap can be very refreshing for someone with narcolepsy or idiopathic hypersomnia. It can therefore make sense to take a short planned nap at a safe and convenient time to prevent a greater need for sleep at a less convenient or more dangerous time, such as when driving. Someone with EDS may well have been prescribed stimulants, but caffeine is widely recommended for drowsy drivers (see Box 4.3). In a nap it is necessary to avoid getting into deep sleep by restricting nap time, using an alarm if necessary and not getting too comfortable. It may take some organization to create opportunities and find a suitable location for a nap: many people retreat to their parked car during breaks, in the way that some smokers do but, ideally, planning naps would be done in conjunction with an employer (see also the Narcolepsy UK website URL in Appendix 7.1).

Kaplan and Harvey (2009) outline an approach to managing excessive sleep in the context of mood disorders based on cognitive behavioural principles; they acknowledge that the approach has yet to be evaluated, but it has intuitive appeal. They stress the importance of goal-setting – not just to sleep for 8 hours, for example, but also to have goals in life, noting 'that "having nothing to get up for" is a key contributor to hypersomnia in patients with mood disorders' (Kaplan and Harvey 2009, p.282). They recommend providing information on the circadian system, and on the importance of light in maintaining sleep in a regular pattern (and recommend regularity throughout the week). They also observe that most mornings, most people have a period where they remain sleepy; this is known as sleep inertia and it is not necessarily a sign that sleep has been poor or that more is required. In the same way that there is not a sudden transition from wakefulness to sleep, neither is there one from sleep to wakefulness. Similarly, Kaplan and Harvey (2009) suggest that to mirror the evening 'wind-down' period there could be a 'wake-up protocol' (p.283), that is, establishing a habit of not hitting the snooze button on the alarm, getting up and, for example, having a shower and taking a brisk walk.

Kaplan and Harvey (2009) also suggest behavioural experiments. For example, to counter the belief that the only way to feel less tired and generate energy is to sleep more, they report the following experiment. On the first day the patient spent 3 hours conserving energy by sleeping or engaging in light tasks, followed by 3 hours of using energy (taking a walk and seeing a friend). On the next day things were done in reverse – using energy first – but the patient found that mood and energy levels were improved, which led to the conclusion that using energy could be equated to generating energy.

8.5 Conclusion

Occupational therapists are not likely to be involved in managing sleep disorders in the absence of other conditions, but many of their patients will have disturbed sleep and will never receive the attention of a specialist in a sleep clinic. The more complex methods that are described here illustrate what can be done to help and will inform the common-sense advice that a therapist can give and can be combined with 'lifestyle advice' discussed in Chapter 6. More specialized assessment and advice may be necessary for people at different stages in life – especially the young and the elderly – or people with various medical conditions. These are the subjects of the remaining chapters.

Notes

1   We do not want to suggest that people who read in bed and get to sleep without difficulty should give it up (although we would still discourage watching television in bed). However, if someone has difficulty getting to sleep we would not recommend reading to pass the time or reading in the hope of making oneself tired. It would be preferable to read elsewhere until sleepy and then go to bed.

2   It is possible that some new thought will come to mind, in which case a notebook by the bed is often suggested and could be helpful; however, while it may be reassuring that nothing will be overlooked, if someone finds they are using the notebook frequently, it would suggest that they are not yet efficient in rehearsal and planning.

Appendix 8.1 Resources and further reading

Assessment scales described in the chapter are available at the following sites:

- *Dysfunctional Beliefs and Attitudes about Sleep* (www.fss.ulaval.ca/cms_recherche/upload/chaire_sommeil/fichiers/dysfunctional_beliefs_and_attitudes_about_sleep__30_items.pdf; for brief version see Morin, Vallières and Ivers 2007)

- Epworth Sleepiness Scale (http://consultgerirn.org/uploads/File/trythis/try_this_6_2.pdf)

- Glasgow Sleep Effort Scale (www.rockygarrison.com/wp-content/uploads/2013/02/Glasgow-Sleep-Effort-Scale.pdf)

- Insomnia Severity Index (www.myhealth.va.gov/mhv-portal-web/anonymous.portal?_nfpb=true&_pageLabel=healthyLiving&contentPage=healthy_living/sleep_insomnia_index.htm)

- Morningness–Eveningness Questionnaire (www.ubcmood.ca/sad/MEQ.pdf)

- Occupational Impact of Sleep Questionnaire (www.jniosh.go.jp/en/indu_hel/pdf/IH_46_6_601.pdf)

- Pittsburgh Sleep Quality Index (www.sleep.pitt.edu/content.asp?id=1484& subid=2316). Other instruments available at this site:
  ◦ Daytime Insomnia Symptom Scale
  ◦ Insomnia Symptom Questionnaire
  ◦ Pittsburgh Insomnia Rating Scale

- See also: Shahed, A., Wilkinson, K., Marcu, S. and Shapiro, C.M. (eds) (2012) *STOP, THAT and One Hundred Other Sleep Scales*. New York, NY: Springer.

- Sleep diary examples:
  ◦ www.sleepfoundation.org/tools-for-better-sleep/images/SleepDiaryv6.pdf
  ◦ www.nhs.uk/Livewell/insomnia/Documents/sleepdiary.pdf
  ◦ http://yoursleep.aasmnet.org/pdf/sleepdiary.pdf

Sleep hygiene and self-management of sleep problems

Mental Health Foundation publications:

- *Sleep Well: Your Pocket Guide to Better Sleep* (www.bris.ac.uk/equalityanddiversity/act/protected/disability/mhfsleepguide.pdf)

- *Sleep Matters: The Impact of Sleep on Health and Wellbeing* (www.mentalhealth.org.uk/content/assets/PDF/publications/MHF-Sleep-Report-2011.pdf?view=Standard)

Harvard University website:

- External factors that influence sleep (http://healthysleep.med.harvard.edu/healthy/science/how/external-factors)

Light:

- Effect of blue light on sleep; software which is designed to adjust the light on a computer screen to eliminate blue light during the evening is available from F.Lux (http://stereopsis.com/flux)

Alcohol:

- Roehrs, T. and Roth, T. (n.d.) *Sleep, Sleepiness and Alcohol Use* (http://pubs.niaaa.nih.gov/publications/arh25-2/101-109.htm)

Caffeine:

- www.mayoclinic.org/healthy-living/nutrition-and-healthy-eating/in-depth/caffeine/art-20049372?pg=2

- www.leeds.ac.uk/lsmp/healthadvice/caffeine/caffeine.htm

- www.fda.gov/downloads/Drugs/ResourcesForYou/Consumers/BuyingUsing MedicineSafely/UnderstandingOver-the-CounterMedicines/UCM205286.pdf

- www.hc-sc.gc.ca/fn-an/securit/addit/caf/food-caf-aliments-eng.php

All websites were accessed on 23 April 2014. See also Appendix 7.1.

Appendix 8.2 Bristol Sleep Profile

Name _____ Date _____

How do these statements apply to you? Circle the one that applies to you

	Never	Sometimes	Often	Always
1. I am satisfied with my sleep.	Never	Sometimes	Often	Always
2. My partner complains that I twitch or move a lot during my sleep.	Never/no partner	Sometimes	Often	Always
3. I dream a lot.	Never	Sometimes	Often	Always
4. I wake a lot during the night.	Never	Sometimes	Often	Always
5. I snore loudly.	Never	Sometimes	Often	Always
6. I am restless during the evening and night.	Never	Sometimes	Often	Always
7. I have very unpleasant or frightening dreams.	Never	Sometimes	Often	Always
8. I take a long time to go off to sleep at night.	Never	Sometimes	Often	Always
9. I wake up terrified, without knowing why.	Never	Sometimes	Often	Always
10. I feel very tired in the morning.	Never	Sometimes	Often	Always
11. When I wake up in the night I can't get back to sleep again.	Never	Sometimes	Often	Always
12. I wake up very easily in the morning.	Never	Sometimes	Often	Always
13. When I get up I feel groggy and muzzy-headed.	Never	Sometimes	Often	Always
14. My sleep is refreshing.	Never	Sometimes	Often	Always
15. I feel very tired during the day.	Never	Sometimes	Often	Always
16. I walk in my sleep.	Never	Sometimes	Often	Always
17. I keep dropping off to sleep during the day.	Never	Sometimes	Often	Always
18. I take tablets to help me sleep.	Never	Sometimes	Often	Always
19. I have a nap during the day.	Never	Sometimes	Often	Always
20. I wake up very early in the morning and can't get back to sleep.	Never	Sometimes	Often	Always
21. I take tablets or medicine during the day.	Never	Sometimes	Often	Always
22. I have to get up to go to the toilet during the night.	Never	Sometimes	Often	Always

Do you have any children under 5?   YES/NO

Name of tablets/medicine if known _____

References

Bastien, C.H., Vallières, A. and Morin, C.M. (2001) 'Validation of the Insomnia Severity Index as an outcome measure for insomnia research.' *Sleep Medicine 2*, 4, 297–307.

Behar, J., Roebuck, A., Domingos, J.S., Gederi, E. and Clifford, G.D. (2013) 'A review of current sleep screening applications for Smartphones.' *Physiological Measurement 34*, R29–R46.

Berglund, B., Lindvall, T. and Schwela, D.H. (1999) 'Guidelines for Community Noise.' Geneva: World Health Organization. Available at http://whqlibdoc.who.int/hq/1999/a68672.pdf, accessed on 31 October 2013.

Bloom, H.G., Ahmed, I., Alessi, C.A., Ancoli-Israel, S. *et al.* (2009) 'Evidence-based recommendations for the assessment and management of sleep disorders in older persons.' *Journal of the American Geriatric Society 57*, 5, 761–789.

Bootzin, R.R and Perlis, M.L. (2011) 'Stimulus Control Therapy.' In M. Perlis, M. Aloia and B. Kuhn (eds) *Behavioral Treatments for Sleep Disorders: A Comprehensive Primer of Behavioral Sleep Medicine Interventions.* London: Elsevier.

Bootzin, R.R. and Rider, S.P. (1997) 'Behavioral Techniques and Biofeedback for Insomnia.' In M.R. Pressman and W.C. Orr (eds) *Understanding Sleep: The Evaluation and Treatment of Sleep Disorders.* Washington, DC: American Psychological Association.

Broomfield, N.M. and Espie, C.A. (2005) 'Towards a valid, reliable measure of sleep effort.' *Journal of Sleep Research 14*, 4, 401–407.

Buysse, D.J., Reynolds, C.F., Monk, T.H., Berman, S.R. and Kupfer, D.J. (1989) 'The Pittsburgh Sleep Quality Index: a new instrument for psychiatric practice and research.' *Psychiatry Research 28*, 2, 193–213.

David, B. and Morgan, K. (2006) 'Occupational and daytime functioning in primary insomnia: a prospective study.' *Journal of Sleep Research 15*, Suppl. 1, S157.

Espie, C.A. (2006) *Overcoming Insomnia and Sleep Problems.* London: Robinson.

Espie, C.A. (2009) '"Stepped care": a health technology solution for delivering cognitive behavioural therapy as a first line insomnia treatment.' *Sleep 32*, 12, 1549–1558.

Espie, C.A. (2011) 'Paradoxical Intention Therapy.' In M. Perlis, M. Aloia and B. Kuhn (eds) *Behavioral Treatments for Sleep Disorders: A Comprehensive Primer of Behavioral Sleep Medicine Interventions.* London: Elsevier.

Espie, C.A., Fleming, L., Cassidy, J., Samuel, L. *et al.* (2012) 'Randomized controlled clinical effectiveness trial of cognitive behavior therapy compared with treatment as usual for persistent insomnia in patients with cancer.' *Journal of Clinical Oncology 26*, 28, 4651–4658.

Espie, C.A. and Kyle, S.D. (2012) 'Cognitive Behavioral and Psychological Therapies for Chronic Insomnia.' In T.J. Barkoukis, J.K. Matheson, R. Ferber and K. Doghramji (eds) *Therapy in Sleep Medicine.* Philadelphia, PA: Saunders.

Forest, G., van den Heuvel, C., Lushington, K. and De Koninck, J. (2012) 'Temperature biofeedback and sleep: limited findings and methodological challenges.' *ChronoPhysiology and Therapy 2*, 59–66.

Foster, R.G. and Wulff, K. (2005) 'The rhythm of rest and excess.' *Nature Reviews Neurosciences 6*, 5, 407–414.

Gooley, J.J., Chamberlain, K., Smith, K.A., Khalsa, S.B. *et al.* (2011) 'Exposure to room light before bedtime suppresses melatonin onset and shortens melatonin duration in humans.' *Journal of Clinical Endocrinology and Metabolism 96*, 3, E463–E472.

Green, A., Hicks, J., Weekes, R. and Wilson, S. (2005) 'A cognitive-behavioural group intervention for people with chronic insomnia: an initial evaluation.' *British Journal of Occupational Therapy 68*, 11, 518–522.

Harvey, A.G. and Eidelman, P. (2011) 'Intervention to Reduce Unhelpful Beliefs about Sleep.' In M. Perlis, M. Aloia and B. Kuhn (eds) *Behavioral Treatments for Sleep Disorders: A Comprehensive Primer of Behavioral Sleep Medicine Interventions.* London: Elsevier.

Hauri, P.J. (2012) 'Sleep/Wake Lifestyle Modifications.' In T.J. Barkoukis, J.K. Matheson, R. Ferber and K. Doghramji (eds) *Therapy in Sleep Medicine.* Philadelphia, PA: Saunders.

Hicks, J., Green, A. and Wilson, S. (2008) 'Bristol insomnia group: Has it made a difference after 10 years?' *Journal of Sleep Research 17*, Suppl. 1, S197.

Horne, J.A. and Östberg, O. (1976) 'A self-assessment questionnaire to determine morningness–eveningness in human circadian rhythms.' *International Journal of Chronobiology 4*, 2, 97–100.

Hudson, N. (2012) 'Recording and Quantifying Sleep.' In A. Green and A. Westcombe (eds) *Sleep: Multiprofessional Perspectives.* London: Jessica Kingsley Publishers.

Jaehne, A., Loessl, B., Bárkai, Z., Riemann, D. and Hornyak, M. (2009) 'Effects of nicotine on sleep during consumption, withdrawal and replacement therapy.' *Sleep Medicine Reviews 13*, 5, 363–377.

Johns, M.W. (1991) 'A new method for measuring daytime sleepiness: the Epworth Sleepiness Scale.' *Sleep 14*, 6, 540–545.

Kaplan, K.A. and Harvey, A.G. (2009) 'Hypersomnia across mood disorders: a review and synthesis.' *Sleep Medicine Reviews 13*, 4, 275–285.

Kelly, J.M., Strecker, R.E. and Bianchi, M.T. (2012) 'Recent developments in home sleep-monitoring devices.' *ISRN Neurology.* doi: 10.5402/2012/768794.

Kyle, S.D., Morgan, K., Spiegelhalder, K. and Espie, C.A. (2011) 'No pain, no gain: an exploratory within-subjects mixed-methods evaluation of the patient experience of sleep restriction therapy for insomnia.' *Sleep Medicine 12*, 8, 735–747.

Lichstein, K.L., Taylor, D.J., McCrae, C.S. and Thomas, S.T. (2011) 'Relaxation for Insomnia.' In M. Perlis, M. Aloia and B. Kuhn (eds) *Behavioral Treatments for Sleep Disorders: A Comprehensive Primer of Behavioral Sleep Medicine Interventions.* London: Elsevier.

Lichstein, K.L., Thomas, S.J. and McCurry, S.M. (2011) 'Sleep Compression.' In M. Perlis, M. Aloia and B. Kuhn (eds) *Behavioral Treatments for Sleep Disorders: A Comprehensive Primer of Behavioral Sleep Medicine Interventions.* London: Elsevier.

Lundh, L.-G. (2005) 'The role of acceptance and mindfulness in the treatment of insomnia.' *Journal of Cognitive Psychotherapy 19*, 1, 29–39.

McLay, R.N. and Spira, J.L. (2009) 'Use of a portable biofeedback device to improve insomnia in a combat zone: a case report.' *Applied Psychophysiology and Biofeedback 34*, 4, 319–321.

Meoli, A.L., Rosen, C., Kristo, D., Kohrman, M. *et al.* (2005) 'Oral nonprescription treatment for insomnia: an evaluation of products with limited evidence.' *Journal of Clinical Sleep Medicine 1*, 2, 173–187.

Morgenthaler, T., Kramer, M., Alessi, C., Friedman, L. *et al.* (2006) 'Practice parameters for the psychological and behavioural treatment of insomnia: an update. An American Academy of Sleep Medicine report.' *Sleep 29*, 11, 1415–1419.

Morin, C.M. and Espie, C.A. (2003) *Insomnia: A Clinical Guide to Assessment and Treatment.* New York, NY: Kluwer Academic.

Morin, C.M., Hauri, P.J., Espie, C.A., Spielman, A.J., Buysse, D.J. and Bootzin, R.R. (1999) 'Nonpharmacologic treatment of chronic insomnia. An American Academy of Sleep Medicine review.' *Sleep 22*, 8, 1134–1156.

Morin, C.M., Vallières, A. and Ivers, H. (2007) 'Dysfunctional beliefs and attitudes about sleep (DBAS): validation of a brief version (DBAS-16).' *Sleep 30*, 11, 1547–1554.

Murphy, P. and Campbell, S. (1997) 'Nighttime drop in body temperature: a physiological trigger for sleep onset?' *Sleep 20*, 6, 505–511.

Natale, V., Drejak, M., Erbacci, A., Tonetti, L., Fabbri, M. and Martoni, M. (2012) 'Monitoring sleep with a smartphone accelerometer.' *Sleep and Biological Rhythms 10*, 287–292.

Ong, J. and Sholtes, D. (2010) 'A mindfulness-based approach to the treatment of insomnia.' *Journal of Clinical Psychology 66*, 11, 1175–1184.

Okamoto-Mizuno, K. and Mizuno, K. (2012) 'Effects of thermal environment on sleep and circadian rhythm.' *Journal of Physiological Anthropology.* doi: 10.1186/1880-6805-31-14.

Payne, R.A. and Donaghy, M. (2010) *Payne's Handbook of Relaxation Techniques*, 4th edn. Edinburgh: Churchill Livingstone Elsevier.

Perlis, M., Aloia, M. and Kuhn, B. (eds) (2011) *Behavioral Treatments for Sleep Disorders: A Comprehensive Primer of Behavioral Sleep Medicine Interventions.* London: Elsevier.

Pigeon, W.R., Sateia, M.J. and Ferguson, R.J. (2003) 'Distinguishing between excessive daytime sleepiness and fatigue: toward improved detection and treatment.' *Journal of Psychosomatic Research 54*, 1, 61–69.

Posner, D. and Gehrman, P.R. (2011) 'Sleep Hygiene.' In M. Perlis, M. Aloia and B. Kuhn (eds) *Behavioral Treatments for Sleep Disorders: A Comprehensive Primer of Behavioral Sleep Medicine Interventions.* London: Elsevier.

Shen, J., Barbera, J. and Shapiro, C.M. (2006) 'Distinguishing sleepiness and fatigue: focus on definition and measurement.' *Sleep Medicine Reviews 10*, 1, 63–76.

Smith, M.T. and Wegener, S.T. (2003) 'Measures of sleep: The Insomnia Severity Index, Medical Outcomes Study (MOS) Sleep Scale, Pittsburgh Sleep Diary (PSD), and Pittsburgh Sleep Quality Index (PSQI).' *Arthritis & Rheumatism (Arthritis Care & Research) 49*, Suppl. 5, S184–S196.

Spielman, A.J., Yang, C.-M. and Glovinsky, P.B. (2011) 'Sleep Restriction Therapy.' In M. Perlis, M. Aloia and B. Kuhn (eds) *Behavioral Treatments for Sleep Disorders: A Comprehensive Primer of Behavioral Sleep Medicine Interventions.* London: Elsevier.

Stepanski, E.J. and Wyatt, J.K. (2003) 'Use of sleep hygiene in the treatment of insomnia.' *Sleep Medicine Reviews 7*, 3, 215–225.

Stores, G. (2007) 'Clinical diagnosis and misdiagnosis of sleep disorders.' *Journal of Neurology, Neurosurgery and Psychiatry 78*, 12, 1293–1297.

Tan, E., Healey, D., Gray, A.R. and Galland, B.C. (2012) 'Sleep hygiene intervention for youth aged 10 to 18 years with problematic sleep: a before–after pilot study.' *BMC Pediatrics.* doi: 10.1186/1471-2431-12-189.

Van Someren, E. (2006) 'Mechanisms and functions of coupling between sleep and temperature rhythms.' *Progress in Brain Research 153*, 309–324.

Wells, G.A., Li, T., Kirwan, J.R., Peterson, J. *et al.* (2009) 'Assessing quaility of sleep in patients with rheumatoid arthritis.' *Journal of Rheumatology 36*, 9, 2077–2086.

Westcombe, A. and O'Dowd, H. (2012) 'Too Tired to Sleep.' In A. Green and A. Westcombe (eds) *Sleep: Multiprofessional Perspectives.* London: Jessica Kingsley Publishers.

Wiedman, J. (1999) *Desperately Seeking Snoozin'.* Memphis, TN: Towering Pines Press.

Wilson, S. (2012) 'Medication and Sleep.' In A. Green and A. Westcombe (eds) *Sleep: Multiprofessional Perspectives.* London: Jessica Kingsley Publishers.

9

CHILDREN'S SLEEP

Jillian Franklin, Jillian Smith-Windsor and Cary Brown

9.1 Introduction

Up to 30% of children experience a sleep problem at some point during their childhood (Liu *et al.* 2005). Children's sleep requirements are high (see Table 9.1), and poor sleep can affect behaviours such as aggression and impulse control, cognitive development (including learning and memory consolidation), mood regulation and attention. It can also affect health and quality of life (Mindell *et al.* 2006). Additionally, in disorders such as fetal alcohol spectrum disorder, where sensory processing functions (e.g. pain perception and tactile defensiveness) are impaired, poor sleep can heighten the negative consequences of the disorder (Fjeldsted and Hanlon-Dearman 2009; Jirikowic, Olson and Kartin 2008). Furthermore, as shown in a study of children with cerebral palsy, sleep deficiency not only affects the child; other family members' sleep, well-being and family harmony can also suffer (Simard-Tremblay *et al.* 2011).

Table 9.1 Sleep needs in childhood

Newborns (0–2 months)	16–20 hours in 24
Infants (2–12 months)	9–12 hours at night + 2–4.5 hours by day
Toddlers (12 months–years)	12–13 hours in 24; naps continue
Pre-schoolers (3–5 years)	11–12 hours in 24; naps continue
School-aged children (6–12 years)	10–11 hours in 24
Adolescents (12–18 years)	9–9.25 hours in 24 (probably have less)

Data from Davis and Owens (2011).

In turn, the family and social environment affect the child's sleep. Sleep can be considered as a dynamic system of interacting components within a complex context of learned behaviours, social forces (e.g. school activity schedules and parents' hours of work), environmental influences (e.g. light, temperature and noise) and biological processes. As discussed throughout this book, the amount of sleep achieved at all stages of the lifespan is to a large extent dependent on the social, cultural and physical environments (see Sadeh *et al.* 2009). As Meadows (2012) puts it, *'No one sleeps alone. How, where, when (and with whom) we sleep are all achieved by other people'* (p.106; original emphasis). This is especially true in the case of children.

While any child may experience sleep problems, the incidence of sleep deficit is noted to be considerably higher among children with neurodevelopmental, medical and psychiatric conditions (Fjeldsted and Hanlon-Dearman 2009; Rodriguez 2007). For example, 50–80% of children with autism spectrum disorders (Goldman *et al.* 2012) and 23% of children with cerebral palsy (Newman, O'Regan and Hensey 2006) are reported to have sleep problems. Children with chronic health conditions are generally less resilient and consequently their sleep problems tend to be more severe, resistant to treatment and can have more profound psychological and emotional impact on day-to-day functioning (Mindell and Owens 2009).

Occupational therapists in paediatric services routinely see children with autism spectrum disorder, fetal alcohol spectrum disorder, Down syndrome and cerebral palsy. Although sleep problems are common for these children, a recent Canadian study found that most therapists are unaware of the need and the resources to assess for sleep problems and are unable to provide evidence-based non-pharmacological sleep interventions (Brown *et al.* 2012). This lack of awareness of sleep issues is also found in other health care professions such as primary care physicians and nurses (Meltzer and Mindell 2006). Time constraints and other pressing needs are cited by some health care workers as reasons that make it difficult to prioritize patients' sleep (Lee and Ward 2005). As a consequence, problems with sleep often remain unaddressed. The purpose of this chapter is therefore to provide a foundation so that occupational therapists can help manage common sleep problems in young children. Evidence-based sleep assessment tools and interventions pertinent to occupational performance issues are reviewed, and a case study is integrated throughout the chapter (see Boxes 9.1–9.3) to illustrate the role of the occupational therapist working with a child experiencing a sleep problem. The Model of Human Occupation (Kielhofner 2008) is applied to provide a theoretical framework for approaching sleep problems from a perspective relevant to children's occupational performance needs.

BOX 9.1 Case study: part 1

Annie is a 7-year-old with a diagnosis of cerebral palsy. She loves spending time with her friends and is very interested in music. She wants to play the piano in her school's talent show, but she has difficulty stroking the appropriate keys due to high tone in her hands. Because of her strong desire to play in the show like the rest of her friends, she is frustrated with her inability to perfect her piano piece.

Jane, Annie's occupational therapist, is working with her on the fine motor skills needed to help achieve this goal. Upon further investigation, Jane learns that Annie has strong flexion contractures in her knees and hips which cause her pain during the night. Annie shares that she has trouble sleeping because of these contractures and she is often very tired while at school. This pain has affected Annie's sleep routine because she puts off going to bed knowing she will not be able to fall asleep. Instead, she stays up late playing computer games. Annie's parents report that she often complains of daytime sleepiness and that the first thing she wants to do after school is take a nap.

9.2 Special considerations in children's sleep

Unlike most adults, children do not control their own schedules or make their own choices about sleep-related activities, foods and environments. In working with children, therapists need to understand parents' values, beliefs and behaviours in relation to a child's sleep and sleep-influencing daytime activity. A sleep-deprived child is less likely than a well-rested child to benefit to the same extent from treatment interventions for the condition that initially triggered the referral to therapy. It is important to remember that, because they may not recognize that their sleep is abnormal or may not understand the effects that sleep deprivation can have on their daily activities, self-report of sleep problems by children is unlikely. Because young children lack such insight, it would not be usual for them to tell their parents about a sleep difficulty (Givan 2004). Although it is unlikely that a child will be referred to occupational therapy specifically for a sleep disorder, it is possible that sleep problems will become evident during therapy for other conditions. This can be seen in the case example where Annie was referred to occupational therapy because cerebral palsy affected her fine motor skills, but during assessment it became clear that her goal of playing the piano at the school concert was also hindered by sleep deprivation.

The literature (see Chapters 5 and 6) points to a reciprocal relationship between sleep and daytime functioning. This bidirectional relationship is exemplified by Annie's situation where, first, pain disrupted her sleep, and then insufficient sleep affected her daytime functioning and imposed stress on her and her family. This stress, added to the ongoing night-time pain, interfered even more with Annie's ability to sleep, which compounds her stress, and so forth, in an increasingly negative cycle. The outcome of the interaction between pain, sleep and function also affects Annie's parents – and of course, Annie's parents have sleep-related beliefs and values that, in turn, influence Annie's sleep environment and routines.

BOX 9.2 Case study: part 2

Annie's disrupted sleep decreases her motoric control and balance, metabolic processes, new learning, emotional regulation and many other elements important to achieving her full occupational performance potential. Daytime sleepiness also causes Annie to take long naps which decrease her sleep drive at bedtime and further disrupt her sleep-wake cycle. Annie has become a 'night owl' and experiences great difficulty as well as emotional stress in getting up in time for school each day.

It is recommended that children 6–12 years of age have 9–10 hours of sleep in order to remain awake and alert during the day (see Table 9.1; Mindell and Owens 2009). Schoolwork, extracurricular activities and other responsibilities place increased demands on children's time and can delay bedtimes. Behaviours such as excessive napping, dozing off during car rides or while watching television and persistent complaints of daytime sleepiness are indicators of potential sleep deprivation, observation of which should trigger more detailed evaluation (Mindell and Owens 2009). Poor sleep in school-aged children can also cause mood swings, hyperactivity and cognitive problems, which, in turn, can have a negative impact on school performance (Meltzer and Mindell 2006). Substance abuse and aggressive behaviours in adolescents have also been closely linked to a childhood history of sleep problems (Wong, Brower and Zucker 2009). Children with medical conditions and disabilities are at additional risk of sleep problems; early assessment and intervention can minimize long-term complications and reduce the risk of related health conditions such as diabetes, depression, sensory processing problems and poor academic performance.

9.3 Common sleep disturbances in children

Children are susceptible to most sleep disorders that can be experienced by adults, although there are differences. For example, a child is unlikely to suffer from the parasomnia rapid eye movement (REM) behaviour disorder, but will be more likely than an adult to experience non-REM parasomnias such as sleepwalking or sleep terrors (which, typically, will be grown out of). A further difference is that in adult insomnia the difficulty may relate to the individual's own action, whereas in childhood insomnia the parent's actions have a significant influence. It has been argued that the classification of childhood insomnia as a sleep disorder is an example of medicalization of what is 'a lack of consistency and appropriate regulation by parents at bedtime and throughout the night' (Jones and Ball 2012, p.98). Five childhood sleep disorders of note are described here: obstructive sleep apnoea, behavioural insomnia of childhood, excessive daytime sleepiness, sensory processing dysfunction and circadian-rhythm disorders.

Obstructive sleep apnoea

The estimated prevalence of paediatric obstructive sleep apnoea (also see Chapter 7) in the US is 1–4% (Lumeng and Chervin 2008), and some studies have recorded rates as high as 60% in children who have a diagnosis of obesity (Narang and Mathew 2012). A study of 108 Spanish children with Down syndrome reported the prevalence of sleep-disordered breathing as 64.7% in boys and 38.5% in girls (de Miguel-Díez, Villa-Asensi and Alvarez-Sala 2003). Marcus *et al.* (2012) cite studies where reported incidence ranged from 31 to 100% in children with Down syndrome. In a review of the literature Meltzer *et al.* (2010) determined that childhood obstructive sleep apnoea often goes unreported and under-diagnosed. It is likely that several factors contribute to this. First, the child is unaware of snoring or having pauses in breathing (because they do not trigger a full awakening). Second, parents may not realize that snoring is an indicator of a potential problem. Third, the paediatrician may be unaware of the significance of the condition (Davis and Owens 2011). Night-time signs and symptoms to be aware of include loud snoring, frequent awakenings, bedwetting and unusual sleeping positions (e.g. kneeling, sitting, hyperextension of the neck); daytime features include excessive sleepiness, irritability, hyperactivity, impaired concentration and attention, and poor school performance (Gasparini *et al.* 2012). Children with suspected obstructive sleep apnoea should be referred to a respiratory specialist. Occupational therapists can contribute to management through collaboration with a nutritionist and working with parents to increase physical activity levels in order to help weight reduction when the child is obese, strategizing with the parents about ways to increase acceptance of the continuous passive airway pressure (CPAP) mask if the child is on CPAP therapy (see Chapter 7) and by discussing potential environmental factors that may exacerbate breathing problems (for example, bedding choices and allergens).

Behavioural insomnia of childhood

A range of behavioural problems may precipitate or exacerbate sleep problems in children. In turn, sleep deficiency can increase the risk, and perpetuate the existence, of behavioural problems. It is important to help identify environmental, physiological and sensory processing factors that, although unrecognized, can be contributing to the development and maintenance of behavioural problems. For example, if a child has sensory processing problems such that the contact of bedding on his or her skin causes agitation, going to bed can become associated with this unpleasant sensation and the child will resist bedtime. Addressing the underlying negative tactile sensitivity may resolve the bedtime resistance to a great extent. Early attention to these factors can go a long way to preclude establishing negative bedtime associations and behaviours.

In Annie's case the occupational therapist was able to help the parents recognize that Annie's bed was also causing her pain at night and that this was a reversible contributing factor to what – until then – had been labelled a behavioural problem.

Occupational therapists working with families where the child has sleep problems should be aware of common behavioural insomnias, but it would be unwise to initiate more complex behavioural management interventions without additional training and/or collaboration with experienced coworkers. (For a more detailed discussion of behavioural sleep conditions and interventions readers should consult Mindell and Owens 2009, Morgenthaler *et al.* 2006, Owens 2011 and Owens, Palermo and Rosen 2002.) The *Encyclopaedia of Early Childhood Development* (EECD; see Appendix 9.1) identifies the two most common behavioural sleep problems in childhood as being fundamentally psychosocial. The first problem, sleep-onset association disorder, occurs when a child learns to fall asleep only when certain conditions are met. For example, a child who always falls asleep on the couch with his parents while they watch television will associate the couch with sleep and can develop a strong resistance to initiating sleep alone in his own bed. Other examples include a child who will only sleep when he has a juice bottle or when he is being held. Children who strongly associate certain activities with sleep can experience problems with self-soothing such that they cannot return to sleep when they wake in the night and the associated activity is not available. The other common problem is limit-setting sleep disorder. In this case, sleep initiation is the problem, as opposed to night-time wakening, and to avoid sleep the child might employ strategies that are often disruptive to the rest of the family. Bedtime can become an emotionally charged event that parents dread. Information brochures and links to evidence-based lay-language resources for managing these common behavioural issues are provided on the EECD website. The basic principles of managing these types of behavioural problems include:

- Exploring non-pharmacological interventions early before behaviours become well established and family harmony is disrupted.

- Implementing extinction or gradual extinction. This involves a planned withdrawal of parental attention so that children learn to sleep in their own beds and to self-soothe. This can be an emotionally charged process and some assistance in setting up the plan is encouraged.

- Establishing specific and predictable bedtime routines that include pleasant, gentle activities such that parents can praise the child for taking part in getting ready for bed.

- Establishing a system of bedtime rewards when indicated. This can consist of tokens towards a treat when a child goes to sleep and stays in bed until morning without a fuss.

- Using transition objects (such as special blankets and cuddly toys) that are reserved for night-time only. This helps the child develop an association between these items and the transition to bed and sleep. These special objects are helpful when the child wakes in the night and needs to self-soothe back to sleep.

Excessive daytime sleepiness

Although excessive daytime sleepiness is a feature of narcolepsy and other hypersomnias, the most common cause of childhood excessive daytime sleepiness is insufficient night-time sleep. The prevalence of daytime sleepiness in school-aged children is difficult to determine because of inconsistent uses of the term in epidemiological studies (Mindell and Owens 2009). The primary complaint of excessive daytime sleepiness is the overwhelming urge to fall asleep, particularly during times of decreased activity and environmental stimulation. A careful assessment and involvement of other team members is important because of the complexity of excessive daytime sleepiness. In some unusual situations medication alone is indicated; in others behavioural and environmental changes, such as increased daytime activity, modified bright-light exposure or education for parents about childhood sleep needs, are sufficient. In yet other cases combinations of medication, environmental and behavioural change are required. Because the most common cause of excessive daytime sleepiness is insufficient night-time sleep, an assessment of the child's daily activity and sleep patterns should be the starting point. A sleep diary can be helpful to gather this information (see Sleep for Kids in Appendix 9.1). In adolescents excessive daytime sleepiness may be a consequence of the disconnect between hormonal changes during puberty (contributing to the adolescent's inability to initiate sleep until after midnight), early school start times and increased social activities. For some teenagers this becomes a period of chronic sleep deficiency. Millman *et al.* (2005) provide a detailed overview of excessive daytime sleepiness in youth and the evidence base for interventions.

Sensory processing dysfunction

As previously mentioned, children with developmental delay and sensory processing problems are at high risk of sleep problems (Fjeldsted and Hanlon-Dearman 2009; Franklin *et al.* 2008; Goodlin-Jones *et al.* 2008; Jirikowic *et al.* 2008). These children present additional challenges because of their altered sensory processing where even something as simple as the texture of pyjamas, or the feel of a toothbrush in the mouth, can present a significant obstacle to sleep. Children who have sensory processing disorders have problems with neurocognitive self-regulation and therefore are sensitive to daytime stimulation, including sound, light and activities, that would not cause hyperarousal in a typically developing child. Therapists use a combination of sensory integration techniques, environmental modification, anti-reflux positioning and, at times, deep-pressure techniques to promote sensory normalization. A paediatric occupational therapist should be consulted to help develop the most suitable programme for each child. (For more details see Goodlin-Jones *et al.* 2008 and Reynolds, Lane and Thacker 2012.)

Circadian-rhythm disorders

Circadian-rhythm disorders (see Chapter 7) result from a discrepancy between one's biological clock and the environmental demands dictating night-time sleep (Grigg-Damberger 2004). Children with circadian-rhythm disorders tend to wake up and sleep earlier or later than average, to have an irregular sleep-wake cycle or have a non-24-hour sleep-wake cycle. Circadian-rhythm disorders have been particularly noted in children with autism spectrum disorder, and some researchers speculate that recognizing social and environmental cues, including those that signify sleep, is also an important component of maintaining the circadian drive (Goodlin-Jones *et al.* 2008). For example, a child with autism spectrum disorder may not recognize that when other members of the family get ready for bed, this is a cue that he or she also should prepare for bed. Not recognizing social cues can interfere with initiating calming activities that prepare the body for sleep.

Circadian regulation is most influenced by exposure to light at the blue end of the spectrum. Research shows that routine exposure to daylight in sufficient quantities helps maintain the neurochemical processes required to regulate the sleep drive. Conversely, and of great concern, exposure to bright blue-spectrum light in the evening suppresses production of the melatonin* required to initiate and maintain sleep. Children who receive little natural daylight exposure, and who use blue-spectrum light-emitting electronic devices such as laptops, tablets and televisions prior to bedtime, are at particular risk (Durand, Gernert-Dott and Mapstone 1996; Owens 2009).

9.4 Factors affecting occupational performance

The Model of Human Occupation (Kielhofner 2008) is a useful theoretical perspective from which to approach managing children's sleep problems. The four areas – volition, habituation, performance capacity and environment – offer a framework for assessment and suggest opportunities for intervention and are discussed in depth below.

Volition

Kielhofner (2008) describes volition as 'the motivation for occupation' (p.12). This can be any occupation that a child might engage in throughout the course of the day, such as going to school or sleeping. Annie, for example, will select occupations based on the value they hold in relation to her interests and abilities. Her volition is reflected in her interest in music, the value she places on being like other children her age and her feelings of frustration about being unable to concentrate long enough to sit through a piano lesson. Kielhofner (2008) argues that once we experience competency in a given occupation, we will have positive feelings towards that occupation and choose to engage in it again. If a child does not experience competency – or has a bad experience, as in the case where there is a sleep disturbance – negative feelings towards sleep could develop. For example, a child with sleep terrors (see Chapter 7) may resist going to bed because of fear associated with sleep. Similarly, children who are the first to be put to bed in a household may display refusal behaviours because they do not want to feel left out when other family members are still awake (Mindell *et al.* 2009). This can also contribute to negative feelings towards sleep, as the child's family may be engaging in occupations (such as playing or watching television) that he or she finds more appealing than being in bed. Parents can diminish the negative association of bedtime and increase a child's volition for sleep by associating it with an enjoyable activity such as reading a story or reminding them of being able to do valued activities in the morning. Parents' volition is also an important consideration. Interventions often require a time commitment on the part of parents and may disrupt the whole family (Meltzer *et al.* 2010). Understanding parents' values and beliefs about sleep will help the therapist and parents to work together and identify and prioritize acceptable, pragmatic interventions. This process increases the chances that change will be achieved and built on a sense of self-efficacy as opposed to parental failure.

Habituation

'Habituation allows persons to cooperate with their environments to do the routine actions that make up everyday life' (Kielhofner 2008, p.52). This includes both daily routines and those leading up to and involving sleep. Establishing a consistent bedtime routine can be sufficient to improve a child's sleep disturbances in some cases (Mindell *et al.* 2009). Poor sleep habits developed in childhood may carry forward through life and could contribute to poor health and diminished quality of life. A sleep schedule requires allotting an age-appropriate amount of time for sleep and getting up at the same time each day. There are numerous obstacles to developing effective sleep habits or having good sleep hygiene. The pressures of busy lives with social, sports and shopping activities often scheduled for evenings can interfere with a child's sleep schedule. As children do not control their own schedule for the most part, parents need to understand the rationale for sleep hygiene. Changing habits is better facilitated through positive achievements, as opposed to censure, and parents may need help to alter their child's sleep habits in incremental steps that do not lead to feelings of failure or guilt for either child or parent(s).

Performance capacity

The capacity to perform depends on one's musculoskeletal, neurological and cardiopulmonary body systems, along with cognitive abilities, such as memory. When we engage in occupations, we exercise these capacities (Kielhofner 2008). Sleep is essential for physiological, cognitive and emotional processes (see Chapter 5) and, because childhood is a period of rapid growth and development, children's ability to achieve adequate sleep is more easily disrupted than that of adults. While adults have recourse to fatigue counter-measures, such as caffeine and other stimulants, and are able to modify their environment (specifically light, noise and temperature) to decrease the risk of sleep deprivation, this is not the case for children. Sleep in children with chronic health conditions can be particularly vulnerable because many conditions are also painful (Newman, O'Regan and Hensey 2006) or may require use of stimulant medications such as those prescribed for children with conditions such as attention deficit hyperactivity disorder (Owens 2005). We see this in the case example of Annie where her capacity for new learning during piano lessons, and in the classroom, is significantly affected by her sleep deprivation. Additionally, her neuromuscular limitations cause pain leading to sleep-related anxiety, discomfort in bed and an inability to independently modify the amount of light and noise in her bedroom.

Environment

The impact of the environment on the occupation of sleep is complex. The sociocultural environment plays an important role in children's sleep as it does in adults' sleep (see Chapter 4). For example, co-sleeping and communal sleeping is common in many cultures and, although children having their own bedroom is a preference in North America and much of Europe, this is not a universal value (Liu *et al.* 2005; Mindell and Owens 2009). The socioeconomic status of a family may also dictate sleeping arrangements, as there may be limited space in the house for children to have their own room or bed. Where co-sleeping and shared bedrooms are the practice, the occupational therapist needs to use creativity to help parents identify strategies to promote a quiet, dark sleep environment.

Both cultural and social aspects of a family must be considered when recommending interventions for families who co-sleep. Co-sleeping has become quite controversial and it is important to present parents with an opportunity to discuss their practice in a non-judgemental fashion so that parents remain open to discussion and to learning about best-practice recommendations. Burns (2009) provides a detailed overview of the controversy and the current evidence base as it relates to the proposed benefits and negative consequences of co-sleeping. Numerous health policy makers have produced position statements and guidelines on infant sleep positions including co-sleeping. The National Health Service (NHS) in the UK and the Canadian Pediatric Society are two examples (URLs to these documents are in Appendix 9.1). All health care providers need to familiarize themselves with the current health authority recommendations in their areas and ensure they can help parents understand them.

In addition to these individual environmental influences there are other, more universal influences within the physical environment. Three key components of the physical environment that need to be considered are light, noise and temperature. Each component is briefly mentioned here and discussed in detail later in this chapter.

Light

Pre-bedtime blue-spectrum light exposure (such as televisions, electronic tablets, laptops and computers) and night-time light exposure (for example, nightlights, street lighting coming through curtains and hallway lighting showing under the bedroom door) interferes with sleep. Environmental blue light interacts with sleep centres in the brain and triggers the suppression of the sleep hormone melatonin (Wood *et al.* 2013).

Noise

Ambient household noise can be a barrier to sleep. The World Health Organization recommends that for uninterrupted sleep, noise levels should remain under 30 decibels; however, normal conversation at a range of 1–1.5 metres (approximately 3–5 feet) falls into the 60-decibel range. In situations where keeping the decibel level low is not realistic, some research suggests that using sounds slightly louder than 30 decibels that have a consistent non-moderating pitch (such as a fan or air conditioner) can be effective in blocking intermittent, alerting, background noise (Berglund, Lindvall and Schwela 1999).

Temperature

Body temperature influences the sleep centre of the brain to trigger arousal or sleep. Although the evidence base is not abundant, it is typically recommended that bedrooms be kept slightly cool to avoid core body temperature warming (Mindell and Owens 2009). The theoretical basis for this recommendation is that elevated core body temperature interferes with the physiological processes required for circadian regulation. (For more details see Chapter 3 and also Lack *et al.* 2008.) Researchers have recently suggested that sleep deprivation itself interferes with the body's ability to achieve thermoregulation during sleep (Romeijn *et al.* 2012), and the consequent discomfort interferes with deep sleep. The most useful source of information at this point is parental observation of the child to see if bedding is thrown off or if the child appears restless and overly warm to the touch during sleep.

9.5 Assessment of children's sleep problems by occupational therapists

Therapists should always include one or two simple questions about sleep in any assessment they do. Usually asking 'Does your child have any problems falling asleep?' and 'Does your child sleep through the night?' is a good start to identifying difficulties that might need more investigation (Moore 2012). If more investigation seems warranted, parents or caregivers can keep a sleep diary for 1–2 weeks, and there is a range of sleep diaries from which parents can select (see Appendix 9.1). These resources can be modified by occupational therapists depending on the particular needs of their client. Where serious sleep problems are suspected the therapist should use a parental or self-report sleep diary in conjunction with other objective and/or standardized sleep assessments to obtain a more comprehensive picture.

There are several sleep assessment tools, varying in degree of complexity and comprehensiveness, available to clinicians. The 'BEARS' is a practical paediatric sleep-screening tool that assesses five domains: **B**edtime problems, **E**xcessive daytime sleepiness, **A**wakenings during the night, **R**egularity or duration of sleep, and **S**noring. Parents are asked about problems in each specific domain and a 'yes' response indicates that there may be a need for further investigation (Owens and Dalzell 2005). The Children's Sleep Habits Questionnaire (CSHQ) helps identify both behavioural and medically based sleep problems in school-aged children (Owens, Spirito, and McGuinn 2000). The CSHQ is widely used in research and in paediatric sleep clinics. The Sleep Disturbance Scale for Children (SDSC) (Bruni *et al.* 1996) is a 26-item questionnaire using a five-point Likert scale to rate common sleep-disorder symptoms. This scale is useful for identifying the type of sleep difficulties the child experiences and what type of intervention may be useful. (The URLs to free, downloadable versions of these three assessment tools are in Appendix 9.1.) A fourth assessment, known as the SNAKE (because of its full title in German),[1] was developed and psychometrically tested by a German and UK collaboration to address the paucity of resources specific to children with severe psychomotor impairment (Blankenburg *et al.* 2013). The SNAKE can be accessed in the appendix of Blankenburg *et al.* (2013). Occupational therapists who require a detailed review of the range and psychometric properties of available paediatric parental or child self-report tools to help guide selection of appropriate assessment and outcome tool for their setting should refer to Lewandowski, Toliver-Sokol and Palermo (2011). An open-access version of their review is available online.

When objective measurement of sleep is required, actigraphy provides a convenient, cost-effective and non-invasive means of recording a child's sleep-wake cycle (Ancoli-Israel *et al.* 2003). An actigraph is a small device that can be worn on the wrist or ankle. For children where there is a concern that they may tamper with the monitor, Sadeh's (2011) detailed review of actigraphy and children discusses sewing the monitor into a pyjama pocket or the cuff of a sock. This can interfere with the reliability of readings, so parents and therapist may need to do some creative problem-solving if actigraphy is considered.

In Annie's case, Jane decided to use the CSHQ in addition to a sleep diary kept by Annie and her mother. The combination of these results showed that Annie had the most difficulty with initiating sleep and experienced anxiety around falling asleep. Once Jane had identified specific problem areas she was able to select appropriate interventions and monitor the outcomes.

9.6 Management of children's sleep problems by occupational therapists

Sleep disturbances in some children resolve on their own if left untreated, although for many children, and particularly those with other health conditions, this is unlikely (Meltzer *et al.* 2010). This section provides an overview of management approaches within the broad categories of educational, environmental and behavioural strategies. Much of the evidence base for these strategies has been introduced earlier in the chapter and the preceding sections should be read prior to this section. Therapists should consider introducing the most straightforward, pragmatic strategies first so that parents and children build self-efficacy and see some degree of positive change. In a systems approach to intervention, environmental and educational strategies are often the most straightforward and would be addressed first in an effort to reduce the need for demanding and often stressful behavioural interventions.

Educational strategies

Educating parents about the relationship between sleep and positive developmental outcomes is an important step that should precede all interventions. When parents have a clear understanding of the basics of sleep physiology and how sleep impacts behaviour and health they are able to participate in the problem-solving and planning required to help their child achieve restorative sleep. Parent and child sleep education websites and books for this purpose are listed in Appendix 9.1.

Environmental strategies

Sleep hygiene can be considered the cornerstone of environmental modification and consists of developing good sleep habits and an environment that is conducive to sleep. Sleep hygiene includes the physical sleep setting, sleep schedule and sleep practices (e.g. pre-bedtime routine), all of which influence effective sleep. The sleep hygiene principles discussed here are also relevant in behavioural interventions and should be kept in mind while reviewing that section.

Sleep hygiene and the principles of stimulus control (see Chapter 8) recommend that the bedroom be reserved for sleeping only. It is important to create a non-stimulating environment for sleep and to avoid associating the bedroom with waking activities (such as play or watching television) which might also increase arousal; however, this can be a challenge for most families because children routinely use their bedrooms for study and leisure as well as sleep. The occupational therapist can help parents and children devise ways to reduce the amount of stimulation in the immediate area of the bed while still recognizing that the bedroom may need to fulfil several functions. For example, the use of screens or the rearrangement of furniture could help to delineate an area that is reserved strictly for sleep. Importantly, if at all possible, the bedroom should not become associated with punishment, as sending children to their room for bad behaviour may reinforce negative associations and increase bedtime resistance.

Children's use of electronic devices, such as televisions, computers and tablets, in the bedroom before bed will contribute to decreased quality and quantity of sleep because their screens expose the user to bright, blue-spectrum light which suppresses melatonin. Wood *et al.* (2013) determined that a popular brand of laptop, held at a 10-inch viewing distance from the cornea, provided 40 lux additional to ambient room lighting. A recent US study of 18–30-year-olds (Gooley *et al.* 2011) found that exposure to 200 lux of light, which is the equivalent of a normally lit room but insufficient for comfortable reading, delivered prior to bedtime delayed melatonin onset in 99% of participants and suppressed melatonin levels over the night by more than 50% in many of the participants. Laptop light-filtering software is available and should be considered for children and adults where pre-bed use of laptops is essential (see F.Lux information in Appendix 9.1).

Although it is important to eliminate light sources when possible, many children will be uneasy in complete darkness and a nightlight with an automatic timer or a motion detector can be an option. Nightlights should have bulbs that filter out white- and blue-spectrum light. The red light bulbs used by photographers in darkrooms (available through photography suppliers) and LED red bulbs available at specialty lighting stores are two options.

In addition to lighting, noise and temperature, comfortable bedding and physical positioning contribute to effective sleep. For some children allergens are an issue and problems with breathing interfere with restorative sleep. (The National Sleep Foundation website has more information on this topic; see Appendix 9.1.) Finally, for some children, assessment of positioning and recommendations about postural management equipment is required (Ponsonby *et al.* 2004; Wynn and Wickham 2009). In Annie's case, this was carried out in conjunction with an outing to a mattress store to try different mattresses and wedges to ensure she could maintain the most comfortable position throughout the night. Modification of bedding to promote pain-free sleep must be carefully considered and then monitored so that interventions do not contribute to other problems such as joint contractures. For example, placing pillows under Annie's knees might help with comfort at night but will increase her risk for knee-flexion contractures; the therapist therefore needs to balance the complexities of these issues. Optimal positioning decreases Annie's risk of developing postural deformities that will interfere with both her functional abilities and sleep.

In summary, the general principles of sleep hygiene for children include:

- decreasing arousing games and activity at least 60 minutes before bed

- making relaxing activities, such as a story or listening to gentle music, a part of the bedtime routine

- restricting fluids and heavy snacks before bedtime; a light snack or 55–85 ml (2–3 oz) of juice or milk is fine

- restricting the use of any electronic devices (e.g. television, laptops, tablets and games) at least 60 minutes before bed

- not using the bedroom for punishment as it may create a negative association that prevents the desire to go to bed.

A brochure of children's sleep hygiene practices can be downloaded from the Sleep for Kids website (see Appendix 9.1). Sleep hygiene and environmental modification recommendations are based on ideal situations and are not always practical or achievable for some families. Applying a systems approach, such as the Model of Human Occupation, will help the therapist see where pragmatic, realistic opportunities to intervene exist. For example, it may not be acceptable to parents to remove a nightlight from the child's room, but they may be willing to use a motion-activated one instead of a consistent light source.

Behavioural strategies

For some children behavioural programmes (such as sleep restriction and extinction) are indicated, and excellent resources to guide therapists in working with these types of interventions are available. For example, the workbook series *When Children Don't Sleep Well* includes both a therapist- and a parent workbook (Durand 2008a, 2008b). However, occupational therapists new to sleep management issues should be cautious when considering behavioural interventions because they are often very stressful to the child and the family. These skills can be developed within the scope of occupational therapy practice and therapists are encouraged to network with more experienced mentors so that they have sufficient support and guidance in planning and carrying out a behavioural sleep programme. Additionally, because the evidence base for some behavioural programmes is quite sparse, therapists working in this area need to keep themselves updated as the research advances.

A recent review of non-pharmacological sleep interventions for youth with health conditions found that of 31 behavioural intervention studies critiqued, none was of strong methodological quality and only seven were of moderate quality (Brown *et al.* 2013). Interventions that have been demonstrated to be effective in some children may not directly translate for children who have more complex needs; however, this does not mean that the interventions are not effective, but rather could mean that we need to do more research in the specific client populations (such as children with sensory processing problems). The more common behavioural interventions, detailed in Durand (2008b) and Weiss and Corkum (2012), are outlined below.

Interventions for sleep anxiety

Progressive muscle relaxation is a method of systematic contraction and relaxation of muscle groups. Progressive muscle relaxation should be performed in the child's bed immediately prior to their bedtime. Gentle massage can also be incorporated into children's bedtime routine to help with relaxation. Sybil Hart's book *Lullaby Massage: Rhyme and Touch Massage for Infants and Children* (Hart 2009) is a useful massage guide for parents. This book describes various massage techniques with accompanying rhymes developed especially to help children from age 6 months on get to sleep.

Interventions for difficulties falling asleep

When children have difficulties falling asleep, it is usually due to an inconsistent bedtime, inconsistent pre-bed routine, or requiring a parent or other external stimulus to be present while falling asleep (Meltzer *et al.* 2010). There are several approaches to help establish consistent sleep patterns for children.

STANDARD EXTINCTION

Standard extinction involves letting the child 'cry it out'. The child remains in the bed/bedroom and the parent does not respond to his or her cries or protests, and the child eventually falls asleep. This is intended to teach the child to self-soothe and usually begins to take effect after approximately 1 week (Mindell and Owens 2009). While standard extinction can be an effective treatment, many parents find it difficult to ignore their child when in distress (Mindell *et al.* 2006) and they may need additional support. As a caution to therapists, this intervention, along with graded extinction, may not be appropriate for children who are unsafe when left unattended, or for those parents who do not feel comfortable ignoring their child's cries.

GRADED EXTINCTION

Graded extinction is similar to that of standard extinction but graded by the parent progressively increasing the amount of time between responses to their child's cries. In order to implement graded extinction, the parents first establish an initial time interval (usually 3–5 minutes) that they will wait before checking when the child first cries. If the child is still crying and/or protesting after the established interval time, the parent briefly enters the room to soothe the child. Parents are instructed to not pick up the child and to keep their visit brief, as the goal is for the child to fall asleep independently, without the parent in the room. If the child's protests continue, the parent must wait the length of the initial time interval before going back into the bedroom. This should continue until the child falls asleep. For each night thereafter, the initial time interval before checking on the child is increased, usually by 2 or 3 minutes (Durand 2008b).

SLEEP RESTRICTION

Sleep restriction involves initially shortening the child's overall sleep time by keeping them out of bed and awake longer into the night. This makes the child drowsy, and they eventually learn to fall asleep without resistance. Once the child is accustomed to falling asleep without protesting, their bedtime can be progressively adjusted to achieve an age-appropriate number of hours of night-time sleep. When implementing sleep restriction, an accurate sleep diary or actigraph helps establish the child's usual time for sleep onset. Once this has been identified, a new bedtime should be set half an hour later than sleep-onset time as the child will likely be able to fall asleep in this time frame. It is important that the child stay awake until the bedtime has been reached, give or take 15 minutes. Once the child falls asleep within this time frame for two consecutive nights, the bedtime should be moved earlier by 15 minutes. Parents should then keep the child up again until the new bedtime. If the child does not fall asleep within a 15-minute window of being put to bed, he or she should be kept up an hour later than their bedtime, then repeat the steps until the desired bedtime is reached. Throughout the process, parents should consistently wake the child up at the same time each morning and should not allow the child to nap during the day. Durand (2008b) cautions that during the implementation of sleep restriction, the child might experience sleepwalking, sleep talking and/or sleep terrors due to sleep deprivation.

BOX 9.3 Case study: part 3

Jane determined from the sleep history, sleep diary and CSHQ (Owens *et al.* 2000) that Annie's bedtime varied because of her fear of going to sleep: she puts off going to bed knowing she will have pain during the night. Annie also uses her laptop in bed before trying to fall asleep. Her anxiety and use of the laptop contributes to wide fluctuations in her sleep-onset and wake schedule. Jane explained to Annie and her parents that the bright, blue-spectrum light Annie is exposed to while playing computer games before bed suppresses her body's ability to produce the melatonin needed for sleep (Cain and Gradisar 2010). Annie's parents were surprised by this and thought that would be a good place to start making changes.

Jane also explained that a regular bedtime routine would help improve Annie's overall ability to sleep. Jane suggested that, in place of computer games, they develop a bedtime routine involving getting ready for bed, then listening to soft music for 20 minutes before the lights are turned out. Jane also showed Annie's parents an electronic software program that can be downloaded to reduce the intensity of blue-spectrum light exposure Annie received from her laptop in the evenings (see Appendix 9.1). Annie and her parents also worked through the games and information on the Sleep for Kids website (see Appendix 9.1), which Annie shared with her classmates at school as well. Annie's mother decided to change her routine so that she no longer took Annie to the grocery store late in the evening. That way Annie had a more consistent bedtime and was not exposed to arousing sounds and lights close to the time she needed to sleep. Annie and her dad also planned monthly trips to the library to stock up on story books they could read together instead of watching a television show before bed.

A further measure that Jane suggested was the use of gentle massage to help with Annie's comfort and anxiety before bed. Jane showed Annie's parents some massage techniques, which they began to incorporate into her music. Annie and her parents looked for sleep massage books online and found *Lullaby Massage* (Hart 2009), which they liked. They also found a book called *What to Do When You Dread Your Bed* (Huebner 2008) which Annie described as 'exceptional!'

Bedtime positioning required some trial and error, but Jane and Annie were able to problem-solve their way to a comfortable and neutral position that Annie could maintain throughout the night. Jane took photos of the ideal position and left them with Annie's parents so they were able to help comfortably position her each night before bed. While Annie's flexion contractures persisted, her pain was significantly reduced, and this, in turn, helped to calm her anxiety about sleep.

Over the following weeks Annie, her parents and Jane all began to notice a difference. Annie was more focused and alert during sessions, and she reported no longer feeling the need to nap after school. Not only did Annie's piano playing improve, but her school grades also went up. Annie invited Jane to the school's talent show to hear her play as proof of how much better she was feeling.

9.7 Conclusion

This chapter provides occupational therapists with the basic knowledge and resources to identify children at risk of sleep deficiency, an introduction to evidence-based non-pharmacological sleep interventions for children and guidance about when to consult other team members. By considering sleep as a dynamic system with highly interrelated volitional, habituation, performance capacity and environmental components, therapists can apply their core occupational therapy process skills to effecting pragmatic and meaningful change for children with sleep problems and their families.

Key points

- Sleep is a lifelong occupation, and taking sleep hygiene measures can be both preventative and part of the management strategy for existing sleep problems. Where there are problems, early intervention can make a significant contribution to future health, well-being and productivity.

- Basic sleep-screening questions should be incorporated into paediatric assessments regardless of the reason for referral.

- Pragmatic, cost-effective, standardized screening and assessment tools are available. Providing parents and children with sleep education first will help them to take an active, self-management role.

- Sleep hygiene with particular focus on light exposure, activity, temperature and sound should be addressed first before moving, if needed, to more demanding behavioural-change strategies.

Note

1   Schlaffragebogen für Kinder mit Neurologischen und Anderen Komplexen Erkrankungen = Sleep questionnaire for children with severe psychomotor impairment.

Appendix 9.1 Resources for managing sleep problems
Organizations
- American Academy of Sleep Medicine (www.aasmnet.org)
- Autism Treatment Network, *Strategies to Improve Sleep in Children with Autism Spectrum Disorders: A Parent Guide* (www.autismspeaks.org/science/resources-programs/autism-treatment-network/tools-you-can-use/sleep-tool-kit)
- British Sleep Society (www.sleepsociety.org.uk)
- Canadian Sleep Association (www.canadiansleepsociety.ca)

- FASD Sleep and Research Project, University of British Columbia, Canada, Resources for working with children with FASD (www.chroniccare4sleep.org/Clinical%20Tools.html)
- National Association of School Psychologists (UK) (www.nasponline.org/resources/health_wellness/sleepdisorders_ho.aspx)
- National Health Services (UK) (www.nhs.uk/livewell/childrenssleep/pages/childrens sleephome.aspx)
- National Sleep Foundation (US) (www.sleepfoundation.org)

Assessment tools

- BEARS (accessible free at www.meritsleep.com/Web_Data/bears%20screen%20tool%20 (peds)%2020090721.pdf)
- Children's Sleep Habits Questionnaire (CSHQ; the abbreviated CSHQ can be downloaded with instructions free at www.education.uci.edu/childcare/pdf/questionnaire_interview/ Childrens%20Sleep%20Habits%20Questionnaire.pdf)
- Sleep Disturbance Scale for Children (can be accessed free at www.julielowmd.com/Sleep_ Disturbances_Scale_for_Children.pdf, or search 'Sleep Disturbance Scale for Children')
- SNAKE: Parental report questionnaire for children with severe psychomotor impairment (available in the appendix of Blankenburg *et al.* 2013; full citation in list of references)

Resources for parents and therapists

- Canadian Pediatric Society co-sleeping information (www.cps.ca/en/documents/ position/safe-sleep-environments-infants-children)
- *Encyclopedia on Early Childhood Development* (www.child-encyclopedia.com/en-ca/child-sleeping-behaviour/what-can-be-done.html)
- F.Lux: downloadable blue-spectrum light filter for computers (http://stereopsis.com/flux)
- National Health Service co-sleeping information (UK) (www.nhs.uk/conditions/ pregnancy-and-baby/pages/sleep-problems-in-children.aspx#close)
- Sleep for Kids (www.sleepforkids.org/html/learn.html)
- SleepRight: evidence-based sleep resources and information for children with physical and mental health problems (www.sleepright.ualberta.ca)

All websites were accessed in May 2014.

Books

Culbert, T. and Kajander, R. (2007) *Be the Boss of Your Sleep.* Minneapolis, MN: Free Spirit Publishing.

Durand, V.M. (2008a) *When Children Don't Sleep Well: Interventions for Pediatric Sleep Disorders: Parent Workbook.* New York, NY: Oxford University Press.

Durand, V.M. (2008b). *When Children Don't Sleep Well: Interventions for Pediatric Sleep Disorders: Therapist Guide.* New York, NY: Oxford University Press.

Hart, S. (2009) *Lullaby Massage: Rhyme and Touch Massage for Infants and Children.* Amarillo, TX: Hale Publishing.

Owens, J.A. and Mindell, J.A. (2005) *Take Charge of Your Child's Sleep: The All-in-One Resource for Solving Sleep Problems in Kids and Teens.* New York, NY: Marlow.

Shapiro, L.E. (2008) *It's Time to Sleep in Your Own Bed.* Oakland, CA: New Harbinger Publications Inc.

References

Ancoli-Israel, S., Cole, R., Alessi, C., Chambers, M., Moorcroft, W. and Pollak, C.P. (2003) 'The role of actigraphy in the study of sleep and circadian rhythms.' *Sleep 26,* 3, 342–392.

Berglund, B., Lindvall, T. and Schwela, D.H. (1999) *Guidelines for Community Noise.* Geneva: World Health Organization. Available at http://whqlibdoc.who.int/hq/1999/a68672.pdf, accessed on 23 September 2013.

Blankenburg, M., Tietze, A.L., Hechler, T., Hirschfeld, G. *et al.* (2013) 'Snake: the development and validation of a questionnaire on sleep disturbances in children with severe psychomotor impairment.' *Sleep Medicine 14,* 4, 339–351.

Brown, C.A., Kuo, M., Phillips, L., Berry, R. and Tan, M. (2013) 'Non-pharmacological sleep interventions for youth with chronic health conditions: a critical review of the methodological quality of the evidence.' *Disability and Rehabilitation 35,* 15, 1221–1255.

Brown, C., Swedlove, F., Berry, R. and Turlapati, L. (2012) 'Occupational therapists' health literacy interventions for children with disordered sleep and/or pain.' *New Zealand Journal of Occupational Therapy 59,* 2, 9–17.

Bruni, O., Ottaviano, S., Guidetti, V., Romoli, M. *et al.* (1996) 'The Sleep Disturbance Scale for Children (SDSC). Construction and validation of an instrument to evaluate sleep disturbances in childhood and adolescence.' *Journal of Sleep Research 5,* 4, 251–261.

Burns, C.E. (2009) 'Sleep and Rest.' In C.E. Burns, M.A. Brady, A.M. Dunn, C.G. Blosser and N.B. Starr (eds) *Pediatric Primary Care: A Handbook for Nurse Practitioners,* 4th edn. St Louis, MO: Saunders.

Cain, N. and Gradisar, M. (2010) 'Electronic media use and sleep in school-aged children and adolescents: a review.' *Sleep Medicine 11,* 8, 735–742.

Davis, K.F. and Owens, J.A. (2011) 'Sleep Disorders in Children.' In A.Y. Avidan and P.C. Zee (eds) *Handbook of Sleep Medicine,* 2nd edn. Philadelphia, PA: Lippincott Williams & Wilkins.

de Miguel-Díez, J., Villa-Asensi, J.R. and Alvarez-Sala, J.L. (2003) 'Prevalence of sleep-disordered breathing in children with Down syndrome: polygraphic findings in 108 children.' *Sleep 26,* 8, 1006–1009.

Durand, V.M. (2008a) *When Children Don't Sleep Well: Interventions for Pediatric Sleep Disorders: Parent Workbook.* New York, NY: Oxford University Press.

Durand, V.M. (2008b) *When Children Don't Sleep Well: Interventions for Pediatric Sleep Disorders: Therapist Guide.* New York, NY: Oxford University Press.

Durand, M.J., Gernert-Dott, P. and Mapstone, E. (1996) 'Treatment of sleep disorders in children with developmental disabilities.' *Journal of the Association for Persons with Severe Handicaps 21,* 3, 114–122.

Fjeldsted, B. and Hanlon-Dearman, A. (2009) 'Sensory processing and sleep challenges in children with fetal alcohol spectrum disorder.' *Occupational Therapy Now 11*, 5, 26–28.

Franklin, L., Deitz, J., Jirikowic, T. and Astley, S. (2008) 'Children with fetal alcohol spectrum disorders: problem behaviors and sensory processing.' *American Journal of Occupational Therapy 62*, 3, 265–273.

Gasparini, G., Saponaro, G., Rinaldo, F.M., Boniello, R. *et al.* (2012) 'Clinical evaluation of obstructive sleep apnea in children.' *Journal of Craniofacial Surgery 23*, 2, 387–391.

Givan, D.C. (2004) 'The sleepy child.' *Pediatric Clinics of North America 51*, 1, 15–31.

Goldman, S.E., Richdale, A.L., Clemons, T. and Marlow, B.A. (2012) 'Parental sleep concerns in autism spectrum disorders: variations from childhood to adolescence.' *Journal of Autism and Developmental Disorders 42*, 4, 531–538.

Goodlin-Jones, B.L., Tang, K., Liu, J. and Anders, T.F. (2008) 'Sleep patterns in preschool-age children with autism, developmental delay, and typical development.' *Journal of the American Academy of Child and Adolescent Psychiatry 47*, 8, 930–938.

Gooley, J.J., Chamberlain, K., Smith, K.A., Khalsa, S.B.S. *et al.* (2011) 'Exposure to room light before bedtime suppresses melatonin onset and shortens melatonin duration in humans.' *Journal of Clinical Endocrinology and Metabolism 96*, 3, E463–E472.

Grigg-Damberger, M. (2004) 'Neurologic disorders masquerading as pediatric sleep problems.' *Pediatric Clinics of North America 51*, 1, 89–115.

Hart, S. (2009) *Lullaby Massage: Rhyme and Touch Massage for Infants and Children.* Amarillo, TX: Hale Publishing.

Huebner, D. (2008) *What to Do When You Dread Your Bed.* Washington, DC: Magination Press.

Jirikowic, T., Olson, H.C. and Kartin, D. (2008) 'Sensory processing, school performance, and adaptive behavior of young school-age children with fetal alcohol spectrum disorders.' *Physical and Occupational Therapy in Pediatrics 28*, 2, 117–136.

Jones, C.H.D. and Ball, H.L. (2012) 'Medical Anthropology and Children's Sleep: The Mismatch Between Western Lifestyles and Sleep Physiology.' In A. Green and A. Westcombe (eds) *Sleep: Multiprofessional Perspectives.* London: Jessica Kingsley Publishers.

Kielhofner, G. (2008) *Model of Human Occupation: Theory and Application*, 4th edn. Philadelphia, PA: Lippincott Williams & Wilkins.

Lack, L.C., Gradisar, M., Van Someren, E.J., Wright, H.R. and Lushington, K. (2008) 'The relationship between insomnia and body temperatures.' *Sleep Medicine Reviews 12*, 4, 307–317.

Lee, K.A. and Ward, T.M. (2005) 'Critical components of a sleep assessment for clinical practice settings.' *Issues in Mental Health Nursing 26*, 7, 739–750.

Lewandowski, A.S., Toliver-Sokol, M. and Palermo, T.M. (2011) 'Evidence-based review of subjective pediatric sleep measures.' *Journal of Pediatric Psychology 36*, 7, 780–793. Available at www.ncbi.nlm.nih.gov/pmc/articles/PMC3146754, accessed on 3 December 2014.

Liu, X., Liu, L., Owens, J.A. and Kaplan, D.L. (2005) 'Sleep patterns and sleep problems among schoolchildren in the United States and China.' *Pediatrics 115*, Suppl. 1, S241–S249.

Lumeng, J.C. and Chervin, R.D. (2008) 'Epidemiology of pediatric obstructive sleep apnea.' *Proceedings of the American Thoracic Society 5*, 2, 242–252.

Marcus, C.L., Radcliffe, J., Konstantinopoulou, S., Beck, S.E. *et al.* (2012) 'Effects of positive airway pressure therapy on neurobehavioral outcomes in children with obstructive sleep apnea.' *American Journal of Respiratory and Critical Care Medicine 185*, 9, 998–1003.

Meadows, R. (2012) 'Beyond Death's Counterfeit: The Sociological Aspects of Sleep.' In A. Green and A. Westcombe (eds) *Sleep: Multiprofessional Perspectives.* London: Jessica Kingsley Publishers.

Meltzer, L.J., Johnson, C., Crosette, J., Ramos, M. and Mindell, J.A. (2010) 'Prevalence of diagnosed sleep disorders in pediatric primary care practices.' *Pediatrics 125*, 6, e1410–e1418.

Meltzer, L.J. and Mindell, J.A. (2006) 'Sleep and sleep disorders in children and adolescents.' *Psychiatric Clinics of North America 29*, 4, 1059–1076.

Millman, R.P., The Working Group on Sleepiness in Adolescents/Young Adults, and AAP Committee on Adolescence (2005) 'Excessive sleepiness in adolescents and young adults: causes, consequences, and treatment strategies.' *Pediatrics 115*, 6, 1774–1786.

Mindell, J.A., Kuhn, B., Lewin, D.S., Meltzer, L.J. and Sadeh, A. (2006) 'Behavioral treatment of bedtime problems and night wakings in infants and young children.' *Sleep 29*, 10, 1263–1276.

Mindell, J.A. and Owens, J.A. (2009) *A Clinical Guide to Pediatric Sleep: Diagnosis and Management of Sleep Problems*, 2nd edn. Philadelphia, PA: Lippincott Williams & Wilkins.

Mindell, J.A., Telofski, L.S., Wiegand, B. and Kurtz, E.S. (2009) 'A nightly bedtime routine: impact on sleep in young children and maternal mood.' *Sleep 32*, 5, 599–606.

Moore, M. (2012) 'Behavioral sleep problems in children and adolescents.' *Journal of Clinical Psychology in Medical Settings 19*, 1, 77–83.

Morgenthaler, T.I., Owens, J., Alessi, C., Boehlecke, B. *et al.* (2006) 'Practice parameters for behavioral treatment of bedtime problems and night wakings in infants and young children.' *Sleep 29*, 10, 1277–1281.

Narang, I. and Mathew, J.L. (2012) 'Childhood obesity and obstructive sleep apnea.' *Journal of Nutrition and Metabolism*, Article ID 134202. Available at http://dx.doi.org/10.1155/2012/134202, accessed on 21 October 2014.

Newman, C.J., O'Regan, M. and Hensey, O. (2006) 'Sleep disorders in children with cerebral palsy.' *Developmental Medicine and Child Neurology 48*, 7, 564–568.

Owens, J.A. (2005) 'The ADHD and sleep conundrum: a review.' *Journal of Developmental & Behavioral Pediatrics 26*, 4, 312–322.

Owens, J.A. (2009) 'A clinical overview of sleep and attention-deficit/hyperactivity disorder in children and adolescents.' *Journal of the Canadian Academy of Child and Adolescent Psychiatry 18*, 2, 92–102.

Owens, J.A. (2011) 'Update in pediatric sleep medicine.' *Current Opinion in Pulmonary Medicine 17*, 6, 425–430.

Owens, J.A. and Dalzell, V. (2005) 'Use of the "BEARS" sleep screening tool in a pediatric residents' continuity clinic: a pilot study.' *Sleep Medicine 6*, 1, 63–69.

Owens, J.A., Palermo, T.M. and Rosen, C.L. (2002) 'Overview of current management of sleep disturbances in children. II. Behavioral interventions.' *Current Therapeutic Research 63*, Suppl. B, B38–B52.

Owens, J.A., Spirito, A. and McGuinn, M. (2000) 'The Children's Sleep Habits Questionnaire (CSHQ): psychometric properties of a survey instrument for school-aged children.' *Sleep 23*, 8, 1043–1051.

Ponsonby, A.-L., Dwyer, T., Trevillian, L., Kemp, A. *et al.* (2004) 'The bedding environment, sleep position, and frequent wheeze in childhood.' *Pediatrics 113*, 5, 1216–1222.

Reynolds, S., Lane, S.J. and Thacker, L. (2012) 'Sensory processing, physiological stress, and sleep behaviors in children with and without autism spectrum disorders.' *OTJR: Occupation, Participation and Health 32*, 1, 246–257.

Rodriguez, A.J. (2007) 'Pediatric sleep and epilepsy.' *Current Neurology and Neuroscience Reports 7*, 4, 342–347.

Romeijn, N., Verweij, I.M., Koeleman, A., Mooij, A. *et al.* (2012) 'Cold hands, warm feet: sleep deprivation disrupts thermoregulation and its association with vigilance.' *Sleep 35*, 12, 1673–1683.

Sadeh, A. (2011) 'The role and validity of actigraphy in sleep medicine: an update.' *Sleep Medicine Reviews 15*, 4, 259–267.

Sadeh, A., Mindell, J.A., Luedtke, K. and Wiegand, B. (2009) 'Sleep and sleep ecology in the first 3 years: a web-based study.' *Journal of Sleep Research 18*, 1, 60–73.

Simard-Tremblay, E., Constantin, E., Gruber, R., Brouillette, R.T. and Shevell, M. (2011) 'Sleep in children with cerebral palsy: a review.' *Journal of Child Neurology 26*, 10, 1303–1310.

Weiss, K.E. and Corkum, P. (2012) 'Pediatric behavioural insomnia –"good night, sleep tight" for child and parent.' *Insomnia Rounds 1*, 5. Available at http://css-scs.ca/downloadfolder/150-005_Eng.pdf, accessed on 13 October 2014.

Wong, M.M., Brower, K.J. and Zucker, R.A. (2009) 'Childhood sleep problems, early onset of substance use and behavioral problems in adolescence.' *Sleep Medicine 10*, 7, 787–796.

Wood, B., Rea, M.S., Plitnick, B. and Figueiro, M.G. (2013) 'Light level and duration of exposure determine the impact of self-luminous tablets on melatonin suppression.' *Applied Ergonomics 44*, 2, 237–240.

Wynn, N. and Wickham, J. (2009) 'Night-time positioning for children with postural needs: What is the evidence to inform best practice?' *British Journal of Occupational Therapy 72*, 12, 543–550.

10

OLDER ADULTS' SLEEP

Julie Boswell, Jennifer Thai and Cary Brown

10.1 Introduction: sleep in the ageing population

The prevalence of sleep problems in older adults (65 years and older) is cited as between 30 and 43% and appears to be even higher in those living with co-morbidities (Ancoli-Israel 2009). Studies have demonstrated that older adults commonly experience a decrease in total sleep time and sleep quality (Cole and Richards 2007). Decreases in sleep quantity and quality are largely associated with natural changes in sleep architecture* and the higher prevalence of medical co-morbidities in the ageing population (Cole and Richards 2007). Logically, this may not cause much concern for active, well, older adults; however, with increased co-morbidities and advanced age the ability to remain resilient in spite of sleep problems can be compromised. This chapter focuses primarily on the sleep issues of older adults with multiple co-morbidities who are most vulnerable, least able to communicate their needs and present more complex intervention challenges to health care providers. (Problems relating specifically to dementia are discussed in Chapter 14.)

Sleep deficiency in older adults can hinder function and significantly impact quality of life. In older adults, poor sleep has been identified as a risk factor for morbidity, falls, diabetes, cardiovascular problems, depression, physical injury, increased use of medication, altered cognition, pain perception, certain dementias and poor psychosocial functioning (Cricco, Simonsick and Foley 2001; Foley *et al.* 2004; Lunde *et al.* 2010; St George *et al.* 2009; Stone, Ensrud and Ancoli-Israel 2008; Wolkove *et al.* 2007a). Furthermore, sleep problems can have a significant effect on participation in occupations, healthy routines and self-identity. Older adults are seldom referred to occupational therapy for sleep problems; however, sleep problems are so prevalent that therapists should be aware of basic sleep physiology, the relationship between sleep and ageing, and the importance of incorporating sleep-screening questions into assessments, regardless of the client's presenting condition.

This chapter presents contributing factors for sleep problems in older adults, reviews sleep assessment for older adults and presents a range of evidence-based non-pharmacological sleep interventions. At the end of the chapter there is an appendix of resources to provide further information. A case study (see Box 10.1) is provided to illustrate occupational therapy involvement in identifying and intervening in typically occurring older adult sleep problems.

During the course of adulthood there are naturally occurring changes that contribute to greater difficulty in achieving restorative sleep: an increase in non-rapid eye movement* stages N1* and N2* is seen while stage N3 decreases (see Chapter 3). Consequently, there is less of the deep sleep required for physiological healing and neurochemical production (Cole and Richards 2007). The production of sleep-inducing melatonin* also decreases with age, further altering circadian rhythms (Ancoli-Israel 2009). These changes in older adults typically lead to increased difficulty in initiating and maintaining sleep and in achieving sufficient restorative sleep. Additionally, older adults can develop early-to-bed–early-to-rise sleep patterns that, while adaptive in traditional agrarian societies, are problematic in more industrialized settings where social and leisure activities are often scheduled after the end of the workday (Ancoli-Israel 2009). It can be particularly difficult when older adults want to be involved in social activities with family members who are busy at work or school during the day. In this way early-to-bed patterns can unintentionally contribute to social isolation and diminished function and well-being.

Older adults often have coexisting ailments and use multiple medications which can contribute to or compound sleep deficiency (Cooke and Ancoli-Israel 2006; Foley *et al.* 2004; Song *et al.* 2010). Sleep disruption and co-morbid conditions often assume a bidirectional relationship such that many health conditions interfere with restorative sleep while, at the same time, non-restorative sleep is a risk factor for numerous adverse health conditions (Cole and Richards 2007).

The most common sleep problem experienced by older adults is the same as in younger persons: insomnia. Insomnia is characterized by difficulty falling asleep and/or maintaining sleep, or having poor sleep that affects daytime functioning (Wolkove *et al.* 2007b). Insomnia often manifests as restless nights, daytime fatigue and daytime napping, and can affect multiple domains of daily life including cognitive and physical ability, emotional management and mental health (Ancoli-Israel 2009). Insomnia is classified as *primary insomnia* or *secondary insomnia* and can be further categorized based on presenting features. As highlighted in Chapter 7, categorizing primary and secondary insomnia is somewhat problematic and there is some controversy. In general, primary insomnia is considered as an entity in its own right, as opposed to secondary insomnia which arises as a consequence of an existing circumstance (Wolkove *et al.* 2007a). For example, pain from illness or disturbed sleep as a side effect of specific medications can result in secondary insomnia. Secondary insomnia is suggested to be more prevalent than primary insomnia among the ageing population and is reported more in women than in men (Byles, Mishra and Harris 2005; Cricco *et al.* 2001; Nau *et al.* 2005). Insomnia affects multiple areas of functioning and a comprehensive assessment is necessary to determine what factors are interfering with the client's ability to have restful and restorative sleep.

10.2 The role of occupational therapy

Occupational therapists should aim to incorporate basic sleep-screening questions into all assessment regardless of the reason for referral. Although sleep disturbances are experienced by 40–65% of community-living older adults and an estimated 80% of those living in institutions, primary care physicians do not often ask patients about sleep (Ancoli-Israel 2009). A 2012 survey of over 2000 Canadian health care professionals specializing in older adult care found that very few were aware of sleep assessment tools or the range of evidence-based non-pharmacological sleep interventions appropriate for this group (Brown *et al.* 2014). Additionally, as many as 70% of all adults with insomnia do not discuss their poor sleep with a health care professional (Reeve and Bailes 2010). Reeve and Bailes (2010) suggest that this reluctance to seek help results in reduced likelihood of early detection of sleep-related medical conditions, increased risk of self-medicating with alcohol and over-the-counter remedies, and ultimately may exacerbate existing sleep problems. Other researchers have also noted this reluctance to seek medical help for sleep problems and similar forms of self-medication (Ellis, Hampson and Cropley 2007; Morin *et al.* 1993; Venn and Arber 2012).

Falls prevention programmes are an example of one area of practice where occupational therapists could, and should, integrate basic sleep screening and apply their knowledge of the bidirectional relationship between sleep and other health conditions that affect mobility. Falls often result in functional impairments and diminished well-being. Falls are well documented to be associated with sleep disturbances and sleep problems are an identified risk factor for falls (St George *et al.* 2009; Stone *et al.* 2008). For example, in one study older adults experiencing poor sleep were found to be three times more likely to experience recurrent falls (St George *et al.* 2009). Fear of falling can cause avoidance of daily activities and consequently decrease an individual's functioning and quality of life. Additionally, fear of falling or the consequences of falling can exacerbate poor sleep because of pain, decreased daylight exposure, medication and altered environment (e.g. hospitalization or decreased mobility in the home).

A recent study in Philadelphia found that older adults were unlikely to discuss their sleep problems with physicians and most commonly used watching television, listening to the radio and reading to help them fall asleep. Nearly half of the participants had used alcohol or over-the-counter sleeping aids at some point to manage their sleep deficiency (Gooneratne *et al.* 2011). Many participants (40.1%) reported using pain medication to help them sleep and stated that prescription medication that was specifically intended for sleep was the most effective. The authors pointed out that many medications can have side effects and can contain caffeine, which has detrimental effects on the sleep and health of older adults. Although pharmacological intervention can be beneficial for managing short-term insomnia in some instances, the risk of side effects and negative functional consequences can be significant. A recent study of long-term care facility residents found that the side effects of non-benzodiazepine sleep medication included decreased mobility and increased risk of falls and fractures (Berry *et al.* 2013). Other authorities in the field have identified that night-time wandering, impaired cognitive functioning, confusion, anxiety, depression, excessive sedation and daytime fatigue are also potential side effects (Ancoli-Israel 2009). Medication side effects can also be compounded by environmental factors. For example, night-time noise and staff activity in long-term care facilities can serve to further disorient a resident experiencing confusion as a medication side effect. Environmental factors are often simple to modify and should be considered when addressing medication regimes. (The influence of the environment is discussed in depth later in this chapter and in greater detail in Chapter 18.) Additional factors that can compound some sleep medications' negative side effects include daytime fatigue, diminished attention and poor memory as well as decreased activity and participation in daily activities. Finally, some older adults' use of alcohol as a sleep aid separately or in conjunction with medication can present a further sleep challenge, decrease cognitive acuity and increase the risk of adverse medication interactions (Gooneratne *et al.* 2011).

Non-pharmacological sleep interventions should be employed even when sleep medication is indicated (David *et al.* 2010; Reeve and Bailes 2010). Non-pharmacological approaches may also correspond better with older adults' belief systems. For example, Venn and Arber (2012) found that study participants aged 65 years and older believed that relying on sleep medication was a form of addiction and thus immoral. They also found that those who took sleep medication often felt a diminished sense of control. Researchers propose that health care providers' apparent lack of awareness about evidence-based non-pharmacological alternatives contributes to the underuse of these pragmatic interventions (Brown *et al.* 2013; Gooneratne *et al.* 2011; Nau *et al.* 2005).

10.3 Factors affecting sleep occupational performance

Sleep involves multiple, interacting biopsychosocial components. One way that can help occupational therapists organize their understanding and intervention so as to make the best use of the opportunities afforded by a complex biopsychosocial system like sleep is by applying the Model of Human Occupation (MoHO) (Kielhofner 2008). This model can be used to frame the relationship between sleep, occupational performance and well-being. The case study of Mrs Wilson (introduced in Box 10.1) illustrates the application of the MoHO to sleep and is discussed in more detail below.

BOX 10.1 Case study: part 1

Mrs Wilson is a 79-year-old woman who lives with her husband in a three-bedroom home that they have owned for the past 50 years. She has three children (and four grandchildren) who have moved to different cities across the country. Mrs Wilson has been referred to occupational therapy by her family physician for a home assessment due to recent falls. During the home visit Mrs Wilson reports that in the past year, her energy and ability to concentrate have significantly declined. She says that even with drinking coffee and taking a nap, she barely has enough energy to make it through the day. The therapist notes that Mrs Wilson looks upset as she states that recently she's really been feeling her age. She says that she used to be active, lively and social, but now she is not.

Mrs Wilson shows the therapist around her house. In the bedroom, the bedside table has several coffee mugs, medication bottles, newspapers, a book, a television remote control and a plate. Her bed has numerous pillows and three blankets. There is a space heater on Mrs Wilson's side of the bed and a fan on her husband's side. There are thin curtains covering the window that overlooks a busy street. On the dresser, there is a television and a telephone. The therapist decides she should investigate further to see if poor sleep may be contributing to Mrs Wilson's falls and decreased well-being. The therapist decides to follow this up in more detail at the next visit.

Components of the Model of Human Occupation

Volition

Volition is the subsystem of the MoHO that relates to the drive or motivation of an individual to participate in an activity. The volitional domain contributes to decision-making leading to action or inaction (Kielhofner 2008). To engage with Mrs Wilson around volition the occupational therapist would explore her interests, values and the activities that might relate to unhealthy sleep practices. Older adults, in the same manner as everyone else, may disregard the effects of poor sleep or unfavourable sleep habits in favour of other activities such as late-night television viewing and decreased daytime activity.

The therapist would also explore sleep self-efficacy with Mrs Wilson: Does she feel like she has any control in her sleep practices? Does she become frustrated and anxious when bedtime approaches because she feels insomnia is inevitable? Does she avoid going to bed at a set bedtime and stay up until she falls asleep on the couch?

The culture and social values of industrialized countries can also contribute to the prevalent, but incorrect, belief that sleep problems are just a part of ageing and there is nothing to be done (Ellis *et al.* 2007; Morin *et al.* 1993; Venn, Meadows and Arber 2013). The social undervaluing of sleep may cause people to dismiss the issue, delay seeking help, or attempt to self-treat; however, the ability to practise one's values and maintain control over one's life can be a significant motivation for addressing sleep problems. Venn and Arber (2012) found that older adults delayed seeking help for disrupted sleep until the point where it interfered with their ability to maintain independence and autonomy in their lives. Like people in other age groups, older adults' restorative sleep is highly influenced by their own sleep practices. To establish sleep-supporting practices older adults need both the information and the motivation to guide their decision-making. Occupational therapists should remember that changing long-standing sleep practices is not easy, and learning new techniques to promote better sleep takes time and support. Because change is motivated by values and beliefs, volition can play a significant role in any sleep management strategy.

Habituation

Habits are behaviour patterns formed through repetition that eventually become second nature in daily routine. Habituation is highly context dependent and affected by personal, social and cultural expectations (Kielhofner 2008). Habits can be a good indicator of health. For instance, Ohayon and Vecchierini (2005) found that a short sleep duration (less than 4.5 hours), late bedtime (after 1 a.m.), early waking time (before 5 a.m.), long sleep duration (greater than 9.5 hours) and long sleep onset latency* (greater than 80 minutes) were associated with poor health in older adults. Individuals may not intentionally engage in behaviours that have negative consequences for their sleep but, over time, habits can form which have significant implications for an older adult's ability to achieve restorative sleep.

Discussing habits and preferences with clients also provides insight into a person's sense of identity. As Kielhofner (2008) points out, most people develop sets of behaviours and habits that support their occupational performance needs and role demands. For example, in the case study (see Box 10.1 and 10.2), while Mrs Wilson was still in the workforce she woke up at 5 a.m., drank coffee throughout the day and worked long hours. In retirement, her habit of waking at 5 a.m. continued even though she did not need to follow a work schedule. Additionally, she began taking hour-long naps during the afternoon. Her husband was concerned that the long naps indicated that she was not well. Mrs Wilson declared, however, that she was not sick and, as a retiree, could finally rest when and how she pleases. Midday napping became habituated into her daily routine because of her belief that rest was part of retirement and the value she placed on having this autonomy over her daytime activities.

In order to maximize any intervention's success it is helpful for the therapist to first help the client understand basic sleep biology and science. When clients understand the scientific rationale for recommendations they are better able to generalize the information to other circumstances and assume more control for changes to promote their own healthy sleep habits and practices. Therapists should also consider the important influence that environmental cues and triggers have on the success or failure of behaviour change (Marteau, Hollands and Fletcher 2012). Older adults' beliefs and habits built over long periods of time may require careful attention to best support sleep-friendly changes. For example, older couples that have been sleeping in the same bed for the majority of their lives may be reluctant to try sleeping separately even though sharing a bed interferes with each other's sleep. Values related to marriage and social norms may be perceived as conflicting with the sleep-promoting choice of separate bedrooms. Participating in new sleep-promoting habits may become especially challenging for older adults when they are simultaneously adjusting to major life changes (e.g. life after retirement, moving to supportive housing, loss of a partner through divorce or death) (Wolkove *et al.* 2007b). To help clients establish and sustain sleep-supporting habits the therapist should consider including other family members in sleep education and problem-solving.

Performance capacity

Performance capacity is an individual's ability to execute the activities that make up occupation (Kielhofner 2008). The ability to execute activities involves objective components (i.e. performance of bodily systems) and subjective experiences. In older adults symptoms associated with certain conditions (such as arthritis, dementia, cancer, cardiopulmonary diseases, diabetes, mental health conditions, obstructive sleep apnoea and parkinsonism), or medications (such as antidepressants, beta-blockers, chemotherapy, analgesics, antipsychotics and blood pressure medications), can significantly contribute to sleep problems (Ancoli-Israel 2009); therefore, physical and psychiatric diagnoses, and effects of medication, should be assessed for their contribution to sleep disruption. For example, a common condition in older men and women is *nocturia* which is a frequent night-time waking caused by the need, or sensation of need, to pass urine (Wolkove *et al.* 2007a). Wolkove *et al.* (2007a) conclude from their review of the literature that nocturia frequently leads to disordered sleep, increased risk of falls, daytime fatigue and decreased health-related quality of life. They also point out that obstructive sleep apnoea (OSA), more prevalent in the ageing population, males and people with obesity, is highly associated with nocturia.

OSA is characterized by a disruption of airflow during sleep due to the base of the tongue or the palate obstructing the airway and is associated with hypertension, stroke, ischaemic heart disease and non-restorative sleep. In addition, night-time blood oxygen desaturation, known as 'nocturnal oxygen desaturation', commonly occurs with OSA. Chronic desaturation is associated with cognitive impairment in older adults (Wolkove *et al.* 2007a). Researchers repeatedly comment that OSA is under-diagnosed (Ancoli-Israel 2009; Punjabi 2008) and particularly in the older adult population (Bombois *et al.* 2010). Also older adults may not seek assessment and treatment for OSA because the features of OSA (fatigue, daytime drowsiness, decreased concentration and morning headache) may be mistaken for those of other common conditions such as cardiac problems and diabetes. Consequently, many treatable cases of OSA go undiagnosed and untreated. Sleep companions may be the best source of information and often report hearing loud snoring followed by periods of silence. Continuous positive airway pressure (CPAP) is generally used to treat clinically significant OSA, but for some older adults the CPAP mask is uncomfortable, too complex to use or a nuisance (Wolkove *et al.* 2007a). Occupational therapists can play a role in helping clients with OSA to problem-solve around these comfort issues. For example, an older adult (and possibly the spouse) may need additional help in breaking down the steps in caring for the equipment so that the task is less daunting.

These medical conditions and OSA are examples of only a few of the many physiological age-related changes that threaten sleep quality and quantity such that an older adult's sleep-wake cycle becomes out of synchronization with the individual's environment (Ancoli-Israel 2009). For example, in the case study Mrs Wilson tells the therapist that she often experiences early awakenings (between 3 and 5 a.m.) and she believes this is related to arthritic aches and pains. Waking this early can cause discord in scheduling for the rest of the day and Mrs Wilson now needs to rest mid-afternoon to manage the feeling of tiredness she experiences.

Emotional well-being also contributes to performance capacity and healthy sleep. Issues that are common to older adults include spousal death, retirement and social isolation. These factors also increase the risk for depression which, as mentioned previously, is highly associated with insomnia (Wolkove *et al.* 2007a).

Older adults in institutional settings commonly experience sleep disturbances that can be attributed to the organizational and physical environment. The organizational environment includes matters relating to policies and procedures such as cleaning schedules, meal times and night-time toileting routines that can to a great extent negatively affect a resident's ability to have proper sleep (AMDA 2007). Features of the physical environment that commonly interfere with restorative sleep include light, noise, temperature, air quality and sleeping equipment (e.g. bed, pillows, blankets). Because bright, blue-light exposure, activity, noise and temperature are critical variables in effective sleep, therapists should consider these features of the environment to be of primary importance for evaluation and remediation. Evidence-based guidelines for designing effective institutional sleep environments for sound (Berglund, Lindvall and

Schwela 1999) and light (Society of Light and Lighting 2008) exist, and occupational therapists should work in consultation with architects and design engineers to achieve effective outcomes. Several organizations around the world focus on developing best practice guidelines to assist in institutional design promoting more effective sleep. These organizations include the Society of Light and Lighting in the UK and the Centre for Health Design in the US (see Appendix 10.1 and Chapter 18 for more discussion).

10.4 Assessing sleep in older adults

Sleep assessments and tools to identify beliefs, habits and behaviours that interfere with sleep are not, in themselves, age specific; however, older adults often have more complex sleep problems as a consequence of the increasing co-morbidities and changing life circumstances that accompany ageing. This section reviews some of the widely used and accessible assessment tools that may be of use to occupational therapists. New tools are constantly in development and therapists should check periodically for these emergent resources.

The prevalent, but inaccurate, belief in industrialized societies is that poor sleep is the norm for older adults and that there is nothing that can be done. Consequently, therapists should not assume clients will initiate discussion of sleep-related problems. Rather, occupational therapy assessments for all conditions should include one or two basic screening questions to determine whether the client feels his or her sleep is restorative or whether they feel there are any sleep-related problems. The responses may then prompt additional information gathering (for example, the 12 sleep-history questions listed in the 'Sleep history' section below). Responses to this more detailed information may, in turn, trigger a formal assessment and/or referral to another health care provider. In the case study, for example, when the occupational therapist asked Mrs Wilson about her sleep she stated, 'No one has ever asked me about sleep before. I just assume I have to put up with all this up and down at night. I would be so happy if there was something that could be done to help.' Based on this information the therapist was able to develop a more formal assessment plan.

Common assessment tools

The following section gives a brief introduction to the most common and accessible tools to assess components of sleep in various domains. No single tool addresses all of the biopsychosocial domains, and therapists would benefit from being familiar with the options most relevant to their client's context and occupational performance needs.

Glasgow Sleep Impact Index

The Glasgow Sleep Impact Index (GSII) is similar to the Canadian Occupational Performance Measure (Law *et al.* 1992) that many occupational therapists use in daily practice. The GSII, however, is designed for interdisciplinary use and specifically for sleep issues (Kyle *et al.* 2013).

Abbreviated version of the Dysfunctional Beliefs and Attitudes about Sleep Scale

The brief version of the Dysfunctional Beliefs and Attitudes about Sleep Scale (DBAS-16) consists of 16 statements about sleep and the client self-reports how strongly they agree or disagree with each item on a scale of 1 to 10 (Morin, Vallières and Ivers 2007).

Nocturia, Nocturnal Enuresis and Sleep-interruption Questionnaire (NNES-Q)

The Nocturia, Nocturnal Enuresis and Sleep-interruption Questionnaire (NNES-Q) is a brief assessment that looks at the severity and impact of nocturia (see Appendix 10.1 for details) (Bing *et al.* 2006).

Pittsburgh Sleep Quality Index

The Pittsburgh Sleep Quality Index (PSQI) is a psychometrically tested questionnaire with 19 self-report questions about duration, wakening and subjective perceptions of sleep quality, with five questions for the client's bed partner (if applicable) (Buysse *et al.* 1989). (See Chapter 8 for more details and Appendix 10.1 for the PSQI online version's URL.)

Actigraphy

Actigraphy uses a wristwatch-size monitor that records sleep/activity/light exposure data that are downloaded into a software program for analysis. Actigraphy reports incidence of wake after sleep onset and sleep efficiency (the percentage of time in bed actually spent asleep). Actigraphy also has clinical usefulness as a proxy measure of sleep latency (how long it takes to fall asleep once settled for the night); however, this is of course mediated by the accuracy of recording the time the patient settles in bed for the night and if the patient is able to sustain an unusually high degree of inactivity although still awake. While polysomnography* is considered to be the gold standard for assessment, actigraphy is more pragmatic and affordable within the occupational therapy clinic. Actigraphy has been used with increasing frequency with reliable results for older adults, including those with dementia (Beaudreau *et al.* 2008; Lunde *et al.* 2010).

Sleep diaries

There are numerous downloadable versions of sleep diaries for older adults or their caregivers to complete and therapists can do an internet search for one that has the relevant degree of detail for their client group. An example can be found on the How to Sleep Well as You Age website (Robinson, Kemp and Segal 2012 in Appendix 10.1). These self-report instruments are useful to identify patterns of variables that potentially impact restorative sleep as well as how clients perceive their sleep. These are both important dimensions of sleep that are not reflected in actigraphy and other standardized assessment tools.

Sleep history

A sleep history gathers information regarding sleep habits such as sleep onset, duration, frequency of night-time awakenings, timing of going to bed, aggravating or alleviating factors, medication, substance use and family history. Bloom *et al.* (2009, p.764) developed a list of sleep-related screening questions to guide health care workers in primary care:

1. What time do you normally go to bed at night and wake up in the morning?

2. Do you often have trouble falling asleep at night?

3. About how many times do you wake up at night?

4. If you do wake up during the night, do you usually have trouble falling back asleep?

5. Does your bed partner say (or are you aware) that you frequently snore, gasp for air, or stop breathing?

6. Does your bed partner say (or are you aware) that you kick or thrash about while asleep?

7. Are you aware that you ever walk, eat, punch, kick, or scream during sleep?

8. Are you sleepy or tired during much of the day?

9. Do you usually take one or more naps during the day?

10. Do you usually doze off without planning to during the day?

11. How much sleep do you need to feel alert and function well?

12. Are you currently taking any type of medication or other preparation to help you sleep?

Assessing the environment

Ideally the occupational therapist should conduct a home visit in order to observe the sleeping environment for its conduciveness to sleep. An alternative is to ask clients to provide digital images of their sleep environment and carry out basic readings of light, sound and temperature levels themselves or with the assistance of a family member. Lux (light intensity) and decibel levels (sound) can now be measured with smartphone apps, and a number of low-cost options that work with different operating systems are available. Lux and decibel level readings can be interpreted as acceptable or problematic by referring to existing standards for sound from the World Health Organization (Berglund *et al.* 1999) *Guidelines for Community Noise* and the 'Recommended Light Level' table in the online magazine *Engineering ToolBox* (see Appendix 10.1 for access details). The evidence-based rule of thumb is that sounds greater than 30 decibels can interfere with sleep and increase physiological arousal (Berglund *et al.* 1999), and light intensity at 30 lux and higher will suppress the production of the sleep-promoting hormone melatonin (Wood *et al.* 2013). The environment and aspects of occupational performance capacity can also be assessed during a thorough sleep history.

10.5 Interventions to promote healthy sleep in older adults

As previously discussed, occupational therapy can play an important role in recommending non-pharmacological sleep interventions to promote healthy sleep in older adults (Brown *et al.* 2013). Because environmental modifications are often the most pragmatic and least stressful changes for older adults and/or their caregivers to implement, it is appropriate to address these non-pharmacological sleep interventions first. (The URLs to resources are provided in Appendix 10.1.)

Environmental interventions

A growing number of non-pharmacological sleep interventions are documented in the literature and a critical review of the methodological quality of the evidence (Brown *et al.* 2013) found that there is the clearest evidence base for light-based therapies (Alessi *et al.* 2005; Ancoli-Israel *et al.* 2002; Burns *et al.* 2009; Skjerve, Bjorvatn and Holsten 2004; Riemersma-van der Lek *et al.* 2008; Sloane *et al.* 2007). Light-based therapy involves controlling the light in the environment such that persons are exposed to levels of at least 1000 lux (the equivalent of a cloudy day) during the daytime. Lighting of this intensity suppresses melatonin and facilitates the production of neurochemicals, such as serotonin, that promote alertness. Conversely, reducing light exposure in the evenings to less than 30 lux can be used to trigger the production of hormones such as melatonin and thus facilitate sleep. Light-exposure therapies can be designed using light boxes, natural daylight exposure and controlling the timing of exposure to blue-spectrum light from electronic devices such as televisions and computers.

Behavioural changes also mediate the effectiveness of environmental interventions. For example, increased daytime activity can contribute to increased daylight exposure. There is a moderate evidence base for the use of activity, such as walking and social groups, to promote daytime wakefulness (Richards *et al.* 2001, 2005). Integrating evening activities, such as bathing or using a hot water bottle, can also influence the physical environment to induce a sleep-supporting physiological response. Behaviours that modify the ambient temperature or core body temperature are important to sleep as seen in the research on passive body warming to promote sleep for clients with dementia (Mishima *et al.* 2005) and, to a lesser degree, Parkinson's disease (Rutten *et al.* 2012). Passive body warming involves using a warm bath, heating pad or other temporary heat source to artificially raise an individual's core temperature slightly about 60 minutes before bedtime. Because core-temperature cooling triggers feelings of sleepiness, when the heat source is removed core temperature drops and sleep may be more easily initiated. (More details about the evidence and use of the interventions can be found on the Sleep and Dementia Resources website listed in Appendix 10.1.)

Provision of pragmatic evidence-based environmental sleep interventions aligns well with occupational therapists' skills in activity analysis and environmental modification. The international group SomnIA compiled an overview of evidence-informed guidelines and illustrative examples of environmental changes that can be made in both community and institutional settings. (Their report can be accessed through the URL in Appendix 10.1.)

Sleep education

Occupational therapists can support their clients and their clients' caregivers or family members to make better-informed decisions and increase autonomy through providing evidence-based education. Various useful and accessible resources are available (see Appendix 10.1).

Sleep education can include information regarding co-morbidities, age-related changes, medication, sleep abnormalities, sleep hygiene and the importance of bedtime routines and schedule. In the ageing population, it is particularly important to incorporate medication education because of the high prevalence of polypharmacy and risk for adverse medication interactions and side effects. Methods of education should be tailored to clients' learning styles and abilities and, when possible, include family members. While information and understanding are critical components to adopting healthy behaviours, the physical and social environments are strong influences on habits; therefore, it is recommended to educate all household members so as to support good habits and behaviour change.

Sleep hygiene

Sleep hygiene refers to incorporating behaviours conducive to restorative sleep into a client's routine. There is no standard protocol for sleep hygiene and it is often used in conjunction with other interventions. Components of sleep hygiene may include, but are not limited to, physical activity, night-time rituals, sleep scheduling, reduced caffeine, nicotine and alcohol before bed, and controlling the light, sound and temperature in the sleep environment. (Sleep hygiene principles are discussed in more depth in Chapter 8 and therapists can also download sleep hygiene handouts designed with older adults in mind from the American Psychological Association and from the US Geriatric Mental Health Foundation.)

Cognitive behavioural therapy for insomnia

Cognitive behavioural therapy for insomnia (CBT-I) usually includes a number of components (see Chapter 8) including a focus on adapting thoughts, beliefs and cognitions that interfere with healthy sleep behaviours. Negative thoughts and subsequent behaviours can create stress for an individual, often making it even more difficult to fall asleep. For example, in Mrs Wilson's case, her belief that afternoon napping is a positive aspect of retirement is causing some discord between her and her husband and also leading to delayed bedtime with the consequence of feeling unrested and lethargic in the morning. In some studies (for example, Jacobs *et al.* 2004) CBT-I has been shown to be as effective as pharmacotherapy in achieving sleep onset in working-age adults.

Nocturia reduction and safety issues

Occupational therapists can provide information about what types of beverages are more likely to contribute to frequent awakenings because of acting as night-time diuretics and irritants to the bladder. (Information about foods and beverages that have an irritating effect on the bladder, such as asparagus, cabbage, grapes, caffeine and salt, can be found on the Cleveland Clinic website listed in Appendix 10.1.) If this is a significant issue, occupational therapists should work in consultation with a dietician to ensure that a sound dietary plan is developed. Occupational therapists can also help clients problem-solve about safety issues when waking at night. For example, clients may be in the habit of leaving a light on all night so they can safely navigate to the bathroom; however, this persistent light source can trigger suppression of melatonin and consequently interfere with restorative sleep. A sleep-friendly alternative would be to install a motion-activated nightlight that comes on only when the client is getting out of bed.

Obstructive sleep apnoea interventions

Sleep apnoea (discussed in more detail in Chapter 7) has significant health and quality-of-life consequences. Occupational therapists can assume a role in identification of possible sleep apnoea and in referring their clients for further investigation. Scott *et al.* (2003) highlight that the prevalent, but incorrect, societal belief that snoring is not an indication of a potentially serious underlying condition and that nothing can be done to address snoring, continues to dissuade persons from seeking treatment. This research-to-practice gap indicates that occupational therapists, as well as all team members, need to assume a more active role in screening for the possibility of apnoea. Reasons for adhering to continuous positive airway equipment and problem-solving to help clients maintain a side-lying position to reduce airway collapse during sleep can be discussed with older adults by occupational therapists. Simple pragmatic interventions, such as body pillows to support side lying, or having a small ball placed in a pocket sewn onto the back of a pyjamas top so that lying on the back is not comfortable, may be quite effective in helping some clients. (More details about positioning can be found on the University of Maryland Medical Center website; see Appendix 10.1.)

10.6 Summary and conclusion

This chapter reviews common sleep problems experienced by older adults and frames the complex nature of sleep within the occupational therapy Model of Human Occupation. The case study of Mrs Wilson, woven through the chapter and concluded in Box 10.2 below, illustrates the occupational process. A list of resources to assist the occupational therapist in assuming an active role in sleep problems with older adults is also provided. The small body of evidence for managing sleep-related problems experienced by older adults is growing rapidly. Currently, the evidence base is sufficiently strong so that occupational therapists can confidently apply their skills in environmental modification, activity, educational approaches and cognitive behavioural techniques to help manage sleep issues of older adults and their caregivers. Research and knowledge-exchange activities to develop non-pharmacological sleep interventions for older adults is an exciting new area, and the opportunities for occupational therapists to advance practice and clinical research in this area are extensive.

BOX 10.2 Case study: part 2

The occupational therapist identified sleep as a potential problem during her first visit to Mrs Wilson's home. Before she meets with Mrs Wilson again, the therapist prepares a list of screening questions to ask that will help her identify any patterns or changes of circumstance that may indicate the need for more formal assessment. The specific questions are as follows:

1. Does Mrs Wilson have any strategies intended to help reduce her fear of falling at night? Is she taking a sedating medication that could make her less alert when she gets up to toilet during the night? Does she leave lights on so that she feels safer at night but which also interfere with sound sleep?

2. Why was there a decline in her energy? Does Mrs Wilson report any changes to her sleep practices or patterns over that time? For example, in the past 3 years has there been a change to her routine, health or environment that could have negative sleep consequences?

3. How many caffeinated beverages does she drink a day and at what times?

4. When, and for how long, does she nap during the day?

5. What is her current sleep routine?

6. What are her beliefs regarding sleep? (The therapist plans to use the standardized Dysfunctional Beliefs and Attitudes about Sleep scale [Morin, Vallières and Ivers 2007] to gather this information.)

7. What medication does she take and when does she take it? (The therapist will review these medications to see if any influence sleep and alertness. What she finds may indicate the need for a referral to a clinical pharmacist or contacting Mrs Wilson's physician.)

8. Does she or her husband snore?

The therapist also recognizes some additional factors that may be contributing to poor sleep for Mrs Wilson:

- The extra blankets and heater may indicate the bedroom temperature is kept too high for her core body temperature to drop sufficiently to maintain effective sleep.

- The television, fan, heater and other electronics in the bedroom are all possible sources of disturbing noise at night.

- The number of activities on Mrs Wilson's night-table indicate she is not habituated to associate her bed with sleep.

- Pain or discomfort are indicated by medication bottles and the number of extra pillows.

- Light from the street, television and other electronics are sources of melatonin-suppressing blue-spectrum light.

The therapist identifies several possible adaptations to Mrs Wilson's sleep environment that could promote better sleep:

- Install a timer on the heater and television that will shut the electronics off after a certain amount of time to allow for sleep-promoting bedroom cooling and prevent ongoing blue-spectrum light exposure and noise from the television.

- Install thicker curtains to reduce light and noise.

- Purchase a supportive mattress and use wedges for positioning.

- Do leisure activities in the living room instead of the bed and do not go to bed until ready to go to sleep.

When the therapist discusses sleep problems with Mrs Wilson and how they may be related to her falls, she learns more about Mrs Wilson's sleep practices and beliefs. This information presents the therapist with an opportunity to introduce a number of small, pragmatic sleep-promoting changes to Mrs Wilson. Having many options allows Mrs Wilson to have more control and make healthy changes at her own pace and in ways that she sees as relevant to her own context. For example, Mrs Wilson likes to have a cup of tea while video chatting with her grandchildren before bed. She then has a second cup and a light snack while watching television in bed until she is tired enough to fall asleep. When the therapist said there was free software (stereopsis.com/flux) that would help filter melatonin-suppressing bright blue light from her computer screen when she video-chatted with her grandchildren, Mrs Wilson was keen to try this. She was also interested in using a timer to turn off the electronics when she went to sleep.

The therapist and Mrs Wilson made a plan to review a list of other sleep-promoting changes Mrs Wilson could make. They will discuss these changes at the next home visit. These strategies include:

- Learn more about how sleep changes with age and what people can do to promote better sleep.

- Consult the pharmacist about possible adverse drug interactions that could contribute to poor sleep, motivation and/or concentration.

- Create a regular bedtime routine and establish a set time to get up every day.

- Limit liquid consumption before bedtime and have decaffeinated beverages.

- Get as much natural light exposure during the day as possible and learn more about why this matters.

- Avoid watching television in the bedroom, especially before sleeping.

- Limit naps to no more than 30 minutes early in the day.

- Complete a sleep diary to monitor changes in sleep based on recommendations.

- With her grandchildren, play the online sleep awareness games on the Science: Human Body & Mind – Sleep, BBC interactive website (see Appendix 10.1). Mrs Wilson selected this activity so that the whole family could enjoy themselves while learning more about how to have healthy sleep.

Appendix 10.1 Further resources

- Age UK: insomnia and ageing plain-language article and podcast (Sept 2012; www.ageuk.org.uk/health-wellbeing/conditions-illnesses/getting-a-good-nights-sleep)

- American Academy of Sleep Medicine: *Practice Guidelines* (www.aasmnet.org/practiceguidelines.aspx)

- American Psychological Association: *Psychology Topics: Sleep* (www.apa.org/topics/sleep/why.aspx)

- Canadian Sleep Society: *Sleep in Older Adults* (http://giic.rgps.on.ca/files/sleep_aging.pdf)

- Carrier, J., LaFortune, M. and Drapeau, C. (2012) *Sleep in the Elderly: When to Reassure, When to Intervene. Insomnia Rounds* (http://css-scs.ca/downloadfolder/150-004_Eng.pdf)

- Centre for Health Design (US) (www.healthdesign.org)

- Cleveland Clinic: information about diuretic foods (http://my.clevelandclinic.org/disorders/overactive_bladder/hic_bladder_irritating_foods.aspx)

- College of Occupational Therapists' free resource, 'Living well through activity in care homes: the toolkit' (www.cot.co.uk/living-well-care-homes)

- Joseph Rowntree Foundation: *Supporting Older People in Care Homes at Night* (www.jrf.org.uk/sites/files/jrf/night-care-older-people.pdf)

- Nocturia, Nocturnal Enuresis and Sleep-interruption Questionnaire (NNES-Q) (www.urosource.com/fileadmin/user_upload/european_urology/PIIS0302283805008328.pdf)

- Pittsburgh Sleep Quality Index: University of Pittsburgh Sleep Medicine Institute (www.sleep.pitt.edu)

- Recommended Lighting Levels (*Engineering Tool Box*; www.engineeringtoolbox.com/light-level-rooms-d_708.html)

- Science: Human Body & Mind – Sleep: BBC interactive website (www.bbc.co.uk/science/humanbody/sleep)

- 'Science of Sleep': documentary, CBS network (www.cbsnews.com/video/watch/ ?id=4181992n)
- Sleep and Dementia Resources (www.sleep-dementia-resources.ualberta.ca)
- Sleep hygiene resources: American Psychological Association (www.apa.org/pi/aging/ resources/guides/insomnia.aspx#) and the US Geriatric Mental Health Foundation (www. gmhfonline.org/gmhf/consumer/factsheets/hlthage_sleep.html)
- Smith M., Robinson, L. and Segal, R. (2014) *How to Sleep Well as You Age: Tips for Overcoming Insomnia and Sleeping Better Over 50* (www.helpguide.org/articles/sleep/how-to-sleep-well-as-you-age.htm#why)
- Society of Light and Lighting (UK) (www.cibse.org/index.cfm?go=page.view&item=68)
- SomnIA: *Optimising Quality of Sleep Among Older People in the Community and Care Homes: An Integrated Approach* (www.somnia.surrey.ac.uk/pdf%20and%20word%20documents/ ndafindings.pdf)
- University of Maryland Medical Center: Sleep apnea background and positioning information (http://umm.edu/health/medical/reports/articles/obstructive-sleep-apnea)

All websites were accessed on in May 2014.

References

Alessi, C.A., Martin, J.L., Webber, A.P., Kim, E., Harker, J.O. and Josephson, K.R. (2005) 'Intervention to improve abnormal sleep/wake patterns in nursing home residents.' *Journal of the American Geriatric Society 53*, 5, 803–810.

AMDA (2007) *Sleep Disorders: Clinical Practice Guidelines.* Columbia, MD: American Medical Directors Association.

Ancoli-Israel, S. (2009) 'Sleep and its disorders in aging populations.' *Sleep Medicine 10*, Suppl. 1, S7–S11.

Ancoli-Israel, S., Martin, J.L., Kripke, D.F., Marler, M. and Klauber, M.R. (2002) 'Effect of light treatment on sleep and circadian rhythms in demented nursing home patients.' *Journal of the American Geriatrics Society 50*, 2, 282–289.

Beaudreau, S.A., Spira, A.P., Gray, H.L., Depp, C.A. *et al.* (2008) 'The relationship between objectively measured sleep disturbance and dementia family caregiver distress and burden.' *Journal of Geriatric Psychiatry and Neurology 21*, 3, 159–165.

Berglund, B., Lindvall, T. and Schwela, D.H. (eds) (1999) *Guidelines for Community Noise.* Geneva: World Health Organization. Available at http://whqlibdoc.who.int/hq/1999/a68672.pdf, accessed on 31 October 2013.

Berry, S., Lee, Y., Cai, S. and Dore, D. (2013) 'Nonbenzodiazepine sleep medication use and hip fractures in nursing home residents.' *JAMA Internal Medicine 173*, 9, 745–761.

Bing, M.H., Moller, L.A., Jennum, P., Mortensen, S. and Lose, G. (2006) 'Validity and reliability of a questionnaire for evaluating nocturia, nocturnal enuresis and sleep-interruptions in an elderly population.' *European Urology 49*, 4, 710–719.

Bloom, H.G., Ahmed, I., Alessi, C.A., Ancoli-Israel, S. *et al.* (2009) 'Evidence-based recommendations for the assessment and management of sleep disorders in older persons.' *Journal of the American Geriatric Society 57*, 5, 761–789.

Bombois, S., Derambure, P., Pasquier, F. and Monaca, C. (2010) 'Sleep disorders in aging and dementia.' *Journal of Nutrition and Healthy Aging 14*, 3, 212–217.

Brown, C.A., Berry, R., Tan, M., Khoshia, A., Turlapati, L. and Swedlove, F. (2013) 'A critique of the evidence-base for non-pharmacological sleep interventions for persons with dementia.' *Dementia: The International Journal of Social Research and Practice 12*, 2, 174–201.

Brown, C.A., Wielandt, P., Wilson, D., Jones, A. and Crick, K. (2014) 'Healthcare providers' knowledge of disordered sleep, sleep assessment tools and non-pharmacological sleep interventions for persons living with dementia: a national survey.' *Sleep Disorders*. doi: http://dx.doi.org/10.1155/2014/286274.

Burns, A., Allen, H., Tomenson, B., Duignan, D. and Byrne, J. (2009) 'Bright light therapy for agitation in dementia: a randomized controlled trial.' *International Psychogeriatrics 21*, 4, 711–721.

Buysse, D.J., Reynolds, C.F., Monk, T.H., Berman, S.R. and Kupfer, D.J. (1989) 'The Pittsburgh Sleep Quality Index: a new instrument for psychiatric practice and research.' *Psychiatry Research 28*, 2, 193–213.

Byles, J.E., Mishra, G.D. and Harris, M.A. (2005) 'The experience of insomnia among older women.' *Sleep 28*, 8, 972–979.

Cole, C. and Richards, K. (2007) 'Sleep disruption in older adults. Harmful and by no means inevitable, it should be assessed for and treated.' *American Journal of Nursing 107*, 5, 40–49.

Cooke, J.R. and Ancoli-Israel, S. (2006) 'Sleep and its disorders in older adults.' *Psychiatric Clinics of North America 29*, 4, 1077–1093.

Cricco, M., Simonsick, E.M. and Foley, D.J. (2001) 'The impact of insomnia on cognitive functioning in older adults.' *Journal of the American Geriatric Society 49*, 9, 1185–1189.

David, R., Zeitzer, J., Friedman, L., Noda, A. *et al.* (2010) 'Non-pharmacologic management of sleep disturbance in Alzheimer's disease.' *Journal of Nutrition and Healthy Aging 14*, 3, 203–206.

Ellis, J., Hampson, S.E. and Cropley, M. (2007) 'The role of dysfunctional beliefs and attitudes in late-life insomnia.' *Journal of Psychosomatic Research 62*, 1, 81–84.

Foley, D., Ancoli-Israel, S., Britz, P. and Walsh, J. (2004) 'Sleep disturbances and chronic disease in older adults: results of the 2003 National Sleep Foundation "Sleep in America" survey.' *Journal of Psychosomatic Research 56*, 5, 497–502.

Gooneratne, N.S., Tavaria, A., Patel, N., Madhusudan, L. *et al.* (2011) 'Perceived effectiveness of diverse sleep treatments in older adults.' *Journal of the American Geriatric Society 59*, 2, 297–303.

Jacobs, G.D., Pace-Schott, E.F., Stickgold, R. and Otto, M.W. (2004) 'Cognitive behavior therapy and pharmacotherapy for insomnia: a randomized controlled trial and direct comparison.' *Archives of Internal Medicine 164*, 17, 1888–1896.

Kielhofner, G. (2008) *Model of Human Occupation: Theory and Application*, 4th edn. Philadelphia, PA: Lippincott Williams & Wilkins.

Kyle, S.D., Crawford, M.R., Morgan, K., Spiegelhalder, K., Clark, A.A. and Espie, C.A. (2013) 'The Glasgow Sleep Impact Index (GSII): a novel patient-centred measure for assessing sleep-related quality of life impairment in insomnia disorder.' *Sleep Medicine 14*, 6, 493–501.

Law, M., Baptiste, S., McColl, M., Opzoomer, A., Polatajko, H.J. and Pollack, N. (1992) 'The Canadian Occupational Performance Measure: an outcome measure for occupational therapy.' *Canadian Journal of Occupational Therapy 57*, 2, 82–87.

Lunde, L.H., Pallesen, S., Krangnes, L. and Nordhus, I.H. (2010) 'Characteristics of sleep in older persons with chronic pain: a study based on actigraphy and self-reporting.' *Clinical Journal of Pain 26*, 2, 132–137.

Marteau, T.M., Hollands, G.J. and Fletcher, P.C. (2012) 'Changing human behavior to prevent disease: the importance of targeting automatic processes.' *Science 337*, 6101, 1492–1495.

Mishima, Y., Hozumi, S., Shimizu, T., Hishikawa, Y. and Mishima, K. (2005) 'Passive body heating ameliorates sleep disturbances in patients with vascular dementia without circadian phase-shifting.' *American Journal of Geriatrics Psychiatry 13*, 5, 369–376.

Morin, C.M., Stone, J., Trinkle, D., Mercer, J. and Remsberg, S. (1993) 'Dysfunctional beliefs and attitudes about sleep among older adults with and without insomnia complaints.' *Psychology and Aging 8*, 3, 463–467.

Morin, C.M., Vallières, A. and Ivers, H. (2007) 'Dysfunctional beliefs and attitudes about sleep (DBAS): validation of a brief version (DBAS-16).' *Sleep 30*, 11, 1547–1554.

Nau, S.D., McCrae, C.S., Cook, K.G. and Lichstein, K.L. (2005) 'Treatment of insomnia in older adults.' *Clinical Psychology Reviews 25*, 5, 645–672.

Ohayon, M.M. and Vecchierini, F.M. (2005) 'Normative sleep data, cognitive function and daily living activities in older adults in the community.' *Sleep 28*, 8, 981–989.

Punjabi, N.M. (2008) 'The epidemiology of adult obstructive sleep apnea.' *Proceedings of the American Thoracic Society 5*, 2, 136–143.

Reeve, K. and Bailes, B. (2010) 'Insomnia in adults: etiology and management.' *Journal of Nurse Practitioners 6*, 1, 53–60.

Richards, K.C., Beck, C., O'Sullivan, P.S. and Shue, V.M. (2005) 'Effect of individualized social activity on sleep in nursing home residents with dementia.' *Journal of the American Geriatrics Society 53*, 9, 1510–1517.

Richards, K.C., Sullivan, S.C., Phillips, R.L., Beck, C.K. and Overton-McCoy, A.L. (2001) 'The effect of individualized activities on the sleep of nursing home residents who are cognitively impaired: a pilot study.' *Journal of Gerontological Nursing 27*, 9, 30–37.

Riemersma-van der Lek, R.F., Swaab, D.F., Twisk, J., Hol, E.M., Hoogendijk, W.J. and Van Someren, E.J. (2008) 'Effect of bright light and melatonin on cognitive and noncognitive function in elderly residents of group care facilities: a randomized controlled trial.' *Journal of the American Medical Association 299*, 22, 2642–2655.

Rutten, S., Vriend, C., van den Heuvel, O.A., Smit, J.H., Berendse, H.W. and van der Werf, Y.D. (2012) 'Bright light therapy in Parkinson's disease: an overview of the background and evidence.' *Parkinson's Disease 2012*. doi: 10.1155/2012/767105.

Scott, S.A., Ah-See, K.B., Richardson, H.C. and Wilson, J.A. (2003) 'A comparison of physician and patient perception of the problems of habitual snoring.' *Clinical Otolaryngology and Allied Sciences 28*, 1, 18–21.

Skjerve, A., Bjorvatn, B. and Holsten, F. (2004) 'Light therapy for behavioural and psychological symptoms of dementia.' *International Journal of Geriatric Psychiatry 19*, 6, 516–522.

Sloane, P.D., Williams, C.S., Mitchell, C.M., Preisser, J.S. *et al.* (2007) 'High-intensity environmental light in dementia: effect on sleep and activity.' *Journal of the American Geriatric Society 55*, 10, 1524–1533.

Society of Light and Lighting (2008) *Lighting Guide 02: Hospitals and Health Care Buildings (Society of Light and Lighting SLL LG2)*. London: Chartered Institute of Building and Service Engineers.

Song, Y., Dowling, G.A., Wallhagen, M.I., Lee, K.A. and Strawbridge, W.J. (2010) 'Sleep in older adults with Alzheimer's disease.' *Journal of Neuroscience Nursing 42*, 4, 190–198.

St George, R.J., Delbaere, K., Williams, P. and Lord, S.R. (2009) 'Sleep quality and falls in older people living in self- and assisted-care villages.' *Gerontology 55*, 2, 162–168.

Stone, K.L., Ancoli-Israel, S., Blackwell, T., Ensrud, K.E. *et al.* (2008) 'Actigraphy-measured sleep characteristics and risk of falls in older women.' *Archives of Internal Medicine 168*, 16, 1768–1775.

Stone, K.L., Ensrud, K.E. and Ancoli-Israel, S. (2008) 'Sleep, insomnia and falls in elderly patients.' *Sleep Medicine 9*, Suppl. 1, S18–S22.

Venn, S. and Arber, S. (2012) 'Understanding older people's decisions about the use of sleeping medication: issues of control and autonomy.' *Sociology of Health and Illness 34*, 8, 1215–1229.

Venn, S., Meadows, R. and Arber, S. (2013) 'Gender differences in approaches to self-management of poor sleep in later life.' *Social Science and Medicine 79*, 1, 117–123.

Wolkove, N., Elkholy, O., Baltzan, M. and Palayew, M. (2007a) 'Sleep and aging: 1. Sleep disorders commonly found in older people.' *Canadian Medical Association Journal 176*, 9, 1299–1304.

Wolkove, N., Elkholy, O., Baltzan, M. and Palayew, M. (2007b) 'Sleep and aging: 2. Management of sleep disorders in older people.' *Canadian Medical Association Journal 176*, 10, 1449–1454.

Wood, B., Rea, M.S., Plitnick, B. and Figueiro, M.G. (2013) 'Light level and duration of exposure determine the impact of self-luminous tablets on melatonin suppression.' *Applied Ergonomics 44*, 2, 237–240.

11

SLEEP PROBLEMS IN PEOPLE WITH LEARNING DISABILITIES

Eva Nakopoulou, Megan Wale and Emma Wood

11.1 Introduction

The World Health Organization (2014) defines intellectual disability as:

> a significantly reduced ability to understand new or complex information and to learn and apply new skills (impaired intelligence). This results in a reduced ability to cope independently (impaired social functioning), and begins before adulthood, with a lasting effect on development.

However, 'learning disabilities' (LD) is the most commonly used term within health and social care services in the UK and is used in this chapter, although other terms, such as 'mental retardation' and 'learning difficulties', may be used elsewhere. Whatever term is used, it is important to acknowledge the wide range of abilities that is represented: some people with mild LD live fairly independently and go to work, whereas those with profound and multiple LD have most or all of their needs met by others. Another consideration is the age range encompassed within the LD population, including both children and adults, and increasingly older adults, as more people with LD are living into old age. This chapter focuses on adults with LD, although in the absence of literature on adults, the section on autism spectrum condition relates more to children.

As noted, people with LD might live independently and without close supervision, partly as a consequence of the NHS and Community Care Act (Department of Health 1990), which led to the closure of large residential institutions. Despite moves away from institutionalization in the UK and other countries, with the encouragement of social inclusion, provision for people with LD is not always readily available and this can lead to social isolation. For example, an individual with mild LD who lives independently might receive little or no formal support and may lack the intrinsic motivation, structure of daily routine or knowledge to ensure that the need for sleep is properly met. Without support, the individual has little chance of identifying the existence of a sleep problem, and might have even less opportunity to deal with it. Similarly, where individuals are cared for in family settings, where the carers themselves might be elderly or have LD, and in residential settings, because of the needs of the group or restrictions posed by staff shift work, priority might not be given to sleep.

It is often found that individuals with LD are more susceptible to physical illness and mental health issues and may have complex behavioural needs. Any of these factors may pose a risk to their health and may be prioritized to the detriment of resolving sleep problems. As Hank, Hicks and Wilson (2012) state, 'with a wide range of sleep difficulties, in the context of a wide range of ability, treatment of sleep problems in people with learning disabilities will depend on careful assessment' (p.200). This chapter therefore looks at sleep issues, occupational performance and sleep, assessment of sleep difficulties and management of sleep problems that affect adults with LD.

11.2 Sleep problems that affect adults with a learning difficulty

It has been suggested that people with LD experience sleep problems as often as the general population (Gunning and Espie 2003); however, Doran, Harvey and Horner (2006) have estimated that 39% of adults with severe LD suffer from insomnia, in comparison with estimates of about 1 in 10 of the general population (Roth 2007). Research also shows that sleep problems in this population correlate with the level of disability (Gunning and Espie 2003) and with the individual's mental health (Didden and Sigafoos 2001). An adult with profound and multiple LD who requires support for postural management and communication is more likely than someone with a mild LD to suffer from sleep problems. For example, an individual with such a level of disability cannot independently change position in bed to be more comfortable and is also unable to communicate the need to do so. There may be several other reasons why sleep problems are more prevalent in the learning-disabled population; these might relate to lifestyle, environment and other medical conditions.

Lifestyle

Evidence indicates that adults with LD often have sedentary lifestyles (Hawkins and Look 2006). Green (2012) has explored the reciprocal association between sleep and balance of activity (see also Chapter 6), and there appears to be evidence that a less active lifestyle could contribute towards sleep problems. Many suggestions have been made with regard to the cause of inactivity in this client group, including a lack of understanding of the benefits of an active lifestyle by both the individual with the LD and their carers (Hawkins and Look 2006). Another major reason is the dependence of many of the learning-disabled population on other people for the organization of a balanced and meaningful routine. They might also depend on others (either family members with a car or others if they are allocated adequate funding for the provision of transport) to access meaningful occupations (Hurst 2009). Moreover, carers might not be aware of schemes and opportunities that are available free, or at low cost, in the community, such as healthy cooking courses and exercise schemes (Hawkins and Look 2006).

The dependency on carers for provision of an appropriate routine, coupled with the lack of awareness of community opportunities, has been further exacerbated in the UK recently with the closure of day centres. Day centres became established following the closure of the long-stay hospitals in the 1980s and 1990s and provided a structured routine for many adults with LD. Although the centres could be seen as a continuation of the institutionalization that occurred in the hospitals, and their closure could therefore be experienced as liberating, many are left with fragmented routines and with fewer hours of support towards participating in meaningful occupations.

Environment

People with LD may have little autonomy with regard to their living conditions, both in terms of their immediate environment and general community inclusion (Goodman and Locke 2009). In the UK, accommodation for adults with LD ranges from temporary settings, such as prisons, hospitals and homeless shelters, to more permanent settings, such as nursing, residential and supported living. Other adults with LD live with family members or independently in the community, perhaps with some support. In many circumstances individuals tend to share the living space with other people: other service users, family members or staff. In most of these cases, personal space is often limited to the individual's bedroom. As discussed in Chapter 8, the principles of stimulus control and sleep hygiene (which are conceived in terms of Western industrial culture) suggest that a bedroom is reserved for sleep (and sex) only, in order that environmental cues promote sleep. This is clearly not an option for individuals in many residential and institutional settings where all or most of their belongings are kept in their bedroom, and where they might also spend much of their waking time.

The bedroom might contain other distractions from sleep in the form of electronic devices. Televisions and electronic games might delay the winding-down process and be over-stimulating, and the light of the screens can also delay sleep (see Chapters 3 and 18). Games and television are waking activities and, again, from the perspective of stimulus control, are not advised in the bed or in the bedroom. Adults with LD might have difficulty understanding how over-stimulation can affect their sleep, and carers might not be aware of the over-stimulation or might not discourage use of televisions or other devices in order to avoid potentially challenging situations or confrontations.

The social environment can present other obstacles for adults with LD who can be very reliant upon their carers for a healthy sleep routine. Carers may be unaware of what constitutes a good sleep routine or they may establish a rigid routine for their own benefit, rather than that of the individual with the LD. Although some individuals will be natural late sleepers ('owls'; see Chapter 3), research shows that early bedtimes are often set for this client group to facilitate staff work schedules or to provide respite for family members (Gunning and Espie 2003; Hylkema, Petitaux and Vlaskamp 2011; Hylkema and Vlaskamp 2009). In terms of the social environment, another point to consider is that people with LD often have to share accommodation with other residents with whom they might not get along; therefore, other residents can also prevent the individual from sleeping by being noisy or having a different routine.

Profound and multiple LD

Profound and multiple LD (PMLD) is a specific area of practice for therapists working with the general LD population, whereby assessment of sleep problems might need greater consideration, as they might be caused by a number of issues. Many people with PMLD require postural care. This is an essential support for those who have difficulties with mobilizing independently as it aims to protect the individual's body shape by avoiding the development of distortions (Postural Care Action Group 2011). Postural management during the night in the form of the use of a sleep system is crucial in this population. A sleep system consists of different pieces of body positioning equipment (such as shaped foam blocks), which help to improve posture in sleep. Occasionally when sleep systems are implemented, the individual might initially have difficulty sleeping; therefore, both the provision of equipment and/or the lack of postural control can cause the sleep disturbances in this population.

Sensory integration (SI) is a term coined by Ayres (2005, p.5), referring to 'the organisation of sensation for use', and is linked to a specific form of assessment and intervention used by SI-trained therapists. Sensory processing is a term used to explain and identify symptoms linked with problems in the registration, modulation and organization of internal and external sensory input, with 'sensory processing disorder' or 'sensory processing difficulties' referring to complications with registering and/or modulating and/or organizing sensory input (Schaaf and Davies 2010). The observed outcome of a sensory processing disorder can be unusual behaviours or motor actions. Some examples could be distressed responses to sensory stimuli (Pfeiffer *et al.* 2005), impatience, anger, nervousness (Kinnealey and Fuiek 1999) or states of high alert (Shochat, Tzischinsky and Engel-Yeger 2009).

Sensory processing difficulties can be a major cause of sleep disturbances especially for adults with PMLD, although there is limited evidence of use of sensory approaches to address the sleep difficulties of the learning-disabled population (Hylkema and

Vlaskamp 2009; Hylkema *et al.* 2011). However, a study completed with healthy adults by Engel-Yeger and Shochat (2012) found that there is a correlation between behaviours linked to low sensory thresholds (such as sensory avoiding or sensory sensitivity) and sleep quality. They conclude their report by recommending to occupational therapists that individuals with sensory processing difficulties should be screened for sleep problems, and vice versa.

An individual with sensory processing difficulties could find sleeping difficult, because of difficulties regulating their sensory system in reaction to sensory stimulation during the daytime. Another example would be an individual with tactile sensitivity who could experience difficulties with going to sleep because of the sensation of the bedding or clothing material. Sleep disturbances in this population have also been linked to epilepsy, nocturnal incontinence coupled with incontinence care and excessive bedtime rituals (Didden and Sigafoos 2001; Espie *et al.* 1998; Hank *et al.* 2012; Hylkema *et al.* 2011).

Other conditions

Sleep apnoea in the LD population

Evidence of prevalence of obstructive sleep apnoea as a cause of sleep disturbance in this population is controversial (Didden and Sigafoos 2001; Espie 2000). Resta *et al.* (2003) and Trois *et al.* (2009) have estimated the prevalence of sleep apnoea in adults with Down syndrome to be over 80%, although both studies involved a very small number of participants. In practice, occupational therapists seldom observe such cases, but a growing number of adults with LD are overweight, and this is likely to increase numbers who have sleep apnoea in the future.

Autism spectrum condition

Much literature refers to autism spectrum disorder, but more recently the term autism spectrum condition (ASC) has been used and is the term used here. The literature relating to children and adolescents with ASC has been reviewed by Aitken (2012), who found that sleep problems are more common than in the rest of the population. For example, Allik, Larsson and Smedje (2006) used parent report and actigraphy[*] to compare the sleep of 32 children (aged 8–12 years) with Asperger syndrome or high-functioning autism and children in a matched control group. It was found that 10 of 32 children had insomnia compared with 0 of 32 in the control group. Furthermore, parents of the children with insomnia reported more autistic and emotional symptoms, and their teachers reported more emotional symptoms and hyperactivity. Tani *et al.* (2003) have shown that insomnia is also more prevalent in adults with Asperger syndrome.

The sleep of 27 high-functioning young adults (aged 16–27 years) with ASC was compared with a group of 78 age- and gender-matched controls in a laboratory study by Limoges *et al.* (2005). Participants spent two nights in a sleep laboratory and completed various questionnaires. Results indicated that people with ASC reported significantly more problems in getting to sleep and remaining asleep than the control group. The researchers found objective differences that corresponded with the subjective data and it was also found that people with ASC had more light sleep (stages 1 and 2) and less deep, slow-wave sleep*. Analysis of the data and comparison with other studies suggested that objective sleep difficulties in people with ASC might not be attributed only to neurological or psychiatric co-morbidity. This led the researchers to conclude that their findings 'form an additional and independent argument in favour of an intrinsic relation between atypical sleep architecture* and the phenotype of autism, at least at an adult age' (Limoges *et al.* 2005, p.1058).

More recent research has examined the relationship between sleep and ASC. In a two-part study Adams *et al.* (2014) considered two questions: first, whether sleep problems exacerbate ASC symptom severity, and second, whether sleep problems are more common as ASC symptom severity increases. They confirmed the findings of others that the presence of a sleep problem (but not the severity of sleep problems) can affect symptoms of ASC, and showed that increased symptom severity increases the likelihood of sleep problems. They concluded that their findings suggest a bidirectional relationship.

Aitken (2012) lists reasons why people with ASC might experience more sleep problems than others (see also Richdale 1999). Possible causes include genetic differences that disrupt the effect of inhibitory neurotransmitters or the production of melatonin*, and diminished awareness of social cues. Another difficulty is where nightmares become associated with sleep and the individual becomes fearful of sleeping (Didden and Sigafoos 2001). This is not a problem exclusive to the ASC population, although Richdale (1999) reports findings that children with autism have an increased likelihood of experiencing nightmares. The social and environmental context might add to difficulties. Clinical experience with this population suggests that there may be excessive bedtime routines, which can cause settling difficulties (Hank *et al.* 2012). Accordingly, Allik *et al.* (2006) in the study cited above noted that children with ASC and insomnia were significantly more likely to be accompanied by someone at sleep onset and to show signs of anxiety at bedtime than children with ASC without insomnia. A further cause for sleep problems in this group observed in clinical practice tends to be sensory processing issues (see above and also Chapter 9). Schreck, Mulick and Smith (2004) conducted a study with children with autism, which not only highlighted the link between sleep problems and behaviour during the daytime, but also suggested that shorter sleep duration resulted in an increase of behaviours which prevented participation in daily occupations. They therefore suggested that potentially sleep problems in children with autism could be used as a predictor of intensified symptoms of autism.

Interventions to improve sleep are dealt with later in this chapter, but the literature relating to sleep problems in ASC mainly concerns children. In a detailed review Vriend *et al.* (2011) consider a range of measures. They note, for example, a suggestion to keep making small variations in the bedtime routine (such as different pyjamas) in order to reduce the risk of establishing rituals that are hard to break. They conclude, however, that sleep hygiene measures alone are not likely to be effective in improving sleep. Other measures include extinction, which involves ignoring disruptions at bedtime and giving no attention until morning (see Chapter 9), faded bedtime, where the child goes to bed at a time when it is likely that she or he will sleep quickly with a gradual move to an earlier bedtime, and sleep restriction (see Chapter 8). Where sleep terrors are a problem, scheduled awakening can be used (see Chapter 8), and Vriend *et al.* (2011) cite one case report where chronotherapy was used for a disrupted sleep-wake cycle (see Box 7.2).

In the absence of research evidence relating to adults with ASC, it will be up to the therapist to adapt measures suggested for children or measures that have been found useful in other groups. It has been established in other chapters that sleep is important for all of us, but if sleep quality is related to symptom severity, it is all the more important to help improve the sleep of people with ASC.

Dementia

The development of medicine and the increase in the quality of life of people with LD have had an impact on the lifespan in this population (Department of Health 2001; Janicki *et al.* 1999). Consequently, more people with LD are suffering from dementia, with the link between Down syndrome and early-onset dementia being already well established (Hogg *et al.* 2000; Kalsy and Oliver 2002; Watchman 2003). Evidence indicates that there are links between sleep disturbances and dementia in the non-learning-disabled population (Gabelle and Dauvilliers 2010; McCurry and Ancoli-Israel 2003); research focusing on people with Down syndrome and Alzheimer's disease highlights problems such as early night waking, wandering at night (Deb, Hare and Prior 2007) and auditory hallucinations and anxiety (Urv, Zigman and Silverman 2008). Furthermore, there is evidence that the early development of sleep problems is related to the rate of progression of Alzheimer's disease (Urv, Zigman and Silverman 2010).

11.3 Occupational performance and sleep

Occupational performance is the accomplishment of the selected occupation resulting from the dynamic transaction between the client, the environment and the activity

(American Occupational Therapy Association 2008). Dating back to the 1890s (Patrick and Gilbert 1896), and as discussed in Chapter 5, there is overwhelming evidence suggesting that inadequate sleep can result in impaired performance. In particular, sound sleep allows us to rest, repair and re-energize, and a lack of it results in concentration issues, low mood, irritability and, ultimately, a weakened immune system (Dinges *et al.* 1999; McCulloch 2011). Research involving healthy adults indicates that sleep deprivation can negatively impact on mood (Pilcher and Huffcutt 1996) and impair psychomotor performance.

Use of a model of practice allows a therapist to conceptualize what happens when problems arise. Many occupational therapy models can facilitate an exploration of the individual's context and highlight potential causes of sleep disturbance; however, in this chapter the Model of Human Occupation (MoHO) is used to make sense of the underlying dynamics of human behaviour and is selected because of its holistic approach (Kielhofner 2008). The four elements of the model – volition, habituation, performance capacity and environment – are examined in turn in relation to the case of a young man. The case example is introduced in Box 11.1.

BOX 11.1 Case example: Alf

Alf is a 28-year-old man with a diagnosis of autism and moderate LD and has complex needs. He has anxiety, psychosis and sensory issues, which are manifested in behaviours that challenge the service. He communicates using non-verbal techniques such as Makaton and pictorial cards. He is currently placed in a medium secure unit because of the risk posed to himself and others, although a more suitable placement is currently being sought.

Support staff requested occupational therapy involvement as Alf was unable to engage in daily routines because of challenging behaviours and an erratic sleep pattern. Alf was having short periods of broken daytime sleep and slept little during night-time hours. After many years in institutionalized environments, Alf was heavily reliant upon regular medication to aid sleep. It was not known whether this reliance was conditioned behaviour or physiological. Staff members often reported that Alf was drowsy during the day. Because of environmental and financial constraints, Alf's diet at the time of the referral consisted of mass-produced, high-calorie, processed food.

Volition: the mechanisms whereby we choose what to do

In terms of motivation, staff reported that Alf was sporadically motivated to engage with them when he was awake, but there appeared to be no pattern to his level of engagement. Alf often chose to sleep for prolonged periods in the daytime despite encouragement from carers to sleep and rest at night. Alf appeared to have little understanding and insight of the impact of his erratic sleep pattern upon his functional ability; as a result, he did not appear motivated to work on adapting this and did not have the capacity to report any problem to those supporting him.

Habituation: the basic structures with which we organize our lives

Alf chose to engage with staff at times and occasionally engaged with the occupational therapist to complete leisure activities based around his sensory needs, although this engagement was sporadic. Owing to Alf's level of aggression and violence, he was restricted from accessing larger spaces where peers were present; thus, his access to the wider facilities and outdoor space was limited. Alf occasionally completed a meaningful daytime routine, which included minimal self-care and increased levels of social communication and engagement with substantial support from staff. He appeared flexible to adapt although, because of his autism, change would need to be on his terms and completed as a very gradual process. This was identified as an area where the occupational therapist would provide guidance and support to staff members providing 24-hour care.

Performance capacity: the means by which we carry out occupational behaviour

Alf was unable to complete everyday tasks because of lack of energy and motivation. Due to his increasing levels of violence and aggression, staff struggled to promote a healthy routine in a safe fashion. Furthermore, Alf lacked insight and therefore lacked motivation to change. Again, his engagement with therapeutic activities and support was sporadic and dependent upon his motivational levels at the time; however, some tasks were left unfinished and some were not initiated without support from staff. As a result of severe lack of sleep, Alf had difficulties engaging with any form of routine. Therapeutic interventions were generally offered by occupational therapists and psychologists who tend to work daytime hours, which resulted in a narrow window of opportunity to engage Alf.

Environment: the physical and social context

Because of being in a hospital environment, Alf was expected to sleep at certain times, although this was not always meaningful for him as an individual. He was also supported by a staff team, whose numbers were reduced at night in order to encourage a healthy sleep pattern for all inpatients. This offered Alf some encouragement to sleep at night but did not always meet his needs if he was awake then.

11.4 Assessment

In assessment of sleep problems in this client group, as in others, it is first necessary to screen for any problems that might need referral. It is also important to consider whether additional assessment tools relating to sleep need to be used or whether existing tools can be amended, but two other issues are of particular relevance to this group: it may be necessary to gain consent and there may be undetected sensory processing problems.

A referral to an occupational therapist, as one member of a multi-disciplinary team, may not be explicitly for issues related to sleep. On one hand, sleep problems may not be noticed by the referrer in the first place and, on the other hand, a referrer may be unaware of how an occupational therapist can help to improve the individual's sleep. Fung *et al.* (2013) argue that occupational therapists should regularly assess their clients' sleep and wakefulness, and recommend the routine use of tools specifically designed to address sleep difficulties. Occupational therapists should be aware of when it might be helpful to have someone referred for assessment for a sleep disorder, such as obstructive sleep apnoea, or whether, for example, sleep difficulties might relate to poor sleep hygiene or unhelpful routines, which can be addressed by the occupational therapist. (For general principles on the assessment of sleep difficulties see Chapter 8.)

In this area of practice, occupational therapists are already using standardized and non-standardized occupational therapy-specific assessment tools and/or tools designed to address the needs of the learning-disabled population. Therefore, this section explores how existing tools used in this area of practice can support the screening of sleep problems. It is then necessary to consider assessment in the context of an identified problem.

Because of the varying degrees of capacity among this client group, occupational therapists need to ensure that they assess the individual's capacity to consent. In dealing with sleep problems occupational therapists need also to ask who is affected by the sleep difficulty: Is it a problem for the individual or is it more of an inconvenience for the carer(s)? Is the therapist acting in the client's best interest? Therefore, before engaging the individual in the therapeutic process, the occupational therapist should consider whether an easy-to-read consent form is appropriate or whether there is a need for the best-interest process. (For further information on the best-interest process in the UK, refer to the Mental Capacity Act, Ministry of Justice 2005.)

Screening for sleep problems in assessment

Many services develop their own occupational therapy initial assessment questions, and it would be a simple matter to include screening questions on sleep by asking the client and/or the carer about sleep. For example, does the client get to sleep easily at night and remain asleep until the morning? However, a commonly used tool in this area of practice in the UK is the *Life Star* which is part of the *Outcomes Star* toolset which aims to support and measure change as a result of intervention (Burns and MacKeith 2012; MacKeith 2011). One of the 10 areas that the *Life Star* covers is 'Your Health', which the occupational therapist can use to screen for sleep difficulties. Therefore, occupational therapists using the *Life Star* on a routine basis can encompass the screening for sleep difficulties without the need of further tools.

Assessment of identified sleep problems

Once a sleep difficulty has been identified, it is useful to consider asking the following questions of the client and/or the carers:

1. How long has the sleep issue been present?

2. How significant is the issue and what are the consequences?

3. Who perceives this as important?

4. What effect might a change in this have?

According to Hylkema and Vlaskamp (2009) other questions worth asking are:

1. Does the client have her/his own bedroom?

2. What is the client's level of functional mobility and level of overall disability?

3. What are the client's daily activities? Specifying the type (sedentary/active) and number of activities completed during the day

4. Does the client have easy access to drinks containing caffeine at any time?

The answers to these questions will support the occupational therapist to focus on potentially using one of the assessment tools discussed below.

Sleep diary

A sleep diary can aid the understanding of sleep disturbances, but there can be many difficulties in using it with this population because of the degree of literacy and comprehension skills required to complete it; however, an easy-to-read sleep diary, together with examples of completed days, can be provided, or a carer could complete the sleep diary on the client's behalf. A sleep diary should aim to gather information such as times of going to bed and getting out of bed, together with perceived hours of sleep. It can also be beneficial to include a section on daytime activities, to attempt to ascertain whether there is a link between quality and quantity of sleep and daytime activity.

Pictorial Epworth Sleepiness Scale

Where a client is observed or reported to be sleepy during the day, a useful measure is the Epworth Sleepiness Scale (Johns 1991). It has recently been adapted by Ghiassi *et al.* (2011) to a pictorial format in order to address the need of individuals with diminished literacy skills. This tool can be used with individuals with LD who can self-report levels of sleepiness throughout the day.

Sensory processing assessments

When the initial occupational therapy assessments indicate that the cause of sleep difficulties is of sensory processing nature, the first assessment to consider is the Sensory Integration Inventory – Revised for Individuals with Developmental Disabilities (Reisman and Hanschu 1992), which was devised for occupational therapists working with adults with LD. Other useful tools when considering sensory modulation difficulties are the Adolescent/Adult Sensory Profile (Brown and Dunn 2002), for when the client can self-report, and the Sensory Profile Caregiver Questionnaire developed by Dunn (1999) when relying on the carer's report (Ohl *et al.* 2012). Although the latter assessment was designed for use with children, it can be useful when relying on carers for reporting sensory difficulties. Completion of these assessment tools is complemented with observations carried out by the occupational therapist while the individual is participating in activities of daily living. Furthermore, the occupational therapist can request the individual's carers to complete a diary devised by the occupational therapist. This diary can highlight the sensory qualities of the activities and their effect on the individual immediately and up to 3 hours later, and monitor whether the carer perceives that the individual had a good quantity and quality of sleep.[1]

Because of the complexities of sensory processing, it is important to eliminate any other factors that could impact upon the sleep-wake cycle and sleep latency*. For example, some behaviours could also be explained by frustration or communication difficulties which are not being addressed effectively.

Volitional Questionnaire

The Volitional Questionnaire (VQ) (de las Heras *et al.* 2007) is an observational tool, with its initial version being validated by Chern *et al.* (1996). It aims to give insight into individuals who are unable to self-report their own volition. It highlights the client's inner drives and indicates how the environment influences one's volition. It can be used when examining the potential link between sleep difficulties and volition.

The Residential Environmental Impact Survey

The Residential Environmental Impact Survey (REIS) was designed for mild to moderate learning-disabled people by Fisher *et al.* (2013), with its initial version being validated by Fisher and Kayhan (2012). The REIS aims to investigate how residents are affected by the community residential facilities and therefore considers how well the client's needs are being met by the home. It can be used when considering whether the environment is contributing towards sleep difficulties, as it examines the sensory, physical and social aspects of the individual's home.

MOHO Exploratory Level Outcome Ratings

The MOHO Exploratory Level Outcome Ratings (MOHO-ExpLOR) is a new assessment currently being developed. It aims to highlight the dynamic consequences of intervention by linking key environmental factors to changes in a person's volition, habituation and performance skills. It is hoped that it will measure the earliest signs of change when occupational performance and participation are severely impaired (Parkinson *et al.* 2014), and therefore it can be a useful tool in the profoundly learning-disabled population. In relation to sleep difficulties this tool briefly explores the individual's level of environmental awareness and whether this environment supports or hinders the individual's sensory processing needs. The tool also considers whether an individual is able to maintain a stable sleep pattern and has sufficient energy to engage in activities, including the postural support required to achieve this.

Polysomnography and actigraphy

It is unusual to assess sleep in a laboratory unless a particular disorder is suspected or needs to be excluded. Polysomnography* is an expensive resource in the UK, and sleeping in a strange place with multiple electrodes attached to the head and the body could be a very unsettling experience for a person with LD. However, a possibility for monitoring the sleep-wake cycle is through actigraphy*, which involves only the wearing of a device like a wristwatch to measure movement over the course of a week or two. Use of actigraphy in the UK has traditionally required a referral to a specialist sleep centre, but devices that monitor movement are now becoming cheaper and more widely available.

11.5 Management of sleep problems of people with LD

For the purpose of this chapter the different approaches have been categorized as pharmacological, environmental, educational and maintaining of a balanced lifestyle, although it should be appreciated that the boundaries are often blurred and more than one approach can be applied at a time.

Pharmacological interventions

Measures to improve sleep cannot be discussed without the use of medication being acknowledged. For occupational therapists, medication is never a first (or any) choice of intervention, but it is one that is readily called upon by others. Occupational therapists working in multidisciplinary teams will work with clients who take medication to aid sleep and may need to support service users in all aspects of treatment, and help them keep to the necessary routines and note any adverse effects of medication.

Medication to aid sleep can be useful in helping to establish a healthy sleep-wake cycle when used over a short period, but it is best used whilst exploring other interventions. As Kripke (2000) suggests, using medication, such as benzodiazepines, to manage sleep disorders should only be a short-term measure for acute insomnia. Furthermore, users of hypnotic medication can become reliant upon it and, after prolonged use, build up a tolerance; it is also possible to become reliant on medication as part of a routine as opposed to the pharmacological effects of the medication itself. To avoid these issues, medication should be used as part of a wider strategy with the aim of its eventual discontinuation. If hypnotic medication has been used on a long-term basis, it should be questioned and alternatives should be sought. Education on the side effects should also be considered in order to raise awareness and potentially increase insight and promote choice.

Environmental interventions

Social environment

The importance of the social environment is illustrated in a case study by Belcher (1995) involving a learning-disabled man, known as Peter, who was moved from a small institution into a community home for three people. The study showed that, following adjustments to the home environment, positive changes could be seen in Peter's sleep pattern. In the original setting he would get up in the night to interact with staff and then compensate for lost sleep with daytime naps; in the community home personal choices were emphasized and the environment was structured to increase the availability of household and community activities. As shown in Chapter 6, daytime activity can have an influence on sleep, but this study also shows that if one has positive interaction with people in the daytime, there is no need to socialize at night.

Similar success was described in a case study by Hylkema and Vlaskamp (2013), concerning an elderly man, known as John, with Down syndrome and Alzheimer's disease. The study showed that adapting John's bedtime to a time that suited him, rather than the staff's shift pattern, improved his sleep efficiency*, although sleep duration was largely unchanged during the study period. The study emphasizes the importance of a person-centred approach in residential facilities with regard to sleep habits.

It has also been observed in clinical practice that buildings and routines are likely to be designed around the needs of the majority rather than those of the individual. Occupational therapists should support and work with carers in order to establish boundaries and routines that are meaningful to the client. The impact of social relationships and how the expectations of others can be placed onto the person with LD should also be considered.

Physical environment

In order to combat difficulties caused by the environment, the following should be considered: window coverings, decoration and presentation of a room, noise levels and the temperature as well as the sleeping space and its comfort. The difficulty with this clientele, as mentioned before, is that the bedroom tends to also be their living space; therefore, while we would normally recommend that the bedroom be used for sleeping and sex only (and thus for sleep it should be unstimulating and promote a sense of relaxation), at the same time we might recommend that the same room be stimulating in order to promote a sense of home, comfort and security. This is a difficult balance that the client, carers and occupational therapist have to strike.

The physical environment may need careful assessment where there are sensory processing issues (see section 11.2).[2] Addressing sensory processing issues in a client-centred manner is within the occupational therapy domain, so the client and their needs should remain at the centre of intervention to promote empowerment and choice.

Interventions linked to sensory processing can be roughly divided into two categories:

1. provision of appropriate level of stimulation during daytime activities and provision of stimulating environments for individuals who regularly experience delay or failure to respond to sensory information (under-reacting)

2. provision of a calming and relaxing environment and appropriate level of stimulation during daytime activities for individuals who over-respond to sensory information (sensory avoiding).

In both cases the occupational therapist is looking for learned patterns of behaviour established by the individual to avoid or seek out sensations in order to restore comfort or provide a sensory input that they can control. These patterns of behaviours have become part of the individual's meaningful routine. The role of the intervention is either to enable the carers to understand and promote these meaningful routines or to enable the client to replace potentially harmful behaviours (such as hitting and biting) with behaviours that provide the same sensory input but are safe to carry out.

The effects of the sensory interventions could be explored with the use of diaries; again, these are based on varying activities and a wide time frame. These diaries are used to recognize patterns of behaviour and reactions to sensory stimulus in order to reassess and make further recommendations.

A key environmental factor in regulating a healthy sleep-wake cycle, as described elsewhere in this book, is light. Short and Carpenter (1998) explore the use of light therapy, which consists of individuals being woken at a set time each day and exposed to natural or artificial sunlight periodically throughout the day. Short and Carpenter (1998) note that 'patients with learning disabilities, especially those with sensory impairments, have fewer social cues to help resynchronize the internal sleep-wake rhythm' (p.144). They report a case study involving a 34-year-old man with profound LD as well as poor visual acuity who had a disrupted sleep pattern. Medication (which had proved ineffective) was stopped and he was woken at a set time in the morning and exposed to direct natural light for at least 2 hours, either by going outdoors or by sitting by a window. Within 2 weeks a normal sleep pattern was established and remained stable. This demonstrates that light therapy can be a very useful tool: it requires little input from the individual and needs only passive engagement. For example, full-spectrum light can be used at breakfast time. This may be a particularly appropriate intervention where individuals are unable to engage actively in behaviour change or in a decision-making process.

The provision of equipment to be used during sleep to correct posture, prevent pressure ulcers or address issues related to incontinence needs to be slow and graded, owing to the disruption it will cause to a person's sleep quality. Within the learning-disabled population this is more pertinent in the initial stages because of barriers to communication related to the level of disability; therefore, gradual provision of equipment needs to take place with close monitoring of possible effects on a person's sleep quality. This can be managed by using sleep diaries completed by support staff and the introduction of the system in a slow and graded manner, all the while responding to the client's needs to ensure a client-centred approach.

Educational interventions

A study carried out in a residential setting for people with LD by Hylkema *et al.* (2011) suggests that education of staff (workshops and lectures) is beneficial and can lead to significant improvement in understanding the sleep needs of the client group. A significant environmental influence in residential settings is the knowledge of clients and staff, and an important part of occupational therapy intervention is therefore education. Similarly, within family homes the education of family members/carers is a significant aspect of an occupational therapist's role.

When considering the social environment of a person, the routines, rituals and boundaries that are imposed on them must be considered, as well as the ones that they impose on themselves. Changing a person's daily routine can impact on their sleep pattern; for example, moving medication to better suit sleep needs can be helpful, as medications can cause drowsiness and be taken more appropriately in the late evening.

As illustrated above in the case example of Peter (Belcher 1995), a more active lifestyle with meaningful daytime occupations, paired with restful evening routines, can encourage a need for rest in the evening and increase the need and/or ability to sleep at night. This could also be supported by moving more sedentary activities to the evenings, such as reading or watching films, to encourage rest and provide a prompt to sleep or a 'bedtime routine'.

In practice, the education offered to staff will vary depending upon the setting, funding and procedures in place regarding how to increase understanding. It could be the role of the occupational therapist to deliver training regarding basic concepts of sleep hygiene, although in other services specialist training programmes may be available. A further illustration of interventions to improve sleep is given in the case example of Madeline (see Box 11.3).

Interventions encouraging a balanced lifestyle

Hylkema and Vlaskamp (2009) conducted a study involving 41 learning-disabled residents from small-scale residential facilities (with 6–10 individuals per unit), with an average age of 36.95 years and a level of LD ranging from moderate to profound. It was found that participants spent an average 11 hours and 19 minutes in bed but only an average of 8 hours and 3 minutes asleep (a sleep efficiency of about 70%). The five types of interventions were: (1) bedtime scheduling, where time of going to bed corresponds to age, acknowledging that a 7-year-old needs more sleep than a 20-year-old; (2) change in daily routine (moving activities to more suitable times); (3) increase in daytime activity; (4) a combination of these; and (5) 'other' – that is, specifically tailored individual interventions: for example, identifying that an individual's daytime activity was sedentary (listening to calming nature sounds) and would better be carried out in the evening prior to bedtime. For the majority of the participants the combination of sleep scheduling, provision of a routine meaningful to the individual and an increase in the number and extent of daily activities was found to be the most effective intervention. It was shown that 80.5% of participants had an improvement in either sleep efficiency or sleep latency following the interventions. Interestingly, results indicated that individuals with epilepsy gained less from the interventions, but it was not clear whether this was related to use of anticonvulsant medication or to the nature of epilepsy itself.

In clinical practice, the negative impact of an imbalanced lifestyle, without provision of appropriate routines, is regularly observed to cause sleep problems in this client group. People with LD are often reliant on their carers for provision of a healthy routine and for maintaining sleep hygiene; it is therefore essential to provide person-specific meaningful occupations. However, people with LD often lack insight, and when planning intervention it cannot be assumed that intrinsic factors, such as motivation and the ability to modify one's own behaviour, can be relied upon. It is therefore useful to consider extrinsic factors to increase a person's motivation to engage in an intervention. For example, a behavioural approach, such as an incentive scheme where the person knows what is expected of them and can anticipate a 'reward' in response to meeting the expectation, could be considered. The reward works best when it is chosen by the person in question and it could be given, for example, when any aspect of sleep hygiene is improved, such as following an appropriate bedtime routine, getting up at a regular time or avoiding daytime naps. However, a behavioural approach should be considered carefully, ensuring that it contributes towards the client's aims and goals, and only following lack of success in using an educational approach. (For an illustration of the ways that interventions may be carried out in practice see Box 11.2, which picks up on the case study of Alf; see Box 11.3 for a further case example.)

BOX 11.2 Case example: Alf
Assessment and intervention

Because of the complexity of Alf's case, the multi-disciplinary team agreed to maintain his current medication in the first instance. Assessment took two approaches. First, with input from a speech and language therapist, Alf completed a Talking Mat (an interactive communication aid)[3] in order to express his likes and dislikes for his daily routine: this indicated that once Alf was able to complete a fixed morning routine, he was then able to participate in other activities during the day. Second, staff kept a sleep diary for 2 weeks, which showed that Alf appeared to sleep in the afternoon as a result of boredom and lack of engagement throughout waking hours. The occupational therapy team addressed this by enhancing the range of activities available for him – including productivity and leisure, getting outdoors where possible for exposure to daylight – in attempting to provide a more meaningful routine. The multi-disciplinary team also explored the impact that Alf's diet was having upon his energy levels and he was provided with a more balanced diet with the intention of reinforcing the improved routines.

Improving sleep patterns in cases such as this is a long-term process. When Alf begins to settle in the new patterns, the team can review his medication and consider other interventions, such as light therapy.

11.6 Conclusion

In conclusion, it is clear that there is a lack of strong evidence in this area of practice, and research is necessary to establish the optimum ways to assess and address sleep problems in adults with LD. It is especially important in this client group to remember that everyone is individual, particularly where there are vast differences within age and ability ranges; it is also necessary to consider expectations of the social environment. Similarly, support networks and resources can vary widely. These factors require occupational therapists to draw on their core skills and natural creativity and to take a holistic approach.

Moreover, this is a largely non-vocal group with a variety of disabilities, and sleep difficulties can easily go undetected and untreated. It is therefore the responsibility of each professional working in this field to enquire regularly about their client's quality of sleep. Occupational therapists are well placed to be making this enquiry, as one of the main reasons for poor quality of sleep in this client group tends to be a lack of meaningful daytime occupations.

BOX 11.3 Case example: Madeline

Madeline is a 21-year-old woman who likes shopping and dancing. She volunteers for 5 hours per week at an animal shelter, which she attends with the support of staff. She has Down syndrome with moderate LD and lives in a group home with three other women who have varying levels of disability. She has her own bedroom, which she uses for sleep and also during the day to carry out activities such as drawing and watching television. The house is staffed full time with one waking-night staff member from 10 p.m. to 7 a.m. because of the complex needs of other clients in the house. Madeline had been referred to community services because of 'challenging behaviour around bedtime' and 'poor sleep', and it was felt that occupational therapy was the most appropriate profession to become involved. At the time she was on no medication to help her sleep.

During the initial interviews with Madeline and her carers the following was reported: the view of staff members was that Madeline was challenging at bedtime, arguing about when to go to bed and waking other residents during the night by being loud. Her sleep pattern interfered with her mornings and hindered her in getting to work on time. Madeline's view was that as an adult she could choose her own bedtime, and that staff members were being unfair about the time she was expected to go to bed. She also stated that it was 'unfair' that staff 'get to stay up all night' and she did not. Her room was near the kitchen, which was used by all residents and staff, including night staff. The room had a large window and multiple electronic devices, such as a television, games station and music system. Madeline showed little understanding of

---

the effect her sleep pattern was having on her daily occupations, and staff felt they needed to ensure that the house rules were being followed. The planned intervention had several aspects.

Educational intervention

An initial teaching session based around sleep hygiene was held, primarily for Madeline but also involving support staff. It was supported by the use of accessible information on sleep hygiene, such as picture cards and leaflets tailored to Madeline's functional and cognitive abilities. Visual prompts, including posters using one key word and one key image, were used as a reminder to reinforce what had been learnt. Because a key issue for Madeline was her lack of understanding of the essential aspects of staff routine, involving being awake throughout the night, in a further session there was discussion on the preparation that staff need in order to remain awake, and the effect it had on them. It was stressed that it was for work and not for fun that staff remained awake. The need to reinforce boundaries was also discussed with staff.

Environmental and lifestyle changes

An important change in routine was staff starting work at 10p.m. to dedicate time early in their shift to spend with Madeline in order to discourage her from staying awake to spend time with them. It was also felt that giving Madeline some responsibility would help. For example, helping staff to prepare the house for night-time by tidying up could help her understand the role of the night staff and also establish routines that, once habituated, would continue to provide cues for Madeline that it is time to sleep. An incentive system was also considered to encourage Madeline to improve her time in bed at night.

Madeline's room was not identified as an issue, although it could not be assumed that her room would support a good sleep pattern; the occupational therapist checked that it was not over-stimulating, too untidy or cluttered, too warm or too cold, and that there was sufficient window covering to obscure natural light or any other outside light. Her computer had software installed to reduce the blue-spectrum light that could suppress melatonin production in the evening.

Evaluation

Madeline's insight lent itself to a client-centred incentive-based approach whereby she enjoyed setting her own goals and was able to select a personalized way of celebrating her achieving these goals. Madeline also benefited from the education regarding staff roles and the reason for them being awake during the night. Staff similarly reported improved routines, with the outcome being that Madeline showed a significant improvement in meeting her responsibility of getting to work on time.

Notes

1 In the UK and Ireland education on the theory and practice of sensory integration is provided by the Sensory Integration Network (www.sensoryintegration.org.uk), which advocates that training is required to be able to interpret competently the results of the assessments and to implement interventions.

2 Advice on creating a sensory-friendly bedroom can be found at www.friendshipcircle.org/blog/2014/04/10/how-to-create-the-right-sensory-environment-for-a-good-nights-sleep (accessed on 9 May 2014). Other useful resources relating to children's sleep may be found in Appendix 9.1.

3 Further information is available at www.talkingmats.com (accessed on 30 April 2014).

References

Adams, H.L., Matson, J.L., Cervantes, P.E. and Goldin, R.L. (2014) 'The relationship between autism symptom severity and sleep problems: Should bidirectionality be considered?' *Research in Autism Spectrum Disorders 8*, 3, 193–199.

Aitken, K.J. (2012) *Sleep Disorders and Autism Spectrum Disorders: A Guide for Parents and Professionals.* London: Jessica Kingsley Publishers.

Allik, H., Larsson, J. and Smedje, H. (2006) 'Insomnia in school-age children with Asperger syndrome or high-functioning autism.' *BMC Psychiatry.* doi: 10.1186/1471-244X-6-18.

American Occupational Therapy Association (2008) 'Occupational Therapy Practice Framework: Domain and Process, 2nd edn.' *American Journal of Occupational Therapy 62*, 6, 625–683.

Ayres, A.J. (2005) *Sensory Integration and the Child*, 25th Anniversary Edition. Los Angeles: Western Psychological Services. (Original work published in 1976.)

Belcher, T. (1995) 'Environmental changes affect sleep patterns: a case study.' *Perceptual and Motor Skills 80*, 3 (Pt 2), 1089–1090.

Brown, C. and Dunn, W. (2002) *Adolescent/Adult Sensory Profile: User's Manual.* San Antonio, TX: Pearson.

Burns, S. and MacKeith, J. (2012) *Life Star: The Outcomes Star for Your Life.* Brighton: Triangle Consulting.

Chern, J.-S., Kielhofner, G., de las Heras, C. and Magalhaes, L. (1996) 'The Volitional Questionnaire: psychometric development and practical use.' *American Journal of Occupational Therapy 50*, 7, 516–525.

Deb, S., Hare, M. and Prior, L. (2007) 'Symptoms of dementia among adults with Down's syndrome: a qualitative study.' *Journal of Intellectual Disability Research 51*, 9, 726–739.

de las Heras, C.G., Geist, R., Kielhofner, G. and Li, Y. (2007) *A User's Manual for the Volitional Questionnaire.* Version 4.1. Chicago, IL: University of Illinois at Chicago.

Department of Health (1990) *The NHS and Community Care Act.* London: HMSO.

Department of Health (2001) *The National Service Framework for Older People.* London: Department of Health.

Didden, R. and Sigafoos, J. (2001) 'A review of the nature and treatment of sleep disorders in individuals with developmental disabilities.' *Research in Developmental Disabilities 22*, 4, 255–272.

Dinges, D.F., Maislin, G., Kuo, A., Carlin, M.M. *et al.* (1999) 'Chronic sleep restriction: neurobehavioural effects of 4hr, 6hr and 8hr TIB.' *Sleep 22*, Suppl., S115–S116.

Doran, S.M., Harvey, M.T. and Horner, R.H. (2006) 'Sleep and developmental disabilities: assessment, treatment, and outcome measures.' *Mental Retardation 44*, 1, 13–27.

Dunn, W. (1999) *Sensory Profile: User's Manual.* San Antonio, TX: Pearson.

Engel-Yeger, B. and Shochat, T. (2012) 'The relationship between sensory processing patterns and sleep quality in healthy adults.' *Canadian Journal of Occupational Therapy 79*, 3, 134–141.

Espie, C.A. (2000) 'Sleep and disorders of sleep in people with mental retardation.' *Current Opinion in Psychiatry 13*, 5, 507–511.

Espie, C.A., Paul, A., McFie, J., Amos, P. *et al.* (1998) 'Sleep studies of adults with severe or profound mental retardation and epilepsy.' *American Journal of Mental Retardation 103*, 1, 47–59.

Fisher, G. and Kayhan, E. (2012) 'Developing the Residential Environment Impact Survey Instruments through faculty–practitioner collaboration.' *Occupational Therapy in Health Care 26*, 4, 224–239.

Fisher, G., Kayhan, E., Arriaga, P. and Less, C. (2013) *The Residential Environment Impact Survey (REIS).* Version 3.0. Chicago, IL: University of Illinois at Chicago.

Fung, C., Wiseman-Hakes, C., Stergiou-Kita, M., Nguyen, M. and Colantonio, A. (2013) 'Time to wake up: bridging the gap between theory and practice for sleep in occupational therapy.' *British Journal of Occupational Therapy 76*, 8, 384–386.

Gabelle, A. and Dauvilliers, Y. (2010) 'Sleep and dementia.' *Journal of Nutrition, Health & Aging 14*, 3, 201–202.

Ghiassi, R., Murphy, K., Cummin, A.R. and Partridge, M.R. (2011) 'Developing a pictorial Epworth Sleepiness Scale.' *Thorax 66*, 2, 97–100.

Goodman, J. and Locke, C. (2009) 'Occupations and the Occupational Therapy Process.' In J. Goodman, J. Hurst and C. Locke (eds) *Occupational Therapy for People with Learning Disabilities.* Philadelphia, PA: Churchill Livingstone Elsevier.

Green, A. (2012) 'A Question of Balance: The Relationship Between Daily Occupation and Sleep.' In A. Green and A. Westcombe (eds) *Sleep: Multiprofessional Perspectives.* London: Jessica Kingsley Publishers.

Gunning, M. and Espie, C. (2003) 'Psychological treatment of reported sleep disorder in adults with intellectual disability using a multiple baseline design.' *Journal of Intellectual Disability Research 47*, 3, 191–202.

Hank, D., Hicks, J. and Wilson, S. (2012) 'Sleep and Psychiatry.' In A. Green and A. Westcombe (eds) *Sleep: Multiprofessional Perspectives.* London: Jessica Kingsley Publishers.

Hawkins, A. and Look, R. (2006) 'Levels of engagement and barriers to physical activity in a population of adults with learning disabilities.' *British Journal of Learning Disabilities 34*, 4, 220–226.

Hogg, J., Lucchino, R., Wang, K. and Janicki, M. (2000) *Healthy Ageing – Adults with Intellectual Disabilities: Ageing & Social Policy.* Geneva: World Health Organization. Available at www.who.int/mental_health/media/en/23.pdf, accessed on 4 November 2013.

Hurst, J. (2009) 'Occupation and Health Promotion.' In J. Goodman, J. Hurst and C. Locke (eds) *Occupational Therapy for People with Learning Disabilities.* Philadelphia, PA: Churchill Livingstone Elsevier.

Hylkema, T., Petitiaux, W. and Vlaskamp, C. (2011) 'Utility of staff training on correcting sleep problems in people with intellectual disabilities living in residential settings.' *Journal of Policy and Practice in Intellectual Disabilities 8*, 2, 85–91.

Hylkema, T. and Vlaskamp, C. (2009) 'Significant improvement in sleep in people with intellectual disabilities living in residential settings by non-pharmaceutical interventions.' *Journal of Intellectual Disability Research 53*, 8, 695–703.

Hylkema, T. and Vlaskamp, C. (2013) 'Improving sleep in a person with Down syndrome and Alzheimer's disease.' *Journal of Sleep Disorders: Treatment & Care 2*, 4, 1–4.

Janicki, M.P., Dalton, A.J., Henderson, C.M. and Davidson, P.W. (1999) 'Mortality and morbidity among older adults with intellectual disability: health services considerations.' *Disability and Rehabilitation 21*, 5–6, 284–294.

Johns, M.W. (1991) 'A new method of measuring daytime sleepiness: the Epworth Sleepiness Scale.' *Sleep 14*, 6, 540–545.

Kalsy, S. and Oliver, C. (2002) *Psychosocial Interventions for People with Down's Syndrome and Dementia.* London: The Foundation for People with Learning Disabilities. Available at www.learningdisabilities.org.uk/content/assets/pdf/publications/psychosocial_interventions.pdf?view=Standard, accessed on 20 October 2013.

Kielhofner, G. (2008) 'The Basic Concepts of Human Occupation.' In G. Kielfhofner (ed) *Model of Human Occupation: Theory and Application*, 4th edn. Philadelphia, PA: Lippincott Williams & Wilkins.

Kinnealey, M. and Fuiek, M. (1999) 'The relationship between sensory defensiveness, anxiety, depression and perception of pain in adults.' *Occupational Therapy International 6*, 3, 195–206.

Kripke, D. (2000) 'Hypnotic drugs: deadly risks, doubtful benefits.' *Sleep Medicine Reviews 4*, 1, 5–20.

Limoges, É., Mottron, L., Bolduc, C., Berthiaume, C. and Godbout, R. (2005) 'Atypical sleep architecture and the autism phenotype.' *Brain 128*, 5, 1049–1061.

MacKeith, J. (2011) 'The development of the Outcomes Star: a participatory approach to assessment and outcome measurement.' *Housing, Care and Support 14*, 3, 98–106.

McCulloch, A. (2011) *Sleep Well – Your Pocket Guide to Better Sleep.* Available at www.bris.ac.uk/equalityanddiversity/act/protected/disability/mhfsleepguide.pdf, accessed on 10 November 2013.

McCurry, S.M. and Ancoli-Israel, S. (2003) 'Sleep dysfunction in Alzheimer's disease and other dementias.' *Current Treatment Options in Neurology 5*, 3, 261–272.

Ministry of Justice (2005) *Mental Capacity Act.* Available at www.legislation.gov.uk/ukpga/2005/9/contents, accessed on 19 December 2013.

Ohl, A., Butler, C., Carney, C., Jarmel, E. *et al.* (2012) 'Brief report: test–retest reliability of the Sensory Profile Caregiver Questionnaire.' *American Journal of Occupational Therapy 66*, 4, 483–487.

Parkinson, S., Cooper, J.R., de las Heras de Pablo, C.G. and Forsyth, K. (2014) 'Measuring the effectiveness of interventions when occupational performance is severely impaired.' *British Journal of Occupational Therapy 77*, 2, 78–81.

Patrick, G.T.W. and Gilbert, J.A. (1896) 'Studies from the psychological laboratory of the University of Iowa: on the effects of loss of sleep.' *Psychological Review 3*, 5, 469–483.

Pfeiffer, B., Kinnealey, M., Reed, C. and Herzberg, G. (2005) 'Sensory modulation and affective disorders in children with Asperger syndrome.' *American Journal of Occupational Therapy 59*, 3, 335–345.

Pilcher, J.J. and Huffcutt, A.I. (1996) 'Effects of sleep deprivation on performance: a meta-analysis.' *Sleep 19*, 4, 318–326.

Postural Care Action Group (2011) *Postural Care: Protecting and Restoring Body Shape.* Available at www.mencap.org.uk/node/13296, accessed on 1 March 2014.

Reisman, J.E. and Hanschu, B. (1992) *Sensory Integration Inventory – Revised for Individuals with Developmental Disabilities: User's Guide.* Hugo, MN: PDP Press.

Resta, O., Foschino Barbaro, M.P., Giliberti, T., Caratozzolo, G. *et al.* (2003) 'Sleep related breathing disorders in adults with Down syndrome.' *Down Syndrome Research and Practice 8*, 3, 115–120.

Richdale, A.L. (1999) 'Sleep problems in autism: prevalence, cause, and intervention.' *Developmental Medicine and Child Neurology 41*, 1, 60–66.

Roth, T. (2007) 'Insomnia: definition, prevalence, etiology, and consequences.' *Journal of Clinical Sleep Medicine 3*, Suppl. 5, S7–S10.

Schaaf, R.C. and Davies, P. (2010) 'Evolution of the sensory integration frame of reference.' *American Journal of Occupational Therapy 64*, 3, 363–367.

Schreck, K.A., Mulick, J.A. and Smith, A.F. (2004) 'Sleep problems as possible predictors of intensified symptoms of autism.' *Research in Developmental Disabilities 25*, 1, 57–66.

Shochat, T., Tzischinsky, O. and Engel-Yeger, B. (2009) 'Sensory hyper-sensitivity as a contributing factor in the relationship between sleep disorders and symptoms of attention deficit/hyperactivity in normal schoolchildren.' *Behavioral Sleep Medicine 7*, 1, 53–62.

Short, C.A. and Carpenter, P.K. (1998) 'The treatment of sleep disorders in people with learning disabilities using light therapy.' *International Journal of Psychiatry in Clinical Practice 2*, 2, 143–145.

Tani, P., Lindberg, N., Nieminen-von Wendt, T., von Nieminen Wendt, L. *et al.* (2003) 'Insomnia is a frequent finding in adults with Asperger syndrome.' *BMC Psychiatry.* doi: 10.1186/1471-244X-3-12.

Trois, M.S., Capone, J.D., Lutz, J.A., Melendres, M.C. *et al.* (2009) 'Obstructive sleep apnea in adults with Down syndrome.' *Journal of Clinical Sleep Medicine 5*, 4, 317–323.

Urv, T.K., Zigman, W.B. and Silverman, W. (2008) 'Maladaptive behaviors related to dementia status in adults with Down syndrome.' *American Journal of Mental Retardation 113*, 2, 73–86.

Urv, T.K., Zigman, W.B. and Silverman, W. (2010) 'Psychiatric symptoms in adults with Down syndrome and Alzheimer's disease.' *American Journal on Intellectual Developmental Disabilities 115*, 4, 265–276.

Vriend, J.L., Corkum, P.V., Moon, E.C and Smith, I.M. (2011) 'Behavioral interventions for sleep problems in children with autism spectrum disorders: current findings and future directions.' *Journal of Pediatric Psychology 36*, 9, 1017–1029.

Watchman, K. (2003) 'Critical issues for service planners and providers of care for people with Down's syndrome and dementia.' *British Journal of Learning Disabilities 31*, 2, 81–84.

World Health Organization (2014) *Definition: Intellectual Disability.* Geneva: World Health Organization. Available at: www.euro.who.int/en/health-topics/noncommunicable-diseases/mental-health/news/news/2010/15/childrens-right-to-family-life/definition-intellectual-disability, accessed on 1 March 2014.

12

SLEEP AND TRAUMA-EXPOSED WORKERS

Nicola Stubbs, Anna Aishford and Cary Brown

12.1 Introduction

Why a chapter specifically about trauma-exposed workers (TEWs)? To answer that question we need first to consider the growing concern expressed in the literature that the traditional conceptualization of trauma, as a directly experienced personal event, is insufficient to understand the prevalence and implications of trauma within society. The *Diagnostic and Statistical Manual of Mental Disorders* (DSM-IV) (APA 2000) defines trauma as the direct personal experience of an event that involves actual or threatened death or serious injury, or other threat to one's physical integrity; or witnessing an event that involves death, injury or a threat to the physical integrity of another person; or learning about unexpected or violent death, serious harm or threat of death or injury experienced by a family member or other close associate (p.463). However, an increasing number of experts in the area of psychological health have pointed out that this definition excludes those who experience secondary trauma by the nature of their work (for example, social workers in refugee camps, emergency responders, those responsible for dealing with body search and recovery) and those persons who have experiences that, although not life threatening, are abjectly terrorizing, profoundly humiliating or degrading (for example, through sexual coercion or bullying in the workplace). Experts in trauma caution that the traditional, more narrow DSM-IV definition contributes to trauma being under-recognized and not treated, leaving traumatized workers unable to fulfil their occupational roles or maintain resilience and well-being (Tehrani 2004). Briere and Scott (2012) propose a more inclusive definition such that 'an event is traumatic if it is extremely upsetting and at least temporarily overwhelms the individual's internal resources' (p.8). Briere and Scott conclude from their review of the trauma literature that close to 50% of Americans experience a significant traumatic experience at some point in their lives. They also review the various biopsychosocial features that influence how an individual responds to that trauma and the range of resultant negative consequences for those who lack the resiliency to cope. They point out that, because of perceived stigma, shame, organizational culture and, at times, lack of insight, many persons who have been traumatized in the workplace do not introduce the topic during health care encounters. The consequences of trauma, and repeated trauma, can be extensive and interfere with all aspects of occupational performance to the extent of the person being unable to attend to his or her own personal care and carry out employment safely and competently.

The trauma associated with serious injuries, such as burns and road crashes, or violence, such as rape and assault, is more readily anticipated by health care workers who are treating the patient for that specific reason. However, most therapists would not necessarily think to explore ongoing trauma exposure with a client referred for another reason. For example, if a worker in a poultry processing plant is referred for low back pain, the therapist would be unlikely to explore if the worker finds killing birds on this scale on a daily basis to be traumatic. A similar example can be presented for those workers who are vicariously exposed to their clients' trauma. While the actual job duties of a school teacher may not be considered highly traumatic, the degree of vicarious trauma exposure that teacher receives, consequent to working with refugee children who were exposed to extensive violence in their home country, for example, can be extensive. As Baird and Kracen (2006) point out, research consistently demonstrates that vicarious exposure to another person's trauma can have a cumulative negative effect significantly interfering with emotional health and resilience.

Occupational therapists' clients have diverse backgrounds and experiences that are not necessarily evident in the reason for referral. For example, a client referred for a flexor tendon injury may have a background of work-related stress that only becomes known as the relationship between therapist and client develops. When this emerges the therapist now expands her or his treatment focus to help the client explore coping strategies and self-care options while still treating the flexor tendon injury.

Although military and law enforcement officers are the first to spring to mind when discussing trauma-exposing work settings, it is important to expand the list to include firefighters, ambulance personnel, rescue workers, meat processing plant workers, trauma and emergency nurses, correctional institution workers, refugee camp staff and those in similar occupations. These highly disparate jobs all share features of actual or potential violence, lack of individual control over the traumatic events one is exposed to and the likelihood that traumatic workplace events will be an ongoing occurrence. Of importance to this book, workers exposed to trauma also often share sleep deficiency as a consequence of this trauma exposure. Sleep deficiency, defined by the National Institutes of Health – National Center on Sleep Disorders Research (NIH 2011) as 'too little sleep, poor sleep quality, and sleep problems' (p.12), is a frequent outcome of traumatizing experiences in job situations with high exposure to harmful and stressful events (Davis and Wright 2007). The evidence suggests that a bidirectional relationship exists between sleep problems and development of mental health conditions following exposure to traumatic events. For example, research shows that chronic sleep deficiency is a risk factor for developing post-traumatic stress disorder (PTSD) and, conversely, insomnia is a common symptom of PTSD (Germain *et al.* 2007; Lamarche and De Koninck 2007). A recent study of over 15,000 American military members concluded that pre-deployment sleep deficiency was a significant risk factor for developing PTSD, depression and other mental health conditions following exposure to trauma during deployment. The researchers recommended that sleep problems be included in the pre-deployment screening battery so as to identify persons at particular risk (Gehrman *et al.* 2013). Therapists should be aware that trauma exposure, while more likely, is not restricted to traditional military and policing occupations. Many work settings, such as schools, hospitals, abattoirs and even restaurants and banks, have the potential to expose workers to trauma. Congruent with Briere and Scott's (2012) conceptualization of trauma, a worker's interpretation of experiences as traumatic and the consequent development of sleep problems can depend on many factors. These factors include: context and meaning of the event, frequency, intensity and duration of traumatizing event(s), level of social support, age of the individual and emotions experienced after the traumatic incident, such as guilt, humiliation or shame (Davis and Wright 2007).

This chapter explains why occupational therapists working with trauma-exposed workers should be attentive to sleep deficiency, discusses how to assess for sleep problems and reviews the evidence for non-pharmacological sleep interventions studied specifically with TEWs. This is not to imply that other evidence-based sleep interventions not reviewed in this chapter would be ineffective, but TEWs potentially have additional issues that could decrease the effectiveness and practicality of sleep interventions that would be routine for others. For example, firefighters and police officers are not always able to follow traditional sleep hygiene principles to the same degree as other workers. We are using the term 'trauma-exposed worker' (TEW) to be congruent with the emerging literature in this area (for example, Frans *et al.* 2005).

The chapter also presents information from a preventative perspective relevant to therapists working with TEWs to decrease their risk of developing sleep problems, as well as treatment interventions for those TEWs exhibiting sleep deficiency. This dual focus is important because early intervention to promote restorative sleep can serve a protective function and help maintain workers' resilience during work-related trauma exposures. Additionally, attending to existing sleep deficiencies can often help speed restoration of function and reduce the severity of co-morbidities.

Unfortunately, to this point there is only a small body of sleep research related to TEWs, and the majority of the limited evidence that does exist is based on studies of military personnel; however, many other professions have work settings with traumatic characteristics similar to those in the military (such as erratic sleep availability, shift work and exposure to and/or use of violence), so we have extrapolated the available evidence to apply across the range of TEWs when appropriate. As the evidence base grows across occupations, we will be better able to understand patterns of commonality and difference so as to better be able to tailor interventions.

12.2 The relationship between trauma exposure and sleep

Trauma-exposed workers share the same risk for, and likelihood of, sleep deficiency as other adults in the general population. However, there are additional features in many trauma-exposing work settings that compound the likelihood of a worker experiencing sleep deficiency. Perhaps the most common feature is that TEWs in many professions often have shift patterns that rotate through all 24 hours and, consequently, have a higher prevalence of sleep deficiency (20.1%) compared with permanent daytime workers (12%) (Ohayon *et al.* 2002). This is important because we now know that fatigue consequent to sleep deficiency plays a major role in workplace accidents. For example, one review found that a number of severe unforeseen events in the US aviation military happen as a result of physical and mental weariness due to exertion and sleep deficiency (Caldwell and Caldwell 2005). Studies in the military have found that the rate of insomnia is particularly high in military members returning from deployment (McLay and Spira 2009; Peterson *et al.* 2008). Sixty-seven per cent of American veterans of the Iraq and Afghanistan wars identify sleep as an occupational performance challenge; only school (97%), relationships (80%), driving (70%) and leisure (70%) were more frequently selected (Plach and Sells 2013). Although the onset of insomnia can often be related to a specific stressful event, we now know it can become chronic with a specific precipitating event difficult to determine. Over time, chronic insomnia becomes associated with emotional stress, decreased insight and less effective coping strategies. Additionally, a relationship has been demonstrated with pre-existing mental health problems (anxiety disorders and depression), separation or divorce from a partner, ageing, low or threatened socioeconomic status, shift work, environmental stimuli, irregular sleep schedules, cigarette smoking, caffeine use, and drug and alcohol misuse (Lee and Ward 2005; Ohayon and Vecchierini 2005; Peterson *et al.* 2008). Research specific to military members reports that those with chronic sleep deficiency report experiencing decreased vitality in everyday tasks, decreased physical activity, increased difficulty regulating their emotions and increased health-related concerns even after deployment (Peterson *et al.* 2008). For TEWs risk factors and stressors are compounded by job demands and lifestyle choices. In the military, for example, prolonged states of hyperarousal (Bramoweth and Germain 2013), climate extremes, jet lag, rotating shifts, loud, alerting noises in an unfamiliar new sleep environment, lack of privacy, uncomfortable beds, aches, pains, or physical problems, safety concerns and worry over family back home are common (Peterson *et al.* 2008). These factors also exist in varying degrees in the work settings of firefighters, police officers and numerous other TEWs.

Insufficient sleep can negatively impact one's ability to complete tasks associated with emotional, social, physical and cognitive well-being (Colten and Altevogt 2006). Quality of life is also affected (Colten and Altevogt 2006; Lamarche and De Koninck 2007; Strine and Chapman 2005). Higher order functions, such as decision-making abilities and reaction times, are critically important for many TEWs; however, they are negatively impacted by lack of sleep. As a result, the risk of serious errors in the workplace is much higher in people with sleep problems (Lamarche and De Koninck 2007). When trauma and insomnia combine, it is not uncommon for individuals to have symptoms such as reduced short-term memory recall, difficulty with learning and acquiring new information, decreased performance in tasks requiring divergent thinking, lessened ability to be mentally responsive and perceptive, and decreased physical ability to perform tasks.

One study of the impact of sleep deprivation and dietary factors on military personnel found that all groups of military professionals demonstrated significant decline in decision-making capacity and job competency after only 4 days of insufficient sleep (Rognum *et al.* 1986). Curry (2005) concluded that ability to function is reduced with less than 4–6 hours of sleep or when awake in excess of 16 hours. Biological consequences of insufficient sleep include: increased resting heart rate and blood pressure, elevated cholesterol levels, pain (for example, back problems, headaches), gastrointestinal problems, compromised immune system function and slower wound healing (Davis and Wright 2007). Individuals who are constantly in a state of hyperarousal due to trauma are also at a statistically significant higher risk of depression (Krystal 2006), diabetes, hypertension (Buxton and Marcelli 2010; McCracken and Iverson 2002), chronic pain and obesity (McCracken and Iverson 2002) than the general population who are not exposed to ongoing hyperarousal. It is important to note that TEWs are also more often at risk than the general population for acquiring physical injuries when engaged in their professional work. The relationship between pain, sleep and hyperarousal is complex; however, both sleep and pain appear to be mediated in the hypothalamic-pituitary-adrenal axis (Goodin *et al.* 2012), and promising research that can help guide practice is growing in this area. For example, a recent study (Goodin *et al.* 2012) revealed that poor sleep quality was significantly associated with participants reporting higher levels of pain severity and having greater cortisol reactivity during induced acute pain in the laboratory. The researchers also found that the increase in production of cortisol resulting from induced pain was a mediator of the relationship between poor sleep and pain severity. In other words, sleep deficiency contributed to increased sensitivity to pain, and pain contributed to the risk of poor sleep. Similar support for this complex relationship between sleep and pain was found in a large-scale British study (Davies *et al.* 2008) where restorative sleep was found to predict resolution of chronic widespread pain, and in a Finnish study where sleep patterns were determined to be predictors of disability from low back pain (Ropponen *et al.* 2013). Although these relationships are complex and much work remains to be done, sleep interventions to improve both sleep and pain in persons with ongoing pain appear to hold promise. (The relationship between sleep and pain is reviewed in detail in Chapter 16.)

A final difference between TEWs and the general population of particular relevance to sleep deficiency is the relationship between pre-existing or work-acquired traumatic head injuries and concussion. The majority of literature relating to this arises from observational studies of military members who have been affected by explosions or other harmful events during combat/training (Evans 2008). Concussion and head injury can arise in other professions where explosions (for example, firefighters) and vehicle crashes (for example, police officers) occur. Additionally, young persons whose recreational activities included contact sports, such as hockey, American football or rugby, in growing numbers bring pre-existing mild traumatic brain injuries (mTBI) into the work setting (Castriotta and Lai 2001). Research has found that, in persons who have experienced mTBI, sleep and circadian regulation is negatively affected by lower evening melatonin* production, reduced slow-wave sleep* and an increased incidence of depression compared with the general population (Shekleton *et al.* 2010). An Israeli polysomnography* study of 26 adults with mTBI found that light, non-rapid eye movement (NREM) sleep* scores were significantly higher, and REM sleep* scores were lower when compared with those of controls (Schreiber *et al.* 2008). Because REM sleep is important for cognitive function, memory and new learning, these findings are particularly of concern given the high cognitive demand of many occupations where trauma is likely to be experienced. This is an emerging area, and occupational therapists are already well positioned to draw on their foundational knowledge of mTBI.

12.3 Occupational therapy theory to guide practice

Framing the issue of sleep deficiency in TEWs within the Model of Human Occupation (Kielhofner 2008) can help occupational therapists conceptualize sleep as part of an interactive biopsychosocial system with multiple points at which the therapist can engage the client and provide relevant interventions. Sleep, like other occupations, is motivated by volitional values and beliefs, shaped by routines comprising habituation, affected by performance capacities of the body and takes place within the context of the environment. This section reviews how the model can help contextualize and guide interventions for TEWs who experience sleep problems.

Volition

Volition includes one's thoughts and feelings about sleep and work, and the importance individuals attach to occupations (Kielhofner 2008). Western industrial societies tend to undervalue sleep and place high value on paid occupation (Pierce and Summers 2011). Societal context also includes workplace cultures and values that shape worker beliefs about sleep. This is especially true in the case of the TEW, where the worker role may provide an important source of identity and where long hours, shift work or stressful conditions may be the norm (Pierce and Summers 2011). Workplace cultures involving role ambiguity, workload variance and group conflict have been found to contribute to sleep deficiency in TEWs (Carey *et al.* 2011). As such, volition can exacerbate sleep deficiency. Insufficient sleep also affects the judgement and decision-making of TEWs. A study of 3545 police officers in Boston, with diagnosed sleep problems, determined that they were more likely to display uncontrolled anger, to be involved in traffic collisions while on duty and to make more administrative errors and safety violations (Rajaratnam *et al.* 2011). In addition to these issues of executive function and emotional regulation, individuals hold personal values and beliefs that influence, and are influenced by, judgement, insight and decision-making habits. Occupational therapists should ask their clients about these cognitive-emotional components to best understand opportunities and barriers to facilitate optimum restorative sleep. For example, a client may hold the belief that sleep is less important than physical activity, and this belief is reinforced by coworkers who also highly value physical fitness. This leads the client to do intensive physical activity late at night before going to bed. Because the activity is so physiologically arousing, the client cannot sleep afterwards. To be most effective, the therapist should work with the client to maintain his value of fitness while demonstrating how the timing of exercise is interfering with restorative sleep. Together they can strategize about alternative times to engage in exercise that will not interfere with sleep efficiency. In some cases the occupational therapist needs to address societal and workplace values as well as attitudes of the individual client. Given the serious consequences of sleep deficiency in TEWs, the occupational therapist may also take an advocacy approach, seeking opportunities to work with police and fire service administration or military units to discuss workplace values and attitudes toward sleep, provide education on consequences of undervaluing sleep and collaborate with the workplace to facilitate a culture that values and understands the interaction between sleep and participation in potentially traumatic occupations.

Habituation

Habituation involves the automatic routines associated with occupation (Kielhofner 2008), in this case, with sleep. The nature of the TEW's job may involve inconsistent temporal and physical cues such as variable scheduling, daytime sleeping, noisy conditions, extreme temperatures or unfamiliar environments that make establishing consistent sleep patterns difficult (Gerber *et al.* 2010). Exposure to routine daily stressors, pre-existing negative sleep behaviours and lifestyle habits (for example, consuming caffeine to sustain performance or drinking alcohol at bedtime to help fall asleep) are interrelated and can often be counter-productive, ultimately leading to even more sleep loss. New habits developed to self-manage sleep deficiency after it is established can also become an issue. The TEW experiencing insufficient sleep may develop patterns of behaviour involving sustained napping during waking hours or chronic anxiety regarding sleep. Additionally, TEWs experiencing frequent nightmares may resist sleep in order to avoid negative emotional and physiological responses.

While a traumatic workplace event may trigger maladaptive habits, this is not necessarily the case. People may have pre-existing sleep hygiene problems, sleep disruption from mTBI or concussion, or undiagnosed conditions such as sleep apnoea, before entering into trauma-exposing professions. Common pre-existing sleep problems, such as insomnia and obstructive sleep apnoea (OSA), in the general population (see Chapter 7) assume an even more significant role for TEWs because sleep deficiency is a risk factor for conditions such as PTSD (Carey *et al.* 2011). Adaptive habits help the TEW to achieve adequate sleep, whereas maladaptive habits may exacerbate sleep difficulties and fatigue. Occupational therapy's role is to provide support as well as environmental, cognitive and behavioural strategies to address persistent maladaptive patterns and habits surrounding sleep. Such interventions may also serve a preventative role because sleep deficiency, as previously mentioned, has been identified as a risk factor for the development of certain psychiatric disorders such as depression, anxiety and PTSD in military members and possibly other TEW populations (Lamarche and De Koninck 2007).

Performance capacity

Performance capacity considers the impact of the physical body on one's lived experience (Kielhofner 2008). Certain bodily states or conditions greatly influence the sleep of TEWs; of particular note is the state of physiological hyperarousal, as this appears to be a key contributor to the experience of insomnia (Bryant *et al.* 2010). The occupations of TEWs often require periods of sustained vigilance, stress and hyperarousal, which are all risk factors for developing sleep deficiency. The occupational therapist must also be aware of the potential impacts on sleep of conditions such as PTSD, mTBI, OSA, depression, anxiety and alcoholism in TEWs. The occupational therapist should be able to flag the suspected presence of co-morbid conditions in the TEW, understand the implications for sleep of those comorbidities and facilitate referral for specialized assessment and treatment when necessary. Because of the relationship between sleep and the physical and cognitive functional outcomes of PTSD, mTBI and OSA, these three conditions are briefly reviewed in this section.

Post-traumatic stress disorder

Key features of PTSD include initial and sleep-maintenance insomnia, reduced sleep efficiency, nightmares and resistance to falling asleep because of fear of nightmares, inability to fall asleep due to increased arousal and increased number of awakenings (Bryant *et al.* 2010). In fact, PTSD has been shown to change the structure of healthy sleep such that individuals with PTSD have more stage 1 sleep*, less slow-wave sleep and higher frequency of REM during REM sleep than individuals without PTSD (Kobayashi *et al.* 2012). Although PTSD is commonly associated with military and law enforcement personnel, a large 2005 demographic study in the US reported a prevalence rate of 3.5% in the general population (Kessler *et al.*). Pragmatically, this means that the likelihood of patients on a therapist's caseload developing PTSD may be higher than one would anticipate, and skills for basic screening are required. PTSD is also known to have a bidirectional relationship with some sleep problems, such that pre-existing problems may facilitate the development of psychiatric illness following a traumatic event. For example, PTSD symptom severity has been found to be directly related to sleep disturbance severity. Treating PTSD in the TEW often involves specialized intervention, and even so, clients often report residual sleep disturbances following treatment.

Mild traumatic brain injury

An mTBI may result from direct trauma to the head through violence or a leisure activity, vehicular accident, fall or proximity to a blast or explosion on the job. Insomnia, hypersomnia and circadian-rhythm disorders are associated with mTBI in the TEW (Sheng, Hou and Dong 2012). Research estimates that 46% of mTBI patients experience sleep deficiency, and researchers highlight that this problem remains largely unrecognized (Castriotta and Lai 2001). Young, active people may also have experienced an mTBI through sports injuries prior to entering a TEW setting. This research is in its early stages, but occupational therapists should remember to ask their clients with sleep problems if they have ever had an mTBI or other head injury.

Obstructive sleep apnoea

Obstructive sleep apnoea, also often undiagnosed, is a blockage of the airway during sleep (see Chapter 7 for more details). It is considered to be prevalent at rates of 5–7% in the general population (Punjabi 2008) and characterized by heavy snoring and gasping, with a demonstrated negative influence on sleep and health. The prevalence of OSA in some populations of police officers (33.6%) (Rajaratnam *et al.* 2011), firefighters who responded to the World Trade Center bombings in 2001 (13.9%) (Webber *et al.* 2011) and active military members (76.8%) (Capaldi, Guerrero and Killgore 2011) far exceeds that of the general population. Researchers (above) speculate this may have to do with the nature of the workplace including irregular mealtimes and poor diets, inability to regulate periods of activity and rest, and organizational cultures where binge drinking is considered appropriate. In addition, TEWs who are chronically sleep deprived have a greater risk of metabolic problems, such as diabetes and obesity, which in turn increase the likelihood of OSA.

Environmental influences on sleep

The environment is occupational therapy's area of expertise and where the profession can make a distinctive and significant contribution, not only to help individual TEWs address acquired sleep problems but, equally important, to work with policy makers and employers, when possible, to promote preventative, sleep-friendly practices in trauma-exposing workplaces that will mitigate the risk of sleep problems and the myriad associated negative consequences. The advocacy and policy skills occupational therapists have developed in other arenas, such as disability rights (Valmae, Cocks and Chenowich 2010), can serve as models to move forward to effect change for persons with sleep deficiency.

The environment includes physical and social spaces, the objects and conditions within them, and the meanings and opportunities that they offer. Such spaces influence an individual's actions, occupational performance, experiences, expectations and demands (Kielhofner 2008). The sleeping environment for the TEW is particularly unusual in that workplace demands may include sleeping or napping in atypical physical and social settings such as fire stations, offices, shared sleeping spaces or temporary shelters. These environmental contexts often involve shift work, frequent moves or deployments away from home, and necessitate increased levels of arousal or vigilance (Peterson *et al.* 2008). For military members prolonged deployments may alter individual sleep-wake cycles and have a negative impact on sleep, both during deployment and extending into the months after returning home (Capaldi *et al.* 2011). Three key environmental influences on sleep are light, temperature and sound. Addressing such environmental influences with TEWs, management and policy-makers may allow the occupational therapist to prevent or minimize future psychological or physical problems associated with poor sleep, as well as help improve the sleep of TEWs with pre-existing issues. The scientific foundation of these environmental influences is introduced below and expanded upon in detail in the section on environmental interventions.

Light is a critical concern for sleep deficiency. Even small changes in evening light exposure or sleeping rhythms have been shown to negatively impact sleep quality, subjective sleepiness and psychomotor performance in healthy individuals, as well as to increase the risk of developing circadian misalignment (Burgess *et al.* 2013). This is common for TEWs who often engage in periods of high activity in the evening or work in variable time zones during training or deployment. Additionally, workplace duties may require use of electronic devices, such as computers, before bedtime. These devices emit blue-spectrum light which suppresses melatonin release (Wood *et al.* 2013). Core body temperature also plays a significant role in sleep. Core body temperature needs to drop slightly to promote melatonin production (Kräuchi 2007). In general, cooler temperatures are associated with less body movement, higher comfort level and a better quality of sleep than are warmer temperatures. TEWs that sleep during the heat of the day, work or train in hot climates, or sleep in temporary or unventilated shelters may experience particularly high ambient temperatures that interfere with sleep. The third important environmental influence is noise. Noisy sleep environments (above 45 decibels, or the equivalent noise level of a typical conversation) have been significantly associated with difficulty falling asleep, multiple awakenings, poor sleep quality, tiredness after sleep and increased use of sleep medication (Muzet 2007). TEWs, in particular, may be required to sleep with high levels of ambient noise such as close proximity to street and airfield traffic, sirens, conversations in shared sleeping spaces and other alerting sounds.

12.4 Assessing sleep from an occupational therapy perspective

Because clients are seldom referred to occupational therapy because of sleep problems, the therapist should always ask clients if they have any problems sleeping as a routine part of any intake interview. After that, more formal assessment of a client's sleep practices and environment allows occupational therapists to target specific interventions at the level of the sleep system (e.g. beliefs, habits, occupational performance components) most acceptable to the client. For instance, measures such as the Dysfunctional Beliefs and Attitudes about Sleep Scale (Morin, Vallières and Ivers 2007) and the Glasgow Sleep Impact Index (Kyle *et al.* 2013) may be used to elucidate motivational aspects, while measures such as the Sleep Hygiene Index (Mastin, Bryson and Corwyn 2006) or a sleep diary may help the therapist to understand sleep habits. By carrying out a sleep activity analysis, including a detailed review of the sleep environment, the occupational therapist can make valuable recommendations to create sleep-promoting spaces. (More details of specific sleep assessment tools are found in Chapter 8.) Assessments of organizational behaviour and culture may be indicated to facilitate the occupational therapist in an advocacy role, encouraging changes within organizations or workplaces that will enhance the sleep quality of workers, thereby improving overall productivity.

12.5 Occupational-therapy-relevant interventions

Non-pharmacological interventions

Stimulus control therapy, sleep restriction therapy, relaxation training, sleep hygiene education, psycho-educational interventions, cognitive therapy and cognitive behavioural therapy have all been reported to have some degree of success in the scant research on non-pharmacological sleep intervention (NPSI) for TEWs (Lavie 2001). There is only a small body of intervention research that focuses on TEWs, and it comes predominately from the military. This research focuses on bright-light therapy for combat-related PTSD (Youngstedt *et al.* 2010), basic sleep hygiene principles (DeViva *et al.* 2005) and biofeedback (Carmichael 2009; McLay and Spira 2009), and overall the findings have been promising. A recent critical review of NPSIs (Brown, Berry and Schmidt 2013) found that the methodological quality of the evidence base for cognitive behavioural approaches (Nappi, Drummond and Hall 2012) and imagery rehearsal (IR) therapy (Kitchiner *et al.* 2012) was relatively robust. The interventions of multi-component therapies, for example, flooding (Cooper and Klum 1989), biofeedback (Tan *et al.* 2010) and mind/body bridging (Nakamura *et al.* 2011), had moderate quality. Flooding in the study by Cooper and Klum (1989) involved exposing a population of Vietnam veterans over repeated sessions to images that became increasingly distressing. The participants were encouraged to talk about the images in depth as further details were added. At the point where participants could talk about the images in depth without excessive anxiety, the treatment was terminated. The mind/body bridging described by Nakamura *et al.* (2011) 'teaches the individual to recognize and become aware of a dysfunctional mind–body state characterized by a heightened sense of self-centeredness, as indicated by ruminative thoughts, involuntary contraction of awareness, body tension, and impaired mental or physical functioning' (p.336).

Brown *et al.* (2013) found that fitness and relaxation training (for example, breathing exercises and self-massage) sleep interventions had the weakest evidence base but warranted further study. A randomized controlled trial of yoga to reduce combat stress and improve sleep found benefits (Stoller *et al.* 2012), and this non-intrusive form of NPSI would also benefit from further, more rigorously designed study. There appears to be a paucity of research looking at environmental modification to address the influence of light, noise, heat and other environmental factors on TEWs, and this is a high-need area for research-active occupational therapists to pursue. (A detailed review of interventions is beyond the scope of this chapter. Readers are referred to the references accompanying the interventions listed below for more details on theoretical basis, intended outcome and process of interventions.)

Psychological, behavioural and educational interventions

Individuals with hyperarousal consequent to trauma exposure may relive past traumatic experiences including all of the emotions felt when the event was occurring. This hyperarousal to stimuli can make falling and staying asleep difficult (Davis and Wright 2007). As mentioned above, there is a range of psychological and behavioural interventions with a promising evidence base (Belleville, Guay and Marchand 2011; Schoenfeld, DeViva and Manber 2012; Zayfert and DeViva 2004). Much of this evidence has been incorporated into the *PTSD Sleep Therapy Manual for Military Members* (Thompson, Franklin and Hubbard 2005) which is a downloadable group therapy manual designed specifically for military personnel. The cognitive behavioural-based intervention that has received the most review to this point for TEWs with sleep problems is IR therapy (Nappi *et al.* 2010). On a cautionary note, the strength of the evidence varies widely and many of these interventions are outside the scope of an entry-level therapist, as they require additional training and should not be carried out without appropriate supervision. TEWs, by nature of the trauma exposure, are a vulnerable population who can react in aggressive and other unanticipated ways unless interventions are delivered by an experienced therapist within a supportive team environment. An additional caution is that when addressing difficulties with sleep, it is important to take into consideration the functional implications of sleep deficiency for the individual and also the family members. TEWs may experience violent reactions and mood swings because of their sleep deficiency, and family member physical and emotional safety should always be considered (Schoenfeld *et al.* 2012).

A final group of behavioural interventions includes psycho-educational approaches to help TEWs understand and apply sleep hygiene principles. Sleep hygiene recommendations are for the most part grounded in the physiology of sleep, which is intrinsically linked to light exposure, temperature, chemical stimulants and activity (see Chapter 8). Individual studies in the general population have shown the benefit of cognitive behavioural therapy for insomnia (CBT-I) interventions compared with medication. A systematic review by Mitchell *et al.* (2012) concluded that, not only was CBT-I effective for treating insomnia when compared with medications, but that its effects may be more long-lasting than medication's effects. Mitchell *et al.* (2012) go on to recommend that CBT-I should be considered as a first-line treatment option for insomnia. However, the literature specific to TEWs is not as conclusive, and a meta-analysis by Kitchiner and colleagues (2012) of the extant literature for studies of trauma-exposed military personnel found no statistically significant differences between the psycho-educational approach of sleep hygiene and CBT-I. Irrespective of which approach the therapist decides to employ, basic sleep physiology education should precede sleep hygiene interventions so that the client understands not only 'what' they should do but is also empowered through understanding the 'why' of any recommendations.

Environmental interventions

Occupational therapists' knowledge and skills can be well used to address sleep deficiency through modifying the sociocultural and physical environment. High-stress jobs often have a culture where workers are expected to be 'tough', and sleep difficulties are viewed as a sign of weakness and taboo to discuss. For example, in the military there is a prevalent belief that sleep difficulties imply a personal failing of not being able to keep up the pace, that is, the interpretation of setting sleep as a value can be that the person is weak in some way, a characteristic contrary to military culture and values. Furthermore, there is pressure on military members to disengage from intrinsic emotional needs, and as such tolerating stress on and off duty is glorified (Beder 2012). As a result, TEWs may experience greater difficulty in expressing their concerns due to the fear of labelling and associated stigma. Effective sleep intervention may require attention to the cultural environment so that the TEW can explore and gain insight into how the environment influences sleep. This opportunity to explore helps TEWs develop sleep-promoting strategies that are realistic to their own context.

Other modifiable elements of the environment include light, temperature and sound. All of these elements have a key influence on sleep physiology and can be manipulated to create more sleep-positive environments. We briefly review each element below.

Light

Therapists should educate TEWs and, when possible, their families and employers about the relationship between light and sleep. Specific environmental interventions include lowering ambient lighting an hour before bedtime and using heavy blinds to block out light entering from windows or door cracks. In large or communal spaces (for example, during deployment), or at the workplace where creating a dark space is impractical, sunglasses, face masks or eye shades can be worn. Blue-spectrum light exposure from televisions, computers and other electronic devices should be minimized toward the end of the day to promote melatonin production. TEWs using self-luminous electronic devices into the late evening or night can wear orange-tinted goggles that block out melatonin-inhibiting blue-wavelength light.[1] Digital-device screens may also be adjusted to imitate natural daylight cycles, with redder wavelength settings available for evening and night use.[2]

TEWs should increase their exposure to daylight to enhance daytime wakefulness when possible. Strategies include reducing time spent wearing sunglasses and spending as much time as possible outside during daytime. A light box with 20-minute exposure at breakfast and lunchtime can also be used to simulate sunlight and suppress melatonin production, which can be especially effective for those individuals engaged in shift work. Workplaces such as the fire and police station should be encouraged to use bright lights at night that mimic daylight environments. Once off shift, workers should expose themselves to dim lights so as to mimic dusk and to increase melatonin production before bedtime. For example, a police officer coming off night shift into the morning light can wear sunglasses on the way home to dampen exposure to bright, melatonin-suppressing, blue-spectrum light. Once at home, the officer should avoid exposure to electronic devices such as laptops, tablets and televisions. He should also keep the blinds closed in order to block the daylight in the 2-hour period prior to his planned bedtime.

Temperature

Circadian rhythms are regulated by temperature, and the core body temperature needs to drop for sleep initiation. Bedding, fans, air conditioners on timers and layered clothing can all help. Computers, laptops, televisions and digital television systems, and other electronic equipment, in addition to being cognitively alerting and emitting blue-spectrum light, can also be a heat source. A useful general rule is to keep all electronic equipment away from the immediate sleeping area and powered down during sleep. TEWs can take a warm bath or shower or use a heating pad for 30 minutes before bed to first raise their core body temperature. When the heat source is removed, the cooling of the body promotes sleep. In some cases TEWs may choose to monitor fluctuations in temperature in the sleep environment to gain objective information about changes in the environment. When necessary, this type of objective information is helpful to employers and workplace health officers who may be able to effect a change in the built environment.

Sound

To enhance sleep in uncomfortable physical spaces where outside noise from generators, sirens, electronic equipment or workstations, aircraft or even explosions in some settings is common, the TEW can be encouraged to use headphones or earplugs when it is practical. Using personal electronic devices to play relaxation music, a white-noise machine or computer tablet white-noise app, or even a low-cost fan with an audible motor can block out excess stimuli and help minimize disruptive noise in the sleep environment. Evidence suggests that music with beats ranging from 60–80 per minute is most conducive to sleep initiation. For a more detailed discussion of the evidence-base regarding the types of music, tempo and beats per minute see

Harris (2014). Shared or multi-use sleeping/socializing spaces should be reorganized so the association between bed and sleep remain clear, and others who share the space should be educated about the value of maintaining a quiet environment. Noisy equipment should also be relocated away from the sleeping space or placed in a room insulated to noise. Room allocation should aim to group TEWs working the same shifts to prevent unnecessary disruptions during the sleep period. In the home environment shift workers might utilize a basement or attic bedroom, where available, to minimize noise from traffic and other daytime activities and reduce daytime light and temperature levels.

Activity level

The occupational therapist should encourage TEWs on night shifts to go to bed as soon as possible after shift end (Srinivasan *et al.* 2010). The more time spent travelling home or completing duties in daylight following a night shift, the more awake the TEW may become, and falling asleep will become more of a challenge. Sunglasses used when travelling between work and home can help reduce bright-light exposure and subsequent melatonin suppression. Caffeinated drinks should be used only early in the shift. It can also be helpful for the TEW to avoid large meals at night or toward the end of a shift. Even though sleeping arrangements are not always ideal for TEWs, they should aim to have a comfortable sleeping surface. Levels of mattress firmness, foam overlays, pillows with varying supports and potentially allergenic bedding should be addressed and tailored by the therapist to provide maximum possible comfort.

12.6 Conclusion

Workers in trauma-exposing jobs have a heightened risk of developing clinical or subclinical sleep problems. Of concern, such problems may result in decreased ability, safety and vitality in everyday tasks, decreased physical activity, increased difficulty regulating emotions, adverse effects on families and overall greater health concerns. By reviewing the role of occupational therapy in sleep intervention for this high-need population, this chapter serves three primary objectives: (1) to raise awareness about disordered sleep in this often neglected client population, (2) to contextualize sleep difficulty in the TEW population and its impact on functionality and (3) to provide the current evidence base and a range of resources to help guide occupational therapy assessment and intervention. The need is pressing for increased clinical awareness and resources as well as more rigorous sleep research for this unique population.

Notes

1   Examples include Uvex S0360X Ultra-spec 2000 Safety Eyewear Orange Frame SCT-Orange UV Extreme Anti-Fog Lens and products found at www.lowbluelights.com/index.asp.

2   A free downloadable filtering program is provided at http://stereopsis.com/flux.

References

American Psychiatric Association (2000) *Diagnostic and Statistical Manual of Mental Disorders*, 4th edn, revised. Washington, DC: American Psychiatric Association.

Baird, K. and Kracen, A.C. (2006) 'Vicarious traumatization and secondary traumatic stress: a research synthesis.' *Counselling Psychology Quarterly 19*, 2, 181–188.

Beder, J. (2012) *The World of the Military: Advances in Social Work Practice in the Military.* New York, NY: Routledge.

Belleville, G., Guay, S. and Marchand, A. (2011) 'Persistence of sleep disturbances following cognitive-behavior therapy for posttraumatic stress disorder.' *Journal of Psychosomatic Research 70*, 4, 318–327.

Bramoweth, A.D. and Germain, A. (2013) 'Deployment-related insomnia in military personnel and veterans.' *Current Psychiatry Reports.* doi: 10.1007/s11920-013-0401-4.

Briere, J. and Scott, C. (2012) *Principles of Trauma Therapy: A Guide to Symptoms, Evaluation, and Treatment*, 2nd edn. Thousand Oaks, CA: Sage.

Brown, C.A., Berry, R. and Schmidt, A. (2013) 'Sleep and military members: emerging issues and nonpharmacological intervention.' *Sleep Disorders.* doi: 10.1155/2013/160374.

Bryant, R.A., Creamer, M., O'Donnell, M., Silove, D. and McFarlane, A.C. (2010) 'Sleep disturbance immediately prior to trauma predicts subsequent psychiatric disorder.' *Sleep 33*, 1, 69–74.

Burgess, H.J., Legasto, C.S., Fogg, L.F. and Smith, M.R. (2013) 'Can small shifts in circadian phase affect performance?' *Applied Ergonomics 44*, 1, 109–111.

Buxton, O.M. and Marcelli, E. (2010) 'Short and long sleep are positively associated with obesity, diabetes, hypertension, and cardiovascular disease among adults in the United States.' *Social Science and Medicine 71*, 5, 1027–1036.

Caldwell, J.A. and Caldwell, J.L. (2005) 'Fatigue in military aviation: an overview of US military-approved pharmacological countermeasures.' *Aviation Space and Environmental Medicine 76*, Suppl. 7, C39–C51.

Capaldi, V.F., Guerrero, M.L. and Killgore, W.D. (2011) 'Sleep disruptions among returning combat veterans from Iraq and Afghanistan.' *Military Medicine 176*, 8, 879–888.

Carey, M.G., Al-Zaiti, S.S., Dean, G.E., Sessanna, L. and Finnell, D.S. (2011) 'Sleep problems, depression, substance use, social bonding, and quality of life in professional firefighters.' *Journal of Occupational and Environmental Medicine 53*, 8, 928–933.

Carmichael, J.A. (2009) 'Post traumatic stress disorder in police and military personnel: assessment and treatment methods from psychophysiology and neuroscience – essential preliminary information.' *Biofeedback 37*, 1, 32–35.

Castriotta, R.J. and Lai, J.M. (2001) 'Sleep disorders associated with traumatic brain injury.' *Archives of Physical Medicine and Rehabilitation 82*, 10, 1403–1406.

Colten, H. and Altevogt, B. (2006) *Sleep Disorders and Sleep Deprivation: An Unmet Public Health Problem.* Washington, DC: National Academies Press.

Cooper, N.A. and Klum, G.A. (1989) 'Imaginal flooding as a supplementary treatment for PTSD in combat veterans: a controlled study.' *Behavior Therapy 20,* 3, 381–391.

Curry, J. (2005) 'Sleep management and soldier readiness: a guide for leaders and soldiers.' *Infantry Magazine 94,* 3, 26.

Davies, K.A., Macfarlane, G.J., Nicholl, B.I., Dickens, C. *et al.* (2008) 'Restorative sleep predicts the resolution of chronic widespread pain: results from the EPIFUND study.' *Rheumatology 47,* 12, 1809–1813.

Davis, J.L. and Wright, D.C. (2007) 'Randomized clinical trial for treatment of chronic nightmares in trauma-exposed adults.' *Journal of Traumatic Stress 20,* 2, 123–133.

DeViva, J.C., Zayfert, C., Pigeon, W.R. and Mellman, T.A. (2005) 'Treatment of residual insomnia after CBT for PTSD: case studies.' *Journal of Traumatic Stress 18,* 2, 155–159.

Evans, R.W. (2008) 'Expert opinion: posttraumatic headaches among United States soldiers injured in Afghanistan and Iraq.' *Headache 48,* 8, 1216–1225.

Frans, O., Rimmö, P.A., Aberg, L. and Fredrikson, M.M. (2005) 'Trauma exposure and post-traumatic stress disorder in the general population.' *Acta Psychiatrica Scandinavica 111,* 4, 291–299.

Gehrman, P., Seelig, A.D., Jacobson, I.G., Boyko, E.J. *et al.* (2013) 'Predeployment sleep duration and insomnia symptoms as risk factors for new-onset mental health disorders following military deployment.' *Sleep 36,* 7, 1009–1018.

Gerber, M., Hartmann, T., Brand, S., Holsboer-Trachsler, E. and Puhse, U. (2010) 'The relationship between shift work, perceived stress, sleep and health in Swiss police officers.' *Journal of Criminal Justice 38,* 6, 1167–1175.

Germain, A., Shear, M.K., Hall, M. and Buysse, D.J. (2007) 'Effects of a brief behavioral treatment for PTSD-related sleep disturbances: a pilot study.' *Behaviour Research and Therapy 45,* 3, 627–632.

Goodin, B.R., Smith, M.T., Quinn, N.B., King, C.D. and McGuire, L. (2012) 'Poor sleep quality and exaggerated salivary cortisol reactivity to the cold pressor task predict greater acute pain severity in a non-clinical sample.' *Biological Psychology 91,* 1, 36–41.

Harris, M. (2014) 'Music as a transition to sleep.' *Occupational Therapy Now 16,* 6, 11–13.

Kessler, R.C., Sonnega, A., Bromet, E., Hughes, M. and Nelson, C.B. (1995) 'Posttraumatic stress disorder in the National Comorbidity Survey.' *Archives of General Psychiatry 52,* 12, 1048–1060.

Kielhofner, G. (2008) *Model of Human Occupation: Theory and Application,* 4th edn. Philadelphia, PA: Lippincott Williams & Wilkins.

Kitchiner, N., Roberts, N., Wilcox, D. and Bisson, J.I. (2012) 'Systematic review and meta-analyses of psychosocial interventions for veterans of the military.' *European Journal of Psychotraumatology.* doi: 10.3402/ejpt.v3i0.19267.

Kobayashi, I., Huntley, E., Lavela, J. and Mellman, T.A. (2012) 'Subjectively and objectively measured sleep with and without posttraumatic stress disorder and trauma exposure.' *Sleep 35,* 7, 957–965.

Kräuchi, K. (2007) 'The human sleep-wake cycle reconsidered from a thermoregulatory point of view.' *Physiology and Behavior 90,* 2–3, 236–245.

Krystal, A.D. (2006) 'Sleep and psychiatric disorders: future directions.' *Psychiatric Clinics of North America 29,* 4, 1115–1130.

Kyle, S.D., Crawford, M.R., Morgan, K., Spiegelhalder, K., Clark, A.A. and Espie, C.A. (2013) 'The Glasgow Sleep Impact Index (GSII): a novel patient-centred measure for assessing sleep-related quality of life impairment in insomnia disorder.' *Sleep Medicine 14*, 6, 493–501.

Lamarche, L.J. and De Koninck, J. (2007) 'Sleep disturbance in adults with posttraumatic stress disorder: a review.' *Journal of Clinical Psychiatry 68*, 8, 1257–1270.

Lavie, P. (2001) 'Sleep disturbances in the wake of traumatic events.' *New England Journal of Medicine 345*, 25, 1825–1832.

Lee, K.A. and Ward, T.M. (2005) 'Critical components of a sleep assessment for clinical practice settings.' *Issues in Mental Health Nursing 26*, 7, 739–750.

Mastin, D.F., Bryson, J. and Corwyn, R. (2006) 'Assessment of sleep hygiene using the Sleep Hygiene Index.' *Journal of Behavioral Medicine 29*, 3, 223–227.

McCracken, L.M. and Iverson, G.L. (2002) 'Disrupted sleep patterns and daily functioning in patients with chronic pain.' *Pain Research and Management 7*, 2, 75–79.

McLay, R.N. and Spira, J.L. (2009) 'Use of a portable biofeedback device to improve insomnia in a combat zone: a case report.' *Applied Psychophysiology and Biofeedback 34*, 4, 319–321.

Mitchell, M.D., Gehrman, P., Perlis, M. and Umscheid, C.A. (2012) 'Comparative effectiveness of cognitive behavioral therapy for insomnia: a systematic review.' *BMC Family Practice*. doi: 10.1186/1471-2296-13-40.

Morin, C.M., Vallières, A. and Ivers, H. (2007) 'Dysfunctional beliefs and attitudes about sleep (DBAS): validation of a brief version (DBAS-16).' *Sleep 30*, 11, 1547–1554.

Muzet, A. (2007) 'Environmental noise, sleep and health.' *Sleep Medicine Reviews 11*, 2, 135–142.

Nakamura, Y., Lipschitz, D.L., Landward, R., Kuhn, R. and West, G. (2011) 'Two sessions of sleep-focused mind-body bridging improve self-reported symptoms of sleep and PTSD in veterans: a pilot randomized controlled trial.' *Journal of Psychosomatic Research 70*, 4, 335–345.

Nappi, C.M., Drummond, S.P.A. and Hall, J.M.H. (2012) 'Treating nightmares and insomnia in posttraumatic stress disorder: a review of current evidence.' *Neuropharmacology 62*, 2, 576–585.

Nappi, C.M., Drummond, S.P., Thorp, S.R. and McQuaid, J.R. (2010) 'Effectiveness of imagery rehearsal therapy for the treatment of combat-related nightmares in veterans.' *Behavior Therapy 41*, 2, 237–244.

National Institutes of Health – National Center on Sleep Disorders Research (2011) *National Institutes of Health Sleep Disorders Research Plan*. Available at www.nhlbi.nih.gov/health/prof/sleep/201101011NationalSleepDisordersResearchPlanDHHSPublication11-7820.pdf, accessed on 22 December 2013.

Ohayon, M.M., Lemoine, P., Arnaud-Briant, V. and Dreyfus, M. (2002) 'Prevalence and consequences of sleep disorders in a shift worker population.' *Journal of Psychosomatic Research 53*, 1, 577–583.

Ohayon, M.M. and Vecchierini, M.F. (2005) 'Normative sleep data, cognitive function and daily living activities in older adults in the community.' *Sleep 28*, 8, 981–989.

Peterson, A.L., Goodie, J.L., Satterfield, W.A. and Brim, W.L. (2008) 'Sleep disturbance during military deployment.' *Military Medicine 173*, 3, 230–235.

Pierce, D. and Summers, K. (2011) 'Rest and Sleep.' In C. Brown and V. Stoeffel (eds) *Occupational Therapy in Mental Health: A Vision for Participation*. Philadelphia, PA: F.A. Davis.

Plach, H.L. and Sells, C.H. (2013) 'Occupational performance needs of young veterans.' *American Journal of Occupational Therapy 67*, 1, 73–81.

Punjabi, N.M. (2008) 'The epidemiology of adult obstructive sleep apnea.' *Proceedings of the American Thoracic Society 5*, 2, 136–143.

Rajaratnam, S.M., Barger, L.K., Lockley, S.W., Shea, S.A. *et al.* (2011) 'Sleep disorders, health, and safety in police officers.' *Journal of the American Medical Association 306*, 23, 2567–2578.

Rognum, T.O., Vartdal, F., Rodahl, K., Opstad, P.K. *et al.* (1986) 'Physical and mental performance of soldiers on high- and low-energy diets during prolonged heavy exercise combined with sleep deprivation.' *Ergonomics 29*, 7, 859–867.

Ropponen, A., Silventoinen, K., Hublin, C., Svedberg, P., Koskenvuo, M. and Kaprio, J. (2013) 'Sleep patterns as predictors for disability pension due to low back diagnoses: a 23-year longitudinal study of Finnish twins.' *Sleep 36*, 6, 891–897.

Schoenfeld, F.B., DeViva, J.C. and Manber, R. (2012) 'Treatment of sleep disturbances in posttraumatic stress disorder: a review.' *Journal of Rehabilitation Research and Development 49*, 5, 729–752.

Schreiber, S., Barkai, G., Gur-Hartman, T., Peles, E. *et al.* (2008) 'Long-lasting sleep patterns of adult patients with minor traumatic brain injury (mTBI) and non-mTBI subjects.' *Sleep Medicine 9*, 5, 481–487.

Shekleton, J.A., Parcell, D.L., Redman, J.R., Phipps-Nelson, J., Ponsford, J.L. and Rajaratnam, S.M. (2010) 'Sleep disturbance and melatonin levels following traumatic brain injury.' *Neurology 74*, 21, 1732–1738.

Sheng, P., Hou, I. and Dong, Y. (2012) 'Sleep disorders after traumatic brain injury.' *Academic Journal of Second Military Medicine University 33*, 11, 1253–1256.

Srinivasan, V., Singh, J., Pandi-Perumal, S.R., Brown, G.M. *et al.* (2010) 'Jet lag, circadian rhythm sleep disturbances, and depression: the role of melatonin and its analogs.' *Advances in Therapy 27*, 11, 796–813.

Stoller, C.C., Greuel, J.H., Cimini, L.S., Fowler, M.S. and Koomar, J.A. (2012) 'Effects of sensory-enhanced yoga on symptoms of combat stress in deployed military personnel.' *American Journal of Occupational Therapy 66*, 1, 59–68.

Strine, T.W. and Chapman, D.P. (2005) 'Associations of frequent sleep insufficiency with health-related quality of life and health behaviors.' *Sleep Medicine 6*, 1, 23–27.

Tan, G., Dao, T.K., Smith, D.L., Robinson, A. and Jensen, M.P. (2010) 'Incorporating complementary and alternative medicine (CAM) therapies to expand psychological services to veterans suffering from chronic pain.' *Psychological Services 7*, 3, 148–161.

Tehrani, N. (2004) *Workplace Trauma: Concepts, Assessment and Interventions.* London: Routledge.

Thompson, K.E., Franklin, C.L. and Hubbard, K. (2005) *PTSD Sleep Therapy Group: Training Your Mind and Body for Better Sleep – Therapist Manual.* Available at www.mirecc.va.gov/visn16/docs/sleep_therapy_group_therapist_manual.pdf, accessed on 22 December 2013.

Valmae, R., Cocks, K. and Chenowich, L. (2010) 'Advocating and Lobbying.' In M. Curtin, M. Molineux and J. Supyk-Mellson (eds) *Occupational Therapy and Physical Dysfunction: Enabling Occupation,* 6th edn. London: Churchill Livingstone.

Webber, M.P., Lee, R., Soo, J., Gustave, J. *et al.* (2011) 'Prevalence and incidence of high risk for obstructive sleep apnea in World Trade Center-exposed rescue/recovery workers.' *Sleep and Breathing 15*, 283–294.

Wood, B., Rea, M.S., Plitnick, B. and Figueiro, M.G. (2013) 'Light level and duration of exposure determine the impact of self-luminous tablets on melatonin suppression.' *Applied Ergonomics 44*, 2, 237–240.

Youngstedt, S., Ginsberg, J., Powell, D., Kline, E. and Zielinski, M. (2010) 'Bright light: a novel treatment for post-traumatic stress disorder.' *Sleep 33*, Suppl., A237.

Zayfert, C. and DeViva, J.C. (2004) 'Residual insomnia following cognitive behavioral therapy for PTSD.' *Journal of Traumatic Stress 17*, 1, 69–73.

13

MENTAL HEALTH, WELL-BEING AND SLEEP

Diana Hurley and Katie MacQueen

13.1 Introduction

Until fairly recently it had been generally considered that sleep problems are simply common symptoms of psychiatric disorders. However, recent studies have investigated sleep problems and psychiatric disorders (Krystal 2012; Kyung Lee and Douglass 2010) and concluded that the relationship between them is more complex than previously thought. These studies support the view that their causation may be bidirectional, suggesting that sleep disorders may be a key trigger for the development of psychiatric illness and that treating them may reduce psychiatric symptomatology.

This further strengthens the case made by Green *et al.* (2005) and Fung *et al.* (2013), that occupational therapists working with people with mental health problems should make it a priority to tackle sleep-related problems, although sleep problems have not, hitherto, been addressed as a routine part of their practice. This chapter proposes that the particular contribution of the occupational therapist in tackling sleep problems should focus on improving overall well-being, lifestyle and health. In other words, rather than focusing purely on methods to improve sleep, occupational therapists should also address what is keeping the individual awake. This refers to the way in which the individual is using their waking time across physical, psychological, social and occupational domains. Occupational therapy interventions aimed at improving the well-being of the individual will naturally complement those aimed at improving sleep and mental health.

Starting with a brief overview of sleep symptomatology associated with a range of common mental health disorders, this chapter explores what sleep science and related theories have to say about how psychological distress gives rise to sleep problems. Research findings which may illuminate our understanding of the association between sleep and mental health are also discussed. The discourse includes 'organizing ideas' about the function of dream sleep in emotional regulation, as proposed by the 'Human Givens' model (Griffin and Tyrrell 2004a) and others. These insights point the way to practical and effective interventions and approaches, complementary to occupational therapy.

The chapter goes on to explore what is meant by 'well-being' particularly with regard to mental health, and also looks at the inter-relationships between well-being, occupational needs and sleep. The term 'recovery', and how it is understood in the field of mental health, is also explored. This approach makes the case that supporting an individual with mental health problems to make progress in their personal 'recovery journey' can contribute to well-being and, thereby, improve sleep.

Finally, the chapter focuses on interventions to alleviate sleep problems, by working on unmet needs in three priority areas of well-being: physical, emotional and occupational. To illustrate this approach for the clinical setting, case study vignettes are given in Appendix 13.1. A suggested intervention is also outlined, comprising core topic areas for inclusion in sleep improvement programmes for use in group and individual settings.

13.2 Sleep problems in psychiatric disorders

Sleep problems are a common feature across the range of mental health conditions, and may be the cause of considerable distress, serving to compound and exacerbate the symptoms of the underlying disorder (Hank, Hicks and Wilson 2012). Symptoms of insomnia have been identified in 20–40% of individuals with mental illness (Soehner and Harvey 2012). In those with mood and anxiety disorder, rates of insomnia were found to be even greater: 50–70% in those with mood disorders and 70–90% in those with anxiety disorders (Sunderjan *et al.* 2010; Uhde, Cortese and Vedeniapin 2009; Van Mill *et al.* 2010). Symptoms of sleep disturbance frequently typify specific conditions but also vary with each individual according to habits, lifestyle, attitudes and beliefs concerning sleep. Additionally, the negative impact of co-morbid physical conditions on mental health and sleep should not be overlooked (Hayashino *et al.* 2010).

Anxiety disorders

People with anxiety-related disorders almost always have difficulty in getting to sleep and staying asleep (Hank *et al.* 2012; Krystal 2012). Nightmares of a distressing nature are common, particularly in post-traumatic stress disorder, and anticipation of nightmares can lead to reluctance to go to sleep. Worry and arousal-provoking behaviours can be key factors in disrupting sleep, and it is suggested that this aspect may be more important than poor sleep hygiene* in this group (Yan *et al.* 2010).

Mood disorders

People with major depressive disorders tend to experience difficulty falling asleep and staying asleep, and report poor sleep quality, distressing dreams and nightmares. They also show more intensive and longer periods in the rapid eye movement (REM)* phase of sleep; early-morning wakening is a characteristic feature. By contrast, in the manic phase of bipolar disorder, there is a decreased awareness of the need for sleep; this can bring its own problems as states of ongoing sleeplessness increase stress upon the physical and mental health of the individual. A recent study by Li *et al.* (2013) has distinguished a possible genetic link between major depression and the internal clock governing the circadian rhythm. In comparative post-mortem studies a dysregulation in the genes involved in establishing and maintaining circadian rhythms was found in the brains of those people who had had major depressive disorder.

There is continuing uncertainty over the extent to which insomnia is a risk factor for the development of depression. That a correlation between insomnia and depression exists has been generally accepted, and a twofold risk was identified in a study by Baglioni *et al.* (2011); however, another more recent study (Skapinakis *et al.* 2013) has questioned the validity of this association. Nevertheless, for occupational therapists, addressing both mental health and sleep problems at an early stage should still be viewed as a worthwhile preventative strategy.

Schizophrenia

Sleep problems are also common in schizophrenia, insomnia being a prominent feature. A factor which can particularly affect people with schizophrenia is the tendency to develop shifts in the circadian rhythm (Hank *et al.* 2012; Krystal 2012) where the individual tends to be awake at night and asleep during the day. This also compounds the risk of social isolation for the individual with schizophrenia.

A recent study by Wulff *et al.* (2012) suggested that the poor sleep patterns associated with schizophrenia (and bipolar disorder) were also due to disrupted functioning of the body clock, linked to a certain gene mutation. The study concluded that the sleep disruption might be causing the onset of these psychiatric conditions. The authors found that young people at high risk of developing bipolar disorder were already showing an abnormal sleep-wake pattern before diagnosis was made. They suggest that if the means could be found to correct this pattern of sleeping by day and staying awake at night, then it may be possible to have a positive effect on the affected individual's mental health. As in depression, there may be a valuable preventative role for occupational therapists in addressing maladaptive daily routines at an early stage.

Another recent study (Waters, Naik and Rock 2013) looked at the links between sleep, fatigue and functional health in psychotic patients. The study classified patients on the basis of their performance on a range of sleep-quality and fatigue measures.

Their conclusions were that (a) the individual's dissatisfaction with sleep was a more important factor than actual sleep dysfunction in producing fatigue symptoms, and (b) fatigue had a particularly detrimental effect on functional health, whether sleep dysfunction was present or not.

Alcohol misuse

Whilst alcohol might help people to get off to sleep, they frequently find themselves awake soon afterwards and unable to *return* to sleep (Stein and Friedmann 2005). This is compounded by the development of tolerance to the sleep-inducing effects of alcohol and may be further complicated by the development of depressive symptoms related to the regular use of alcohol. Despite these rebound effects, up to 67% of people with insomnia report using alcohol to help them get to sleep (Kyung Lee and Douglass 2010). A recent study found that there was a significant association between insomnia symptoms and unhealthy behaviours such as heavy drinking and physical inactivity (Harrio *et al.* 2012). In turn, heavy and binge drinking were also associated with subsequent insomnia symptoms, setting up a negative cycle in people affected. In alcohol dependence, insomnia is common and is characterized by increased sleep latency* and decreased sleep efficiency*, which can persist months after alcohol cessation (Kyung Lee and Douglass 2010).

Sleep in the older adult with mental health problems

Sleep problems in the older person are complex, multi-factorial and frequently compounded by serious medical conditions. It is therefore difficult to address the sleep problems which occur in older adults with mental health disorders in isolation (see Chapter 10 and also Bloom *et al.* 2009). (The reader is referred to Chapter 14 for discussion of sleep problems occurring with dementia.)

13.3 Sleep science and mental health

For some considerable time there has been general agreement that an important function of dreaming is a link in some way with emotional regulation, although it has not been clear exactly how this complex mechanism operates (Krystal 2012; Kyung Lee and Douglass 2010) or how this knowledge can be used to improve treatment for sleep disorders. It has been widely observed that emotional distress results from sleep deprivation but, conversely, depression can be alleviated when REM sleep (when most dreaming occurs) is prevented. In support of this, Krystal (2012) notes that: 'a night of sleep deprivation has been reported to have robust antidepressant effects' (p.1399), and observes that many effective antidepressant medications suppress REM sleep (which is increased in states of anxiety and depression). Sleep deprivation, as a means of preventing REM, is clearly not a practical or clinically desirable form of treatment for depression. Likewise, attempts to relieve psychological distress through analysis of dream content are not known to have provided consistent evidence of effectiveness.

A perspective on dreaming and REM sleep from the Human Givens approach may have further light to shed on these complexities. This conceptualization, based on his analysis of scientific research relating to sleep and mental illness, has been proposed by Joe Griffin, co-founder of the Human Givens therapeutic approach (Griffin 1993; Griffin and Tyrrell 2004b). It has since found support from studies in which brain scans and electroencephalogram* recordings show desensitization to negative emotions (for example, see van der Helm *et al.* 2011). This is also supported in a study by Gujar *et al.* (2010) which describes the way in which REM sleep appears to recalibrate the brain's sensitivity to specific emotions and increases sensitivity to more positive emotions after sleep. Griffin's theory offers an explanation for why we dream and how REM sleep influences our mental health. Called the 'expectation fulfilment theory of dreams', it focuses on the function of REM sleep, during which most of our dream sleep occurs. (An explanation of the architecture of sleep and its various stages is given in Chapter 3.)

The 'expectation fulfilment' theory of dreaming (Griffin and Tyrrell 2004b) proposes that the purpose of dreams is to deactivate undischarged emotional arousal from the previous day. This may include anticipations, worries, fantasies or other preoccupations which have not been acted out or completed in reality – hence the name of the theory. According to this theory, dreams could be described as the brain's attempt to 'take the rubbish out' and clear the mental space necessary for dealing with the emotionally arousing demands of the next day. Most mental illnesses, including depression and anxiety, are associated with a great deal of worrying and emotional thinking along with high autonomic arousal. However, the theory proposes that the resulting intensity of stressful rumination, and REM, overloads the dreaming system and drives the development of states such as depression. As mentioned already, there is increased REM in depression. To summarize, healthy, restorative sleep requires an optimum balance that includes both REM and deep, slow-wave sleep (SWS)*. It is suggested that too much negative introspection leads to the REM sleep phase increasing disproportionately and reduces the amount of SWS during each period of sleep.

Cognitive behavioural approaches, widely accepted to be effective in anxiety and depression, focus on reducing negative and irrational emotional thinking. The expectation fulfilment theory of dreaming, which lies at the heart of the Human Givens approach, may therefore provide an additional basis for understanding how this approach might work. The approach itself goes further in helping individuals affected to understand how negative thinking and rumination are driving their depressed state and identifies the key elements involved in effective interventions (discussed below).

These principles are naturally complementary to both an occupationally driven intervention and to a 'recovery'-focused approach.

13.4 The effect of sleep problems on occupational function

The relationships between daily occupation and sleep are explored in Chapters 5 and 6, and Chapter 6 highlights the potential for activities such as physical exercise and daily routines to influence sleep quality. As noted in those chapters, the direction of causality in those highly complex relationships has not yet been fully understood and more research is needed; however, some research has been carried out in the context of mental health.

Soehner and Harvey (2012) conducted a large-scale survey ($n = 5692$) which assessed performance over a period of 30 days in eight domains of daytime role functioning, including self-care, mobility, cognition, social functioning and various aspects of leisure and productivity across four groups: no anxiety or mood disorder, anxiety disorders only, mood disorders only, and coexisting mood and anxiety disorders. Participants with co-morbid mood and anxiety disorders reported significantly higher rates of severe insomnia than those with anxiety or mood disorders only. Participants with co-existing anxiety and mood disorders were also found to have substantial functional impairment across a range of domains including cognition, social functioning, time out of role, productive role functioning, self-care and mobility. This finding was confirmed by Kallestad *et al.* (2012) who carried out a study involving over 2000 people attending public mental health centres. Participants rated themselves against three dependent variables including 'quality of life', symptom severity and benefit from treatment. They were also rated by clinicians against a further four dependent variables: disorder severity, level of functioning, symptom severity and benefit from treatment. Levels of sleep disturbance were then rated against each of the variables to establish whether there were any significant associations between them. It was concluded that higher levels of sleep disturbance in people with mental health problems were associated with significantly lower quality of life and higher distress in addition to functional impairment. Furthermore, Soehner and Harvey (2012) and Harvey *et al.* (2004) posit that psychological processes which maintain mood or anxiety disorders can mutually sustain or exacerbate insomnia symptoms, and vice versa.

13.5 Well-being and its relevance to mental health, sleep and occupation

It is widely observed that mental health conditions are characterized by a lack of well-being, almost always associated with poor sleep and difficulty in engaging competently in occupations. Failure to engage in self-care, work and leisure occupations can, in turn, affect health and well-being. However, in a critical review of well-being in occupational therapy and occupational science Aldrich (2011) highlighted the lack of clarity and consistency in the meaning and use of the term 'well-being' in the literature. She recommended that occupational therapists be more explicit and nuanced in their use of the term to make the concept more useful in their work. Hayward and Taylor (2011) explored well-being with reference to its importance and relevance to occupational therapy for human health. They argued that the definition of well-being is subjective and unique to each individual and should be consolidated into the underpinning philosophy of occupational therapy. Eklund and Backstrom (2006) also emphasized the importance of perceived control for well-being and occupational performance and indicated strategies that occupational therapists could employ to promote it. Facilitating improved sleep hygiene would be a relevant example.

There are numerous definitions of 'well-being', depending on which perspective one is concerned with, and the term is used in economics, sociology, philosophy, alternative spirituality and health. Baylis (2005) defines well-being as 'a positive and sustainable state in which we can thrive and flourish. At its best, the science of well-being is about exploring how good life can become and how good we can become at living it' (p.246).

Baylis (2005) describes the 'Relationship with Reality' theory and how coping styles are crucial to well-being. He outlines three ways that people cope with real life:

- reality evasion – using escapist fantasy as a short-term means of avoiding pain or challenge (for example, drug abuse, excessive television viewing, computer games)

- quick fixes – avoiding pain or anxiety by indulging in certain behaviours such as eating comfort food or drinking alcohol

- reality investment – solution-seeking attempts such as planning, practising or mentorship to help the individual achieve lasting improvements to their real-life experience.

This is a very useful model on which to base well-being interventions designed to improve sleep quality and overcome life's problems. Commonly, assessment of an individual with sleep-related problems will reveal the over-use of the first two coping styles, and improvements will result from increasing use of the reality investment (e.g. sleep diaries, information giving and solution-focused action). Finally, any discourse on models of well-being would be deficient without mentioning the 'Five Ways to Well-being' evidence-based recommendations for improved mental health (see Box 13.1).

BOX 13.1 The 'Five Ways to Wellbeing'

The 'Five Ways to Wellbeing' encourages people to:

1. connect (talk and listen, be there, feel connected)

2. be active (do what you can, enjoy what you do, move your mood)

3. take notice (remember the simple things that give you joy)

4. keep learning (embrace new experiences, see opportunities, surprise yourself)

5. give (your time, your words, your presence).

Source: NEF (URL in Appendix 13.3)

13.6 Improving sleep quality in the context of mental health conditions

Cognitive behavioural therapy for managing insomnia (CBT-I) is well established and has a sound evidence base (see Chapters 7 and 8). Chapter 8 goes into more detail on CBT-I (and on sleep hygiene) and nothing further needs to be added here. In this chapter, it is emphasized that occupational therapists working with sleep-related problems linked to mental health conditions should consider three crucial aspects of the individual's well-being:

1. physical health and well-being – physical activity, nutrition, management of long-term conditions, such as pain, and tackling addictions

2. emotional needs – the recovery process, universal human needs and resources

3. occupational needs – lifestyle balancing and health-promoting routines, including sleep hygiene.

Physical health and well-being

Physical activity

Physical activity and exercise are widely accepted to have a positive effect on sleep quality (see Chapter 6). It has been found that people with sleep problems are largely sedentary and that this hampers the ability to fall asleep and stay asleep (Loprinzi and Cardinal 2011). However, people who have suffered from insomnia for any length of time may understandably lack energy or sufficient inclination to engage in physical exercise. With education and encouragement, gradual improvements can be achieved, with additional benefits such as stress reduction and increased fitness.

Nutrition

This is another vital area to address in health-promotion terms and is also related to sleep hygiene. For instance, the consumption of heavy meals and stimulating drinks, such as caffeine, or drinking alcohol late at night may impair sleep. Additionally, where the quality of overall nutrition is poor, this will affect general health and well-being. Some ordinarily available foods and drinks, and herbal preparations, such as camomile, are held to have soporific qualities, and knowledge of them may be useful for some people (Idzikowski 2000). Therapists are recommended to address nutritional intake and related issues, such as evening routines associated with food or drink, which may impact on sleep, general health and well-being.

Management of long-term conditions

It should not be forgotten that people with mental health problems may also have co-morbid physical ill health conditions with which they are struggling to cope. In these cases, their mental health issues and sleep problems will be compounded by these difficulties. For example, various conditions, such as chronic back pain, respiratory conditions and obesity, may affect sleep adversely. Furihata *et al.* (2012) found that those who reported sleep problems perceived poorer health status than those who did not. It is necessary to look at the impact that physical conditions may be having on sleep quality and duration and identify how effectively they are being managed.

Addictions

It is well established that alcohol disrupts sleep (see section 13.2) and that a range of other substances have similar effects. Education is often necessary to ensure that the individual fully understands this. For instance, many people take alcohol at night for its 'sleep-inducing' effects, but they may be unaware that alcohol is equally likely to cause them to wake up after only a short period asleep.

Emotional needs, the 'Recovery' approach and the 'Human Givens'

Two useful approaches are introduced in this section, as they are complementary to occupational therapy practice in mental health: the Recovery approach, which is an essential underpinning model for occupational therapy in the mental health field; and the Human Givens approach, which offers insights of special relevance to psychological health and sleep disorders.

The Recovery approach

Many occupational therapists working in the field of mental health have found the Recovery approach to be inspirational, as well as complementing their practice in supporting individuals to overcome barriers to 'doing what they need to do' in order to achieve a satisfying and purposeful lifestyle. The Recovery approach encourages people to retake control over their lives and the challenges they face, rather than seeking professionals and services to 'fix' their problems for them. According to the Recovery model, professionals' skills are there to be 'tapped' by the individual with mental health problems – rather than the professional being dominant, as in the traditional therapeutic relationship (Ashcraft and Anthony 2005; Repper and Perkins 2012).

The focus should be on supporting self-management and helping people to discover, use and develop their own resources and resourcefulness. In so doing, those affected by mental illness can become experts in their own self-care, making informed choices about their care, rather than being passive recipients of imposed interventions. The 'recovery journey' involves striving for improved physical, psychological, occupational and spiritual well-being, despite the challenge of living with a mental illness.

It is suggested that sleep-related problems be addressed using the Recovery model as an ideal underpinning guide. Therapists cannot directly improve the sleep of those they work with; they can only provide the information, support and resources needed for the individual to achieve this for themselves.

The Human Givens approach

The Human Givens model states that, as well as physical needs, humans have evolved with essential emotional needs, adequate fulfilment of which is necessary for mental health (Griffin and Tyrrell 2004a). People are also endowed with certain 'resources' which help them to get their emotional needs met.[1] These resources include long-term memory, imagination, the ability to learn and understand the world through metaphor (pattern matching), the ability to take a detached perspective and the ability to empathize with others. Of special relevance to sleep, the 'dreaming brain' may enable the individual to process unfulfilled expectations and arousals from the previous set of waking hours. When emotional needs are met in balance we can enjoy a state of well-being or emotional health.

It has often been observed by mental health professionals that individuals with mental health and sleep problems frequently have very few of these needs met. Furthermore, their ability to use their resources effectively to meet their needs may also be compromised. As noted above, it is vital to recognize and tackle the issues which are keeping a person with sleep problems awake. In the Human Givens therapy context, individuals are supported first to identify which needs are unmet, and then to activate appropriate resources to meet them. To summarize, although a Human Givens intervention is always individualized, in mental health problems the following basic principles would be prioritized:

- Instil hope.

- Quickly calm, using re-framing and relaxation techniques.

- Encourage physical activity to reduce arousal.

- Reduce negative rumination and/or misuse of imagination.

- Focus attention outwards by encouraging rational, solution-focused thinking.

- Identify unmet emotional needs and/or misused personal resources.

- Agree on solution-focused action.

- Rehearse, in imagination, successful initiation of the solution-focused action, including coping effectively with setbacks.

- Initiate solution-focused action.

Occupational therapists are likely to find that the Human Givens approach harmonizes well with their holistic, practical and person-centred approach to mental health problems. The model enables both the clinician and the individual to identify unmet emotional needs and to mobilize personal resources in a solution-focused intervention. Recent outcome studies have demonstrated the utility and effectiveness of the Human Givens approach in relieving emotional distress in various settings and applications (Andrews *et al.* 2011, 2013; Tsaroucha *et al.* 2012a; Tsaroucha *et al.* 2012b; Yates and Atkinson 2011).

Occupational needs: lifestyle balancing and health-promoting routines

The relationship between sleep quality and participation in healthy routines has been clearly outlined by Green (2012) who cites studies investigating time use as well as productive and social activities (see also Chapter 6). These factors were identified as having a positive influence on sleep. Additionally, occupation and sleep affected each other bidirectionally – sleep being vital for effective occupational performance, and vice versa. Occupational therapists working in mental health settings are involved with people who are experiencing different forms of occupational deprivation and consequent imbalances in their daily and nightly routines. Within the framework of the Model of Human Occupation (MoHO), sleep is defined as a 'habit' and not perceived as an activity that is engaged in purposefully and dynamically (Kielhofner 2008). However, Fung *et al.* (2013) put the case for sleep to be given a greater profile in occupational therapy and recommend approaches that occupational therapists can use in the assessment and intervention of sleep problems. Occupational therapists are increasingly urged to prioritize the use of their skills in enabling people to engage in healthy, balanced and personally valued routines. Indeed, occupational therapists are frequently expected to provide interventions to promote an effective sleep routine by other members of the interdisciplinary team.

In applying MoHO concepts, the aim should be to improve waking lifestyle balance and well-being in daily living to promote, or maintain, corresponding sleep quality and duration. Many of the factors which typically inhibit sleep are common in people with mental health problems, for instance, volitional deficits in the perception of personal control (causation) and the ability to achieve an improved sleep routine. Also some individuals overvalue their need for sleep and overestimate the amount of sleep they need. The environment plays a key role in aiding or inhibiting sleep, and indeed activity during the day. In addition, there may be difficulty in adapting daily routines to incorporate healthy sleep strategies (i.e. habits). For example, inactive lifestyles impact negatively on motor skills and also result in insufficient energy expenditure to promote rest and sleep.

13.7 Conclusion

The evidence points to the strong inter-relationships between sleep and mental health, occupational performance and well-being. It highlights the importance of sleep-related symptoms in exacerbating psychiatric symptoms and identifies poor sleep as a possible underlying cause of some mental health problems. Research in sleep science has pointed to possible explanations for the function of REM sleep in emotional regulation and indicates how these insights relate to effective therapies for sleep problems (e.g. CBT-I and Human Givens therapy). The concepts of well-being and the Recovery approach have also been explored and proposed as useful and relevant perspectives on which to base occupational therapy interventions for sleep problems linked to mental health disorders.

Note

1   Our emotional needs include:

- security (a safe place to be and to grow)
- personal control (a sense of autonomy and control)
- connection (to be connected to the wider community)
- attention (to give and receive attention)
- intimacy (for at least one close and accepting relationship)
- privacy (space to reflect and consolidate experiences)
- self-respect (to have a healthy and balanced sense of self-worth and competence)
- meaning (having purpose and to be stretched).

Appendix 13.1 Case studies

Case study 1: Linda (aged 39 years)

At the time she was referred to occupational therapy for help with sleep, Linda had a diagnosis of depression and had been struggling to sleep at night for about a year. Although she had been given sleeping tablets by her family doctor, she no longer found them effective. Her sleeping problems had started when her husband lost his job, and she would stay awake worrying. She was also unhappy in her marriage, her second, and spoke of experiencing a sense of loss and regret about the death of her first husband, with frequent intrusive thoughts about 'what might have been'. Several years previously she had suffered a major depressive episode with psychotic features when she lost her job as a receptionist at a local hairdresser. She attributed that to being unable to get along with a coworker.

Linda had three children, all now almost grown-up, resulting in the loss of a major role in her life. Additionally, she lacked an active daily routine, having given up exercise, which she said left her exhausted. She was preoccupied with her inability to get another job and with negative ruminations about the past.

Linda was encouraged to complete daily sleep diaries and to focus on improving her physical and emotional well-being and lifestyle. She tended to sleep badly at night and then to stay in bed for much of the day, feeling too exhausted to get up. The importance of sticking to a consistent routine was explained to Linda. She was also encouraged to be more active during daytime hours and resume physical activities. Sleep quality and duration outcomes were modest but nonetheless improved. Linda's mood improved and she began to be able to recognize the pattern of personal 'cause and effect' in relation to her sleeping habits and acknowledge the extent to which she could influence this herself. Linda was encouraged to continue identifying and challenging her negative and self-defeating thinking and to focus on developing her well-being in the 'here and now', rather than on regrets about the past. She was also encouraged to congratulate herself for the improvements she had achieved so far. At the conclusion of treatment, she had expanded her repertoire of social and leisure activities and had also started job-seeking activities.

Case study 2: Iqbal (aged 58 years)

Iqbal was referred to the occupational therapist with a long-standing history of schizophrenia. Over the previous few months he had been experiencing an increasingly disrupted sleep pattern in which he would stay awake for days at a time, pacing about the house all night, and then compensate by sleeping for the next 2–3 days. His personal hygiene, self-care and physical health were poor. He smoked up to 40 cigarettes daily and drank coffee continually during the daytime and cola continually throughout the night. His night was disturbed by nightmares and hallucinations in the form of commands; however, his mental state was stable and he had a supportive mother and sister, upon whom he was dependent. Iqbal's father had died 8 months previously and his death may have triggered Iqbal's increased problems with sleeping. His main coping strategy and leisure outlets were jazz and poetry.

The intervention was aimed at educating Iqbal about sleep hygiene and supporting him to establish a more sleep-friendly routine. He was first asked to complete a sleep diary to establish a baseline and was encouraged to cut out the excessive amounts of coffee and cola. He quickly achieved this. The risks of smoking were explained to him and he was surprisingly successful in stopping almost immediately, with minimal support. His oral health was very poor and he had not visited his family doctor for a health check in some years, but he also agreed to make appointments with both the dentist and doctor. He agreed to take daily walks but was reluctant to develop his limited social and leisure lifestyle.

Iqbal complied well with all the aspects of the intervention aimed at improving his health and well-being and clearly improved according to a number of measures. He clearly felt much better in many ways, and he had managed to make more modest improvements to his sleep routine due to his preferred habit of listening to the radio at night. He acknowledged that he had found this habit hard to change, although he recognized this as his choice. He was reassured that he now knew how to go about changing his sleep routine, should he decide to do so in the future, and was less anxious about it generally. In conclusion, the significant improvements made to his well-being meant that his overall mental health improved and his sleep problems were of less concern to him.

Appendix 13.2 The Sound Sleep course: a suggested psycho-educational programme outline for a group-based intervention for those with sleep disorders in mental health settings

The course described below is designed to focus on promoting 'recovery' and meeting 'occupational needs' across all domains of daily living. Ideally, it should be delivered by an occupational therapist and a peer trainer with lived experience of mental illness and related sleep problems.

Aims

The course aims to:

- educate and inform participants about the nature of sleep and its relationship with their mental, physical and occupational health

- improve the well-being of participants as a foundation for restoring natural, good-quality sleep

- provide participants with a range of behavioural strategies to restore natural sleep quality and quantity

- teach a variety of relaxation and calming strategies to aid sleep induction

- provide participants with coping strategies to improve mood regulation and thus combat disrupted sleep due to emotional arousal

- provide participants with an opportunity to explore alternative personal problem-solving strategies in a group setting

- assist participants to reduce or discontinue inappropriate or iatrogenic usage of sleep medication (as advised by, and in conjunction with the involvement of, their medical practitioner or psychiatrist).

Course content and format

Each session lasts approximately 2 hours, allowing for one short break. The format of the sessions includes information giving, discussion and personal assignments focused on improving sleep quality and quantity. Group members are expected to carry out homework assignments between sessions. Each session begins with feedback from assignments and open discussion of personal progress and learning among group members. Participants taking long-term sleep medication which is no longer helpful to them should be supported to review the benefits and gradually discontinue their medication, if appropriate, and according to a medically supervised process, as part of the course.

Session 1: Myths and facts

Education and information giving – what you need to know about sleep science and your health, including sleep quality and quantity. How lifestyle and daily activities impact on sleep quality. The role of dream sleep and your mental health. Sleep and medication – 'pros and cons', focusing on problems related to long-term use. Improving sleep quality by restoring natural sleep – the principles.

Homework: Introducing sleep diaries to be completed before the next session.

Session 2: Sleep hygiene

Feedback from sleep diaries. Restoring the balance using sleep-friendly daily routines and habits, restricting time in bed, keeping a regular rising time, physical exercise and the role of food and drink. Setting up the environment for sleep.

Homework: Personal sleep hygiene audits and action plans.

Session 3: Well-being

Feedback on group members' progress: sleep hygiene. Laying the foundation for good-quality sleep – improving general health and well-being. Healthy lifestyles. Assessing personal well-being and emotional health.

Homework: Developing individualized well-being action plans.

Session 4: Relaxation and calming techniques

Feedback on group members' progress: well-being action plans. Getting in the mood for sleep using behavioural wind-down routines and relaxation techniques. Developing individualized sleep inductions.

Homework: Personal practice of relaxation techniques (daily ongoing practice required).

Session 5: Managing your emotions

Feedback on group members' progress: relaxation techniques. Mood management, focusing on coping strategies for dealing with strong emotions (e.g. anxiety, anger and low mood) that disrupt sleep. Mindfulness principles and practices.

Homework: 'Emotional Needs Audit' (see Appendix 13.3).

Session 6: Problem-solving

Feedback on group members' progress: Emotional Needs Audit and mood management strategies. Dealing with what may be keeping you awake using objective problem-solving techniques. Developing a range of alternative solutions and strategies to resolve or improve problematic situations.

Homework: Putting identified solutions into practice.

Session 7: Revision

Opportunity for discussion of individual issues, revision and summing up. Evaluation and sleep-quality rating scales including mental health status.

Session 8: Follow-up

Final session to take place 1–3 months post-course to evaluate longer-term progress as above, including changes in use of sleep medication.

Selection criteria

Inclusion

Adult users of mental health services with reported difficulty sleeping of more than 3 months' duration. Open to those with sleep problems in the context of a mental health problem, including quality and quantity of perceived sleep duration. Must be keen to work on problem and open to self-help approach, including undertaking personal assignments between sessions. Commitment to attend all course sessions punctually is essential.

Exclusion

Unresolved/acute psychotic symptoms, risk of violence, aggression or self-harm. Unwilling or unable to participate in group setting. Social/behavioural issues precluding appropriate participation in group setting. (Note: The course would have to be adapted for individuals with cognitive, perceptual, language or learning issues, or a combination of these, precluding full understanding of theoretical concepts covered on the course.)

Appendix 13.3 Further resources

- Emotional Needs Audit (www.hgi.org.uk/ena)
- The Human Givens Institute (www.hgi.org.uk)
- New Economics Foundation: 'Five Ways to Well-being' (www.neweconomics.org/projects/entry/five-ways-to-well-being)
- Mental Health Foundation, *Sleep Matters: The Impact of Sleep on Health and Wellbeing* (www.mentalhealth.org.uk/content/assets/PDF/publications/MHF-Sleep-Report-2011.pdf?view=Standard)
- Espie, C.A. (2006) *Overcoming Insomnia and Sleep Problems.* London: Robinson.

Acknowledgement

The authors thank Dr Mariwan Husni, Consultant Psychiatrist, Harrow Mental Health Service (Central and North West London NHS Foundation Trust), for his support and encouragement for our work on sleep problems in mental health. We particularly appreciate his understanding of the role and value of occupational therapy in this setting.

References

Aldrich, R.M. (2011) 'A review and critique of well-being in occupational therapy and occupational science.' *Scandinavian Journal of Occupational Therapy 18,* 2, 93–100.

Andrews, W., Twigg, E., Minami, T. and Johnson, G. (2011) 'Piloting a practice research network: a 12-month evaluation of the Human Givens approach in primary care at a general medical practice.' *Psychology and Psychotherapy: Theory, Research and Practice 84,* 3, 389–405.

Andrews, W.P., Wislocki, A.P., Short, F., Chow, D. and Minami, T. (2013) 'A 5-year evaluation of the Human Givens therapy using a practice research network.' *Mental Health Review Journal 18,* 3, 165–176.

Ashcraft, L. and Anthony, W.A. (2005) 'A story of transformation: an agency fully embraces recovery.' *Behavioural Healthcare Tomorrow 14,* 2, 15–21.

Baglioni, C., Battagliese, G., Feige, B., Spiegelhalder, K. *et al.* (2011) 'Insomnia as a predictor of depression: a meta-analytic evaluation of longitudinal epidemiological studies.' *Journal of Affective Disorders 135,* 1–3, 10–19.

Baylis, N. (2005) 'Relationship with Reality and its Role in the Well-being of Young Adults.' In F.A. Huppert, N. Baylis and B. Keverne (eds) *The Science of Well-being.* Oxford: Oxford University Press.

Bloom, H.G., Ahmed, I., Alessi, C.A., Ancoli-Israel, S. *et al.* (2009) 'Evidence-based recommendations for the assessment and management of sleep disorders in the older person.' *Journal of the American Geriatrics Society 57*, 5, 761–789.

Eklund, M. and Backstrom, M. (2006) 'The role of perceived control for the perception of health by patients with persistent mental illness.' *Scandinavian Journal of Occupational Therapy 13*, 4, 249–256.

Fung, C., Wiseman-Hakes, C., Stergiou-Kita, M., Nguyen, M. and Colantonio, A. (2013) 'Time to wake up: bridging the gap between theory and practice for sleep in occupational therapy.' *British Journal of Occupational Therapy 76*, 8, 384–386.

Furihata, R., Uchiyama, M., Takahashi, S., Suzuki, M. *et al.* (2012) 'The association between sleep problems and perceived health status: a Japanese nationwide general population survey.' *Sleep Medicine 13*, 7, 831–837.

Green, A. (2012) 'A Question of Balance: The Relationship Between Daily Occupation and Sleep.' In A. Green and A. Westcombe (eds) *Sleep: Multiprofessional Perspectives.* London: Jessica Kingsley Publishers.

Green, A., Hicks, J., Weekes, R. and Wilson, S. (2005) 'A cognitive-behavioural group intervention for people with chronic insomnia: an initial evaluation.' *British Journal of Occupational Therapy 68*, 11, 518–522.

Griffin, J. (1993) 'The origin of dreams: Did Freud and Jung get it wrong?' *The Therapist 1*, 1, 18–22.

Griffin, J. and Tyrrell, I. (2004a) *Human Givens: A New Approach to Emotional Health and Clear Thinking.* Chalvington, East Sussex: HG Publishing.

Griffin, J. and Tyrrell, I. (2004b) *Dreaming Reality: How Dreaming Keeps us Sane, or Can Drive us Mad.* Chalvington, East Sussex: HG Publishing.

Gujar, N., McDonald, S.A., Nishida, M. and Walker, M.P. (2010) 'A role for REM sleep in recalibrating the sensitivity of the human brain to specific emotions.' *Cerebral Cortex 21*, 1, 115–123.

Hank, D., Hicks, J. and Wilson, S. (2012) 'Sleep and Psychiatry.' In A. Green and A. Westcombe (eds) *Sleep: Multiprofessional Perspectives.* London: Jessica Kingsley Publishers.

Harrio, P., Rahkonen, O., Laaksonen, M., Lahelma, E. and Lallukka, T. (2012) 'Bidirectional associations between insomnia symptoms and unhealthy behaviours.' *Journal of Sleep Research 22*, 1, 89–95.

Harvey, A.G., Watkins, E., Mandsell, W. and Shafran, R. (2004) *Cognitive Behavioural Processes Across Psychological Disorders: A Transdiagnostic Approach to Research and Treatment.* Oxford: Oxford University Press.

Hayashino, Y., Yamazaki, S., Takegami, M., Nakayama, T., Sokejima, S., Fukuhara, S. (2010) 'Association between number of co-morbid conditions, depression, and sleep quality using the Pittsburgh Sleep Quality Index: results for a population-based survey.' *Sleep Medicine 11*, 4, 366–371.

Hayward, C. and Taylor, J. (2011) 'Eudaimonic well-being: its importance and relevance to Occupational Therapy for Humanity.' *Occupational Therapy International 18*, 3, 133–141.

Idzikowski, C. (2000) *Learn to Sleep Well: A Practical Guide to Getting a Good Night's Sleep.* London: Duncan Baird.

Kallestad, H., Hansen, B., Langsrud, K., Ruud, T. *et al.* (2012) 'Impact of sleep disturbance on patients in treatment for mental disorders.' *BMC Psychiatry*. doi: 10.1186/1471-244X-12-179.

Kielhofner, G. (2008) *Model of Human Occupation: Theory and Application*, 4th edn. Philadelphia, PA: Lippincott Williams & Wilkins.

Krystal, A.D. (2012) 'Psychiatric disorders and sleep.' *Neurologic Clinics 30*, 4, 1389–1413.

Kyung Lee, E. and Douglass, A.B. (2010) 'Sleep in psychiatric disorders: Where are we now?' *Canadian Journal of Psychiatry 55*, 7, 403–412.

Li, J.Z., Bunney, B.G., Meng, F., Hagenauer, M.H. *et al.* (2013) 'Circadian patterns of gene expression in the human brain and disruption in major depressive disorder.' *PNAS*. doi: 10.1073/pnas.1305814110.

Loprinzi, P.D. and Cardinal, B.J. (2011) 'Association between objectively-measured physical activity and sleep, NHANES 2005–2006. ' *Mental Health and Physical Activity 4*, 2, 65–69.

Repper, J. and Perkins, R.E. (2012) 'Recovery: A Journey of Discovery for Individuals and Services.' In P. Phillips, T. Sandford and C. Johnston (eds) *Working in Mental Health: Practice and Policy in a Changing Environment*. Abingdon: Routledge.

Skapinakis, P., Rai, D., Anagnostopoulos, F., Harrison, S., Araya, R., Lewis, G. (2013) 'Sleep disturbances and depressive symptoms: an investigation of their longitudinal association in a representative sample of the UK general population.' *Psychological Medicine 43*, 2, 329–339.

Soehner, A.M. and Harvey, A.G. (2012) 'Prevalence and functional consequences of severe insomnia symptoms in mood and anxiety disorders: results from a nationally representative sample.' *Sleep 35*, 10, 1367–1375.

Stein, M.D. and Friedmann, P.D. (2005) 'Disturbed sleep and its relationship to alcohol use.' *Substance Abuse 26*, 1, 1–13.

Sunderjan, P., Gaynes, B.N., Wisiewski, S.R., Miyahara, S. *et al.* (2010) 'Insomnia in patients with depression: a STAR*D Report.' *CNS Spectrums 15*, 6, 394–404.

Tsaroucha, A., Kingston, P., Corp, N., Stewart, T. and Walton, I. (2012a) 'The emotional needs audit (ENA): a report on its reliability and validity.' *Mental Health Review Journal 17*, 2, 81–89.

Tsaroucha, A., Kingston, P., Stewart, T., Walton, I. and Corp, N. (2012b) 'Assessing the effectiveness of the "human givens" approach in treating depression: a quasi-experimental study in primary care.' *Mental Health Review Journal 17*, 2, 90–103.

Uhde, T.W., Cortese, B.M. and Vedeniapin, A. (2009) 'Anxiety and sleep problems: emerging concepts and theoretical treatment implications.' *Current Psychiatry Reports 11*, 4, 269–276.

van der Helm, E., Yao, J., Dutt, S., Rao, V., Saletin, J.M. and Walker, M.P. (2011) 'REM sleep depotentiates amygdala activity to previous emotional experience.' *Current Biology 21*, 23, 2029–2032.

Van Mill, J.G., Hoogendijk, W.J., Vogelzangs, N., van Dyck, R. and Penninx, B.W. (2010) 'Insomnia and sleep duration in a large cohort of patients with major depressive disorder and anxiety disorders.' *Journal of Clinical Psychiatry 71*, 3, 239–246.

Waters, F., Naik, N. and Rock, D. (2013) 'Sleep, fatigue, and functional health in psychotic patients.' *Schizophrenia Research and Treatment 2013*. doi: 10.1155/2013/425826.

Wulff, K., Dijk, D.-J., Middleton, B., Foster, R.G. and Joyce, E.M. (2012) 'Sleep and circadian rhythm disruption in schizophrenia.' *British Journal of Psychiatry 200*, 4, 308–316.

Yan, C.M., Lin, S.H., Hsu, S.C. and Cheng, C.P. (2010) 'Maladaptive sleep hygiene practices in good sleepers and patients with insomnia.' *Journal of Health Psychology 15*, 1, 147–155.

Yates, Y. and Atkinson, C. (2011) 'Using Human Givens therapy to support the well-being of adolescents: a case example.' *Pastoral Care in Education 29*, 1, 35–50.

14

SLEEP PROBLEMS IN DEMENTIA

Katie MacQueen, Julie Boswell and Jennifer Thai

14.1 Introduction

Sleep problems in the context of dementia are complex and may be exacerbated by the coexistence of other medical conditions. They could equally be addressed in the chapter on the sleep of older adults, or the chapter on sleep difficulties in the context of mental health problems, but they are considered in this brief chapter which should be read in conjunction with Chapters 10, 13 and 18. Although a number of forms of dementia exist, Alzheimer's disease is the most common and is the one to which most literature refers; it is therefore the main focus of this chapter.

14.2 Scope of problems

As the number of persons living into old age continues to rise in many countries, so will the numbers living with some form of dementia. As well as cognitive decline, someone with dementia, or their carers, might expect sleep problems. Petit, Montplaisir and Boeve (2011) cite estimates of the prevalence of sleep disturbance at about 25% in mild to moderate cases of Alzheimer's disease and about 50% in severe cases. Problems include difficulty falling asleep at night, frequent wakening, early wakening and excessive daytime sleepiness. Iranzo (2010) suggests that there are similar problems in the case of dementia with Lewy bodies, although Zhou, Jung and Richards (2012) indicate that sleep problems are worse, with more disruption to the sleep-wake cycle, more arousals at night and increased daytime sleepiness. (See Zhou *et al.* 2012 for a comprehensive summary of problems in the other dementias.) A further phenomenon experienced by some people with Alzheimer's disease is known as 'sundowning' where disorientation and 'problem behaviour', including agitation and aggression, occurs in the afternoon and evening; there may also be night-time wandering (Hank, Hicks and Wilson 2012). This can present a particular challenge for carers.

Family carers are likely to have disrupted sleep themselves and to become less able to cope or to suffer effects on their health (Lee and Thomas 2011). They may feel a constant need for vigilance and for providing care, have concerns for safety or, in some cases, fear violent behaviours from the person with dementia. Caregiver burden and distress may be factors that precipitate institutionalization (see Ancoli-Israel *et al.* 1994 and Beaudreau *et al.* 2008 for further discussion).

Sleep problems in dementia are also important because of a two-way relationship between dementia and sleep whereby dementia affects sleep, but disrupted sleep is associated with increased functional impairment. For example, comparing measures of sleepiness, functional status and cognitive impairment Lee *et al.* (2007) demonstrated that higher levels of sleepiness were linked with increased functional impairment independent of cognitive impairment. Cricco, Simonsick and Foley (2001) showed in a study of 6400 community-dwelling persons (aged over 64 years) that 'chronic insomnia independently predicts incidence of increased cognitive decline in older men' (p.1187). This suggests a possibility of reducing the functional impact of dementia by promoting improved sleep. It is also possible that the risk of dementia could be diminished by improved sleep (Spira *et al.* 2012).

14.3 Causes, consequences and implications

The causes of sleep problems in dementia are uncertain and probably result from multiple factors such as those listed by Iranzo (2010) in the case of Alzheimer's disease: damage by the degenerative process to areas of the brain that modulate sleep, associated psychiatric disturbance such as depression and agitation, medical problems and side effects of medications. It is also possible that someone with dementia had a pre-existing sleep disorder or co-morbid disorder, such as obstructive sleep apnoea, affecting sleep. In their review of sleep problems in the older person Neikrug and Ancoli-Israel (2010) state that: 'Multiple causes could be responsible for reduced capability to achieve sufficient sleep with age, including medical or psychiatric illnesses, life changes (e.g. retirement, bereavement, decreased social interactions), environmental changes (e.g. placement in a nursing home) and polypharmacy' (p.181). Furthermore, an older person with mental health problems may have long-established poor sleep routines or unhelpful beliefs about the reasons for their poor sleep. All these factors taken together can make it particularly difficult to achieve improvements, and it is important to address the sleep problems which occur in older adults with dementia individually.

People with dementia will be particularly affected by sleep difficulties as their condition might also result in increased confusion, risk of falls and changes in behaviour during the night; these are especially challenging for carers to cope with (Ganesekaran 2013). The emotional and physical burden of the caring role, coupled with lack of sleep for the carer, may lead to a breakdown of their ability to continue to provide care for their loved one, ultimately leading to placement in a residential setting (Arber and Venn 2011). These issues are exemplified in the case study in Appendix 14.1.

Although sleep deficiency in older persons with dementia is a common problem with serious consequences, it is often overlooked by care providers. In a survey involving 1846 health care professionals (about 60% of whom were nursing staff and 6% occupational therapy staff) in primary care, acute care and long-term residential care facilities in Canada, Brown *et al.* (2014) found that awareness of sleep problems and interventions to improve sleep was low and that knowledge varied between professional groups.

14.4 Management of sleep problems

It is important that occupational therapists and other health care professionals *ask* about sleep, and that they do not rely on the client or carer to report a problem. As noted also in Chapter 10, it is commonly believed that reduced sleep is a natural consequence of aging and just to be expected (Venn, Meadows and Arber 2013). This misconception, coupled with decreased help-seeking behaviours from either client or carer, can contribute to the under-diagnosis and non-treatment of sleep problems. (Assessment of sleep problems in general is covered in Chapter 8 and of the sleep problems of older adults in Chapter 10.) As ever, it is important to consider sleep in the context of the 24-hour cycle: it is helpful to ask how much the individual sleeps during the day as well as during the night, and also how the individual spends waking time, how much there is regularity of activity and how much exposure there is to daylight or full-spectrum artificial light. In the case of dementia, it is particularly important to assess the impact of sleep problems on the carer's sleep. Where the client is in residential care, it may be necessary to take account of the routines of the facility and its environment.

Medical treatment of sleep problems in the context of Alzheimer's disease is 'challenging' according to Iranzo (2010, p.125) and requires an individual approach. Accordingly, in their review of sleep problems in people with dementia, Deschenes and McCurry (2009) conclude that non-pharmacological treatment options should be the first line of treatment of sleep problems of people with dementia. Furthermore, they have been repeatedly demonstrated as effective for improving restorative sleep among older persons (see Brown *et al.* 2013 and Koch *et al.* 2006 for detailed reviews). While noting that respite care had a positive effect on caregivers' sleep, Lee, Morgan and Lindesay (2007) found a negative effect on the sleep of patients with dementia. They therefore recommend that respite care should target sleep management; however, there is evidence that sleep can be improved both in the home and in institutional care.

Given the levels of insight and engagement that are usually necessary to follow cognitive behavioural strategies (see Chapter 8), intervention to improve the sleep of someone with dementia is more likely to involve behavioural and environmental measures. Nevertheless, it is helpful to have an understanding of cognitive behaviour therapy for insomnia and the science that underpins it in devising individual plans and in educating care staff and family members. (Sleep hygiene and environmental issues are discussed in some detail in Chapters 8 and 18 and are not considered further here.) However, it is important to get the basics right in creating an environment (lighting, heating, ventilation and noise levels) and establishing routines conducive to sleep.

It is also important for the individual to be in the optimum condition, for example, by reducing the risk of falls, particularly if the person has to get up more often in the night (see also Chapter 10) and by working to improve well-being, especially after a transition to another life stage involving loss of roles and social interaction. Educating carers on strategies to manage unpredictable behaviour at night can help further to optimize sleep. Daytime measures include increasing physical activity in daily routines, which is also recommended to reduce the risk of cognitive decline (Forbes *et al.* 2008), and preferably outdoors so as to benefit from daylight when possible. Light is the main natural factor (or zeitgeber⋆) in maintaining circadian rhythms, but engagement in occupation, with structure and regularity, can also reinforce rhythms and promote sleep at night (see Chapter 6). Lastly, a key area for intervention includes the facilitation of opportunities to engage in leisure activities (NICE 2013).

Practical examples of interventions to improve sleep can be found in the work of McCurry and colleagues. McCurry *et al.* (2005) conducted a randomized controlled trial of a multifaceted programme to promote rest and sleep, including education on sleep hygiene, 30 minutes of daily walking and bright-light therapy in people with Alzheimer's disease living with family carers. The combination of interventions led to an average reduction of 36 minutes in time awake at night and five fewer nightly wakenings across the treatment group after two months. In subsequent studies, McCurry *et al.* (2011, 2012) demonstrated the feasibility of training staff of small family-run homes to apply similar methods – daily exercise, exposure to light and improved sleep hygiene (e.g. consistent and later bedtime, consistent rising time and no daytime naps). (More comprehensive reviews of non-pharmacological measures are provided by David *et al.* 2010 and Shub, Darvishi and Kunik 2009.)

14.5 Conclusion

Dementia is an increasing problem as people live longer, and the association with sleep problems is well established. It is important therefore that health professionals and carers be aware of measures that can improve sleep. Occupational therapists in particular are well placed to intervene because of their focus on the environment and on activity patterns. There is sufficient evidence for proposing increases in activity levels, changes in routines and the use of bright light, although protocols are not well established. In any event, it is clear that interventions need to be individually applied.

Appendix 14.1 Case study: Bob (a 73-year-old man with a diagnosis of mixed dementia)

Bob was initially referred to a day assessment unit (DAU) as his wife was under considerable strain caring for him owing to the increasing behavioural and psychological symptoms of his dementia. Bob would spend a large proportion of his day trying to leave the house to walk to his former home two miles away, from where he had moved some years before. His constant demands to leave the house were stressful for the family, but they noted that he slept well when he had been active during the day. Whilst at the DAU Bob would repeatedly ask to leave the building. Initially this was not facilitated as it was considered too much of a risk. His wife reported that he was often anxious and restless when he returned home and took longer to wind down in preparation for sleep. A Model of Human Occupation Screening Tool assessment (Parkinson, Forsyth and Kielhofner 2006) was carried out and a Model of Human Occupation case formulation was developed as follows:

> Bob's motor skills allow him to perform activities. He is for the most part aware of others and interested in being helpful. However, his increasing processing difficulties mean that he does not always have the concentration and sequencing abilities to perform tasks. Beyond self-care activities (for which he needs prompting heavily), Bob's daily routine is chaotic and driven by the need to search for 'home'. His social (home) environment, geographical memory and local environment currently support this, but his family is becoming overburdened by his demands to leave the house. The main factor enabling his wife's ability to care for Bob is his robust sleep routine on days when he is active, allowing her to recuperate from the demands placed on her.

Based on these findings, a person-centred occupational therapy intervention was formulated, incorporating the principles of the 'recovery' approach and underpinned by relevant evidence-based guidelines (Department of Health 2001; Deschenes and McCurry 2009; Forbes *et al.* 2008).

The occupational therapy intervention for Bob therefore aimed to maintain his sleep routine by supporting him to be active in a meaningful way during the day. Bob was supported by DAU staff to walk in the locality in the morning and afternoon. His wife reported that when he returned home, he was less restless, his mood had improved and he slept well. Goals upon discharge and transfer to the local reablement and personalization team recommended that this pattern of support be continued, allowing Bob to take daily walks of 1–2 hours.

Appendix 14.2 Further resources

- Alzheimer's Association (www.alz.org/index.asp)
- Alzheimer's Australia, Sleeping (www.fightdementia.org.au/services/sleeping.aspx)
- Sleep and dementia resources: Bendigo Health Authority, Australia (www.dementia managementstrategy.com/Pages/ABC_of_behaviour_management/Management_ strategies/Sleep_disturbance.aspx)
- Sleep and dementia resources: University of Alberta Sleep and Function Interdisciplinary Group (www.sleep-dementia-resources.ualberta.ca)
- *Sleep Disorders and Alzheimer's Disease: How to Manage Alzheimer's-Related Sleep Disturbance* (http://alzheimers.about.com/lw/Health-Medicine/Conditions-and-diseases/Sleep-Disorders-and-Alzheimers-Disease.htm)
- Sundowning (www.alz.org/care/alzheimers-dementia-sleep-issues-sundowning.asp)
- Understanding pain and dementia: University of Alberta (www.painanddementia.ualberta.ca)

Acknowledgement

The authors acknowledge the editorial contributions of Cary Brown and Andrew Green.

References

Ancoli-Israel, S., Klauber, M.R., Gillin, J.C., Campbell, S.S. and Hofstetter, C.R. (1994) 'Sleep in non-institutionalized Alzheimer's disease patients.' *Aging Clinical and Experimental Research 6*, 6, 451–458.

Arber, S. and Venn, S. (2011) 'Care-giving at night: understanding the impact on carers.' *Journal of Aging Studies 25*, 2, 155–165.

Beaudreau, S.A., Spira, A.P., Gray, H.L., Depp, C.A. *et al.* (2008) 'The relationship between objectively measured sleep disturbance and dementia family caregiver distress and burden.' *Journal of Geriatric Psychiatry and Neurology 21*, 3, 159–165.

Brown, C.A., Berry, R., Tan, M., Khoshia, A., Turlapati, L. and Swedlove, F. (2013) 'A critique of the evidence-base for non-pharmacological sleep interventions for persons with dementia.' *Dementia: The International Journal of Social Research and Practice 12*, 2, 174–201.

Brown, C.A., Wielandt, P., Wilson, D., Jones, A. and Crick, K. (2014) 'Healthcare providers' knowledge of disordered sleep, sleep assessment tools and non-pharmacological sleep interventions for persons living with dementia: a national survey.' *Sleep Disorders*. doi: http://dx.doi.org/10.1155/2014/286274.

Cricco, M., Simonsick, E.M. and Foley, D.J. (2001) 'The impact of insomnia on cognitive functioning in older adults.' *Journal of the American Geriatric Society 49*, 9, 1185–1189.

David, R., Zeitzer, J., Friedman, L., Noda, A. *et al.* (2010) 'Non-pharmacologic management of sleep disturbance in Alzheimer's disease.' *Journal of Nutrition, Health & Aging 14*, 3, 203–206.

Department of Health (2001) *National Service Framework for Older People.* London: Department of Health.

Deschenes, C.L. and McCurry, S.M. (2009) 'Current treatments for sleep disturbance in individuals with dementia.' *Current Psychiatry Reports 11*, 1, 20–26.

Forbes, D., Forbes, S., Morgan, D.G., Markle-Reid, M., Wood, J. and Culum, I. (2008) 'Physical activity programs for persons with dementia.' *Cochrane Database of Systematic Reviews*. doi: 10.1002/14651858.CD006489.pub2.

Ganesekaran, G. (2013) 'The Ageing Body – Body Functions and Structures: Part 2.' In A. Atwal and A. McIntyre (eds) *Occupational Therapy and Older People*, 2nd edn. Chichester: Wiley-Blackwell.

Hank, D., Hicks, J. and Wilson, S. (2012) 'Sleep and Psychiatry.' In A. Green and A. Westcombe (eds) *Sleep: Multiprofessional Perspectives*. London: Jessica Kingsley Publishers.

Iranzo, A. (2010) 'Sleep in Other Neurodegenerative Diseases.' In S. Overeem and P. Reading (eds) *Sleep Disorders in Neurology: A Practical Approach*. Chichester: Wiley-Blackwell.

Koch, S., Haesler, E., Tiziani, A. and Wilson, J. (2006) 'Effectiveness of sleep management strategies for residents of aged care facilities: findings of a systematic review.' *Journal of Clinical Nursing 15*, 10, 1267–1275.

Lee, D., Morgan, K. and Lindesay, J. (2007) 'Effect of institutional respite care on the sleep of people with dementia and their primary caregivers.' *Journal of the American Geriatrics Society 55*, 2, 252–258.

Lee, D.R. and Thomas, A.J. (2011) 'Sleep in dementia and caregiving-assessment and treatment implications: a review.' *International Psychogeriatrics 23*, 2, 190–201.

Lee, J.H., Bliwise, D.L., Ansari, F.P., Goldstein, F.C. *et al.* (2007) 'Daytime sleepiness and functional impairment in Alzheimer disease.' *American Journal of Geriatric Psychiatry 15*, 7, 620–626.

McCurry, S.M, Gibbons, L.E., Logsdon, R.G., Vitiello, M.V. and Teri, L. (2005) 'Nighttime insomnia treatment and education for Alzheimer's disease: a randomized, controlled trial.' *Journal of the American Geriatrics Society 53*, 5, 793–802.

McCurry, S.M., LaFazia, D.M., Pike, K.C., Logsdon, R.G. and Teri, L. (2012) 'Development and evaluation of a sleep education program for older adults with dementia living in adult family homes.' *American Journal of Geriatric Psychiatry 20*, 6, 494–504.

McCurry, S.M., Pike, K.C., Vitiello, M.V., Logsdon, R.G. *et al.* (2011) 'Increasing walking and bright light exposure to improve sleep in community-dwelling persons with Alzheimer's disease: results of a randomized, controlled trial. *Journal of the American Geriatric Society 59*, 8, 1393–1402.

Neikrug, A.B. and Ancoli-Israel, S. (2010) 'Sleep disorders in the older adult: a mini-review.' *Gerontology 56*, 2, 181–189.

NICE (National Institute for Health and Care Excellence) (2013) *Quality Standards for Supporting People to Live Well with Dementia*. London: NICE.

Parkinson, S., Forsyth, K. and Kielhofner, G. (2006) *The Model of Human Occupation Screening Tool (MOHOST) Version 2.0 2006*. Chicago, IL: University of Illinois at Chicago.

Petit, D., Montplaisir, J. and Boeve, B.F. (2011) 'Alzheimer's Disease and Other Dementias.' In M.H. Kryger, T. Roth and W.C. Dement (eds) *Principles and Practice of Sleep Medicine*, 5th edn. St Louis, MO: Elsevier Saunders.

Shub, D., Darvishi, R. and Kunik, M.E. (2009) 'Non-pharmacologic treatment of insomnia in persons with dementia.' *Geriatrics 64*, 2, 22–26.

Spira, A.P., Gamaldo, A.A., An, Y., Simonsick, M. *et al.* (2012) 'Self-reported sleep and ß-amyloid deposition in community-dwelling older adults.' *JAMA Neurology 70*, 12, 1537–1543.

Venn, S., Meadows, R. and Arber, S. (2013) 'Gender differences in approaches to self-management of poor sleep in later life.' *Social Science and Medicine 79*, 1, 117–123.

Zhou, Q.P., Jung, L. and Richards, K.C. (2012) 'The management of sleep and circadian disturbance in patients with dementia.' *Current Neurology and Neuroscience Reports 12*, 2, 193–204.

15

SLEEP DISTURBANCE IN NEUROLOGICAL CONDITIONS

Eva Nakopoulou, Katherine Gaylarde and Andrew Green

15.1 Introduction

Sleep is affected in many medical conditions either through the pain or discomfort of the condition or as a result of treatment, or it may be a direct consequence of the condition itself. It has been observed in Chapter 8 that in the case of cancer, the standard non-pharmacological approaches for insomnia might be beneficial, and other chapters look at managing sleep problems in the context of pain, fatigue and psychiatric disorders. Although sleep disturbance is common in many neurological conditions (including dementia with Lewy bodies and Huntington's disease), this short chapter considers four conditions where sleep disturbance is common: Parkinson's disease, multiple sclerosis, traumatic brain injury and stroke. There is not much evidence of successful management of sleep difficulties in these circumstances, but it is hoped that with greater understanding of the range of problems and their possible causes, therapists might be better placed to help in applying the principles and strategies outlined in other chapters.

15.2 Parkinson's disease

The National Institute for Health and Clinical Excellence (NICE) Clinical Guidelines for Parkinson's disease (PD) recommend that a full sleep history be taken when people report sleep disturbance. Particular care should be taken to identify and manage restless leg syndrome (RLS) and rapid eye movement (REM) sleep disorders (NICE 2006; see Chapter 7).

According to Swick (2012) PD has typically been characterized by the principal motor symptoms: bradykinesia, rigidity, resting tremor and postural instability. However, more recently other non-motor symptoms are being recognized; these include autonomic dysfunction, mood disorders, cognitive impairment, pain, gastrointestinal disturbance, impaired olfaction, psychosis and sleep disorders. Sleep problems include fragmented sleep, daytime sleepiness, sleep-disordered breathing, RLS, nightmares and REM sleep behaviour disorder (Swick 2012; see also Löhle, Storch and Reichmann 2009 and Srinivasan *et al.* 2011). Dhawan *et al.* (2006) observe that problems in sleep were first recognized by James Parkinson, and that sleep disturbance might precede motor symptoms.

Sleep problems are prevalent in PD. In a community sample in Norway 60% of PD patients complained of sleep problems, compared with 33% of members of the healthy matched control group (Tandberg, Larsen and Karlsen 1998), whereas Wulff *et al.* (2010) note that it is estimated that 80–90% of PD patients have a sleep disorder. It has been suggested that the sleep-wake problems seen in parkinsonism are a consequence of degenerative changes in the areas of the brain that regulate sleep and arousal (Trenkwalder and Arnulf 2011). As well as that, symptoms of the disease and medication used in its management might add to the difficulties.

Arnulf, Reading and Vidialhet (2010) note that there is a correlation between the severity of the motor symptoms of PD and the degree of insomnia. Among the causes of sleep disturbance are RLS, which has a close association with PD (Ondo, Vuong and Jankovic 2002), painful dystonia in the later part of the night, bradykinesia and difficulty turning in bed or leaving it to use the toilet. Arnulf *et al.* (2010) point out that dopaminergic medication may act as a stimulant and delay sleep, or in some cases a patient might become hyperactive at night, perhaps engaging in compulsive activities such as gambling (dopamine dysregulation syndrome) (see Lawrence, Evans and Lees 2003). Given the level of nocturnal sleep disturbance, a degree of excessive daytime sleepiness is to be expected, although according to Arnulf *et al.* (2010), PD patients are poor at recognizing sleepiness; napping after lunch is common and in severe cases the degree of sleepiness is similar to that found in narcolepsy – with the result that driving presents a risk (see Frucht, Greene and Fahn 2000 and Hobson *et al.* 2002). Movement problems in sleep include repetitive jerks that resemble periodic limb movements and REM sleep behaviour disorder (RBD) (see Chapter 7). In RBD there can be violent defensive movements which are consistent with dream content and pose a risk to the individual and their bed partner.

In discussing management of insomnia, Arnulf *et al.* (2010) suggest a range of medication options for different symptoms but advise not to overlook simple measures to improve comfort such as the use of sheets and bedclothes that slip easily and aid movement, and keeping items such as medication and water close at hand. Use of a bedpan or bottle may be helpful to avoid leaving the bed where nocturia is a problem, especially if confusion is also an issue.

It might seem unlikely that the cognitive behavioural measures, such as stimulus control and sleep restriction therapy (see Chapter 8), can be applied in their strict forms, but Arnulf *et al.* (2010) still caution against going to bed at a fixed time before becoming sleepy and thereby remaining awake in bed and becoming anxious. As ever, standard sleep hygiene* measures might also be helpful and are recommended in the NICE Guidelines (2006).

Two pilot studies have demonstrated that sleep hygiene and cognitive behaviour therapy for insomnia (CBT-I) might make a difference. First, in a small controlled study in the UK, Leroi *et al.* (2010) used behavioural and educational strategies – 'multi-component sleep therapy' (p.1075') – with patient and carer dyads, while the control group had only a simple sleep hygiene intervention. It was found that both groups had a modest improvement in sleep over the 6-week course, although the sample was too small and the sleep problems too heterogeneous to draw firm conclusions. Second, Rios Romenets *et al.* (2013) conducted a small study in Canada, which compared the effect of a six-session programme of CBT, sleep hygiene and bright-light therapy (30 minutes daily) with the effect of a nightly dose of the tricyclic antidepressant, doxepin. There was some improvement in sleep in the group taking medication, but improvement in the non-pharmacological treatment group was limited; however, the groups comprised only six people and in this initial study treatment protocols were perhaps experimental.

Although the research results are modest, they are an encouraging start and suggest that improvements can be made and that further investigation is warranted. While PD patients are poorly placed to follow a strict CBT-I programme, a modified course may be necessary. In any case, it is still worth being aware of the principles of cognitive behavioural management (described in Chapter 8) in giving individual advice. A further possibility is the use of light therapy (Willis and Turner 2007), which has been shown in a small case series study to improve symptoms, including insomnia.

Where excessive daytime sleep is the problem, it is important that medication be reviewed in case of over-sedation. While the medical team might consider stimulant medication, it is also worth considering planned naps. The patient may need reminding not to drive if prone to sleep attacks, and if there is parasomnia, it is important to review safety in the bedroom.

15.3 Multiple sclerosis

The association between multiple sclerosis (MS) and sleep problems is well established, although Kanbayashi, Reading and Nishino (2010) note that there appears to be no typical nocturnal sleep disorder with MS, but that symptoms of the illness contribute to disturbed and unrefreshing sleep. For example, sleep can be disrupted by pain, spasm, bladder problems or mood disturbance. Brass *et al.* (2010) cite estimates of frequency of sleep disorders ranging from 25 to 54% among people with MS and note that insomnia, sleep-disordered breathing, RLS, narcolepsy, REM sleep behaviour disorder and circadian-rhythm disorders have all been reported.

The likely causes of increased prevalence of sleep problems are complex and uncertain, and have not been fully studied. As noted, some insomnia results from disturbance caused by symptoms. In the case of sleep-disordered breathing, Brass *et al.* (2010) observe that it is possible that medication used to treat pain and spasticity might relax muscle tone in the pharynx, or that inactivity might contribute to weight gain (which can be a factor in obstructive sleep apnoea; see Chapter 7). A further possibility is that damage caused by the disease process itself can lead to sleep problems. This has been suggested in the case of circadian-rhythm problems where the effect of MS on the optic nerves could lead to reduced input to the suprachiasmatic nucleus*, and therefore disturb circadian rhythms. Research findings, however, have not been conclusive (see, for example, Attarian *et al.* 2004 and Taphoorn *et al.* 1993). Brass *et al.* (2010) observe that the usual methods of management of circadian-rhythm disorders (chronotherapy or systematic adjustment of sleep times, phototherapy and melatonin*) have not been studied in the patient group.

One factor that can cause disturbed night-time sleep and, in turn, sleepiness by day, is RLS. The mechanism linking MS and RLS is not known according to Li *et al.* (2012), who examined data from a cohort of over 65,000 female nurses in the US who had participated in a prospective study. It was found that women with MS had a significantly higher prevalence of RLS, and daytime sleepiness which affected daily activity, than those without MS. They note that sleepiness could result from damage to sleep-wake regulating structures in the brain, from sleep disturbance (such as that caused by RLS) or from a side effect of medication.

Good sleep, and rest, is all the more important because fatigue is also a significant symptom in MS; however, perhaps because of the complexity of sleep problems in this group, there is no evidence of standard CBT-I strategies having been tried. Nevertheless, sleep hygiene and sleep management strategies discussed elsewhere in this book should be considered, as well as the following:

- night-time positioning and postural support

- pressure relief

- tone management

- timings for medications

- bladder and bowel routines.

Managing these factors can have an impact on sleep disturbance and help to break a negative cycle of reduced activity during the day (Harrison 2007). This applies for people with a range of acquired and progressive neurological conditions.

15.4 Traumatic brain injury

Ouellet, Savard and Morin (2004) report that 30–70% of traumatic brain injury (TBI) patients experience sleep problems, and this is likely to have a negative impact both on other symptoms and on the rehabilitation process. Verma, Anand and Verna (2007) suggest possible mechanisms by which TBI causes sleep disorders; these include direct and indirect brain injury, pain in the neck and back, weight gain and a pre-existing abnormality which is exacerbated by the trauma to the head. There is also a possibility that undiagnosed conditions that cause excessive daytime sleepiness (EDS), such as narcolepsy and obstructive sleep apnoea, might contribute to the cause of accidental injuries (Castriotta *et al.* 2007). (For a further analysis of the relationship between fatigue and sleep disturbance and aetiological factors in TBI see Ponsford *et al.* 2012.)

Castriotta *et al.* (2007) carried out polysomnography* with 87 adults at least 3 months post-TBI in order to determine the prevalence of sleep disorders. They found that 46% had a sleep disorder. Obstructive sleep apnoea was the most common diagnosis (23%), followed by post-traumatic hypersomnia (11%); the symptom of EDS (as measured with the multiple sleep latency test*) was found in 25% of participants. According to Orff, Ayalon and Drummond (2009) 'one of the most common and well-documented syndromes seen in patients with TBI is insomnia' (p.156), although they note that it is defined by self-report. They observe, however, that insomnia can be a persistent problem for months and years after TBI; it can manifest as long sleep onset latency* or increased waking after sleep onset. (See also Parcell *et al.* 2006, and see Zeitzer, Friedman and O'Hara 2009 for more information on insomnia in the context of TBI.)

In terms of consequences of poor night-time sleep, Orff *et al.* (2009) cite evidence that fatigue is present in 43–73% of TBI patients (see also Cohen *et al.* 1992). Fatigue, as opposed to sleepiness, was found to be present 1 month post-injury in about half of 514 participants in a study by Watson *et al.* (2007), who found that more severe head injury was related to greater sleepiness, with about a quarter of respondents reporting sleepiness after a year. Baumann (2010) notes that as well as EDS, 'characterized by recurrent lapses into sleep during the daytime, which are often of relatively short duration' (p.208), some TBI patients can experience hypersomnia which is 'defined by increased sleep need per 24 hours' (p.210).

Daytime sleepiness may result from poor night-time sleep, but it is also possible that it results from a circadian-rhythm disorder which is reported to be associated with TBI. For example, in a study by Ayalon *et al.* (2007) 36% of participants with mild TBI insomnia had a diagnosis of a circadian-rhythm disorder. Just over half of those had delayed sleep phase syndrome while the remainder had an irregular sleep-wake pattern, whereas irregular sleep-wake pattern is rare in the general population (Reid and Zee 2011). Ayalon *et al.* (2007) suggest that there could be damage to the circadian system that does not show in brain scans, or that psychological factors, pain and change in daily routines might also affect circadian rhythms. According to Baumann (2010), it is possible that disruption of circadian rhythms could lead to overestimates of post-traumatic insomnia.

A number of sleep problems are therefore possible after TBI. Unfortunately, treatment options are limited. Although Baumann (2010) indicated that there is no specific treatment for post-traumatic hypersomnia, Kaiser *et al.* (2010) have shown that modafinil can improve post-traumatic EDS (but not fatigue). Because of increased susceptibility of the traumatized brain to hypnotic medications, which may cause additional adverse effects in the daytime, Hank, Hicks and Wilson (2012) suggest that other management should be prioritized. As well as bright light and melatonin for circadian-rhythm disruption (Bjorvatn and Pallesen 2009), it may also be important to encourage regular routines, including physical activity, that might help to promote sleep (see Chapter 6). The management of sleepiness and fatigue is discussed further by Ponsford *et al.* (2012). They note that pharmacological interventions have so far not been shown to be effective, although melatonin might have potential to increase daytime alertness by improving night-time sleep. They suggest that light therapy also holds promise for increasing alertness.

Non-pharmacological approaches to managing insomnia in the context of TBI are reviewed by Zeitzer *et al.* (2009), who note that there is a critical need for research into the management of insomnia specifically in TBI. They report on the one available study (Ouellett and Morin 2007) involving 11 participants with mild to severe TBI. After an 8-week programme of CBT-I, total wake time was halved and sleep efficiency* rose by over 10%. Improvement continued at 3-month follow-up, with an average increase in sleep time of over an hour. Ouellett and Morin (2007) caution that further research is needed but observe that for some participants (such as those not in employment) encouragement of regular routines is important. They add that improving sleep might enhance rehabilitation and increase quality of life for people with TBI and argue for increased access to CBT-I.

15.5 Stroke

Stroke is also associated with sleep disorders such as obstructive sleep apnoea, circadian-rhythm disorders and night-time waking (National Stroke Association 2006). Hermann and Bassetti (2010) note that sleep-disordered breathing and sleep-wake disturbances are each found in up to 50% of stroke patients. Sleep disorders present an associated vascular risk factor which can increase the risk of stroke and, when untreated, may impact on post-stroke rehabilitation and lead to poorer functional outcomes (Wallace, Ramos and Rundek 2012). Damage to areas of the brain that are involved in sleep and arousal regulation may impact on sleep, as well as factors such as medication, depression and anxiety, pain, spasm, inactivity and reduced endurance.

As in the case with TBI, management of sleep problems after stroke is poorly documented. Hermann and Bassetti (2010) observe that compliance with continuous positive airway pressure (CPAP) for sleep-disordered breathing can be low among stroke patients and that further difficulties in using or handling CPAP masks may be caused, for example, by problems related to facial weakness, motor deficits, aphasia and anosognosia. Hermann and Bassetti (2010) suggest no specific non-pharmacological management of other sleep difficulties after stroke except for simple sleep hygiene measures.

15.6 Conclusion

A neurological condition can present particular challenges to sleep since the condition itself, or its consequences, can interfere with sleep mechanisms. Furthermore, where higher-level executive functions, such as initiation, decision-making and ability to self-monitor, are affected, management strategies can be compromised. Referring to TBI (although they could refer to any neurological condition) Agrawal, Cincu and Joharapurkar (2008) argue that a more refined understanding of sleep disorders and their management is needed in order to provide the best care. A comprehensive sleep assessment, which considers all contributing factors, should therefore be offered as part of a rehabilitation programme, and therapists should carefully assess the ability of the person to apply behavioural changes.

This chapter shows that despite the likelihood of sleep disorders in many conditions, very little work has been done in researching management options. It is possible that in the past the conditions highlighted here have been considered so serious that the additional problem of sleep disturbance has been overlooked. However, the existence of co-morbid sleep difficulties is now more widely recognized and their negative consequences are more fully understood, and the challenge for all involved in care is to find ways to help improve sleep. Specifically, occupational therapists can work in a number of ways that are described elsewhere in this book by:

- paying detailed attention to sleep hygiene and environmental factors, adapting as necessary according to the particular condition

- the appropriate application of CBT-I principles, especially discouraging the spending of excessive time in bed

- pacing activity and planning naps in cases of fatigue and excessive sleepiness

- encouraging participation in daytime activities, especially those that reinforce regular rhythms.

Appendix 15.1 Further resources

- National Collaborating Centre for Chronic Conditions (2006) *Parkinson's Disease: National Clinical Guideline for Diagnosis and Management in Primary and Secondary Care.* London: Royal College of Physicians (www.nice.org.uk/guidance/cg35/informationforpublic)

- National Multiple Sclerosis Society and Multiple Sclerosis Society of Canada (2012) *Managing Pain and Sleep Issues in Multiple Sclerosis* (http://mssociety.ca/en/pdf/managing-pain-and-sleep-issues-in-ms-EN.pdf)

- National Stroke Association: *Recovery After Stroke: Sleep Disorders* (www.stroke.org/site/DocServer/NSAFactSheet_SleepDisorders.pdf?docID=1002)

- Parkinson's Disease Foundation: 'Sleep disturbances' (www.pdf.org/en/sleep_disturbance)

All websites were accessed in April 2014.

References

Agrawal, A., Cincu, R. and Joharapurkar, S.R. (2008) 'Traumatic brain injury and sleep disturbances.' *Journal of Clinical Sleep Medicine 4,* 2, 177.

Arnulf, I., Reading, P. and Vidialhet, M. (2010) 'Sleep Disorders in Idiopathic Parkinson's Disease.' In S. Overeem and P. Reading (eds) *Sleep Disorders in Neurology: A Practical Approach.* Chichester: Wiley-Blackwell.

Attarian, H.P., Brown, K.M., Duntley, S.P., Carter, J.D. and Cross, A.H. (2004) 'The relationship of sleep disturbances and fatigue in multiple sclerosis.' *Archives of Neurology 61,* 4, 525–528.

Ayalon, L., Borodkin, K., Dishon, L., Kanety, H. and Dagan, Y. (2007) 'Circadian rhythm sleep disorder following mild traumatic brain injury.' *Neurology 68,* 14, 1136–1140.

Baumann, C.R. (2010) 'Sleep-wake Disorders Following Traumatic Brain Injury.' In S. Overeem and P. Reading (eds) *Sleep Disorders in Neurology: A Practical Approach.* Chichester: Wiley-Blackwell.

Bjorvatn, B. and Pallesen, S. (2009) 'A practical approach to circadian rhythm sleep disorders.' *Sleep Medicine Reviews 13,* 1, 47–60.

Brass, S.D., Duquette, P., Proulx-Therrien, J. and Auerbach, S. (2010) 'Sleep disorders in patients with multiple sclerosis.' *Sleep Medicine Reviews 14,* 2, 121–129.

Castriotta, R., Wilde, M.C., Lai, J.M., Atanasov, S., Masel, B.E. and Kuna, S.T. (2007) 'Prevalence and consequences of sleep disorders in traumatic brain injury.' *Journal of Clinical Sleep Medicine 3,* 4, 349–356.

Cohen, M., Oksenberg, A., Snir, D., Stern, M.J. and Groswasser, Z. (1992) 'Temporally related changes of sleep complaints in traumatic brain injured patients.' *Journal of Neurology, Neurosurgery, and Psychiatry 55,* 4, 313–315.

Dhawan, V., Healy, D.G., Pal, S. and Chaudhuri, K.R. (2006) 'Sleep-related problems of Parkinson's disease.' *Age and Ageing 35,* 3, 220–228.

Frucht, S.J., Greene, P.E. and Fahn, S. (2000) 'Sleep episodes in Parkinson's disease: a wake-up call.' *Movement Disorders 15,* 4, 601–603.

Hank, D., Hicks, J. and Wilson, S. (2012) 'Sleep and Psychiatry.' In A. Green and A. Westcombe (eds) *Sleep: Multiprofessional Perspectives.* London: Jessica Kingsley Publishers.

Harrison, S. (2007) *Fatigue Management for People with Multiple Sclerosis*, 2nd edn. London: College of Occupational Therapists.

Hermann, D.M. and Bassetti, C.L. (2010) 'Sleep Disturbances after Stroke.' In S. Overeem and P. Reading (eds) *Sleep Disorders in Neurology: A Practical Approach*. Chichester: Wiley-Blackwell.

Hobson, D.E., Lang, A.E., Martin, W.R.W., Razmy, A., Rivest, J. and Fleming, J. (2002) 'Excessive daytime sleepiness and sudden-onset sleep in Parkinson disease: a survey by the Canadian Movement Disorders Group.' *Journal of the American Medical Association 287*, 4, 455–463.

Kaiser, P.R., Valko, P.O., Werth, E., Thomann, J. *et al.* (2010) 'Modafinil ameliorates excessive daytime sleepiness after traumatic brain injury.' *Neurology 75*, 20, 1780–1785.

Kanbayashi, T., Reading, P. and Nishino, S. (2010) 'Neuro-immunological Disorders.' In S. Overeem and P. Reading (eds) *Sleep Disorders in Neurology: A Practical Approach*. Chichester: Wiley-Blackwell.

Lawrence, A.D., Evans, A.H. and Lees, A.J. (2003) 'Compulsive use of dopamine replacement therapy in Parkinson's disease: reward systems gone awry?' *Lancet Neurology 2*, 10, 595–604.

Leroi, I., Baker, P., Kehoe, P., Daniel, E. and Byrne, E.J. (2010) 'A pilot randomized controlled trial of sleep therapy in Parkinson's disease: effect on patients and caregivers.' *International Journal of Geriatric Psychiatry 25*, 10, 1073–1079.

Li, Y., Munger, K.L., Batool-Anwar, S., De Vito, K., Ascherio, A. and Goa, X. (2012) 'Association of multiple sclerosis with restless legs syndrome and other sleep disorders in women.' *Neurology 78*, 19, 1500–1506.

Löhle, M., Storch, A. and Reichmann, H. (2009) 'Beyond tremor and rigidity: non-motor features of Parkinson's disease'. *Journal of Neural Transmission 116*, 11, 1483–1492.

National Stroke Association (2006) 'Recovery after stroke: sleep disorders.' Available at www.stroke.org/site/DocServer/NSAFactSheet_SleepDisorders.pdf?docID=1002, accessed on 3 February 2014.

NICE (2006) *Parkinson's Disease: Diagnosis and Management in Primary and Secondary Care*. London: National Institute for Health and Clinical Excellence.

Ondo, W.G., Vuong, K.D. and Jankovic, J. (2002) 'Exploring the relationship between Parkinson's disease and restless legs syndrome.' *Archives of Neurology 59*, 3, 421–424.

Orff, H.J., Ayalon, L. and Drummond, S.P.A. (2009) 'Traumatic brain injury and sleep disturbance: a review of current research.' *Journal of Head Trauma Rehabilitation 24*, 3, 155–165.

Ouellet, M.C. and Morin, C.M. (2007) 'Efficacy of cognitive-behavioral therapy for insomnia associated with traumatic brain injury: a single-case experimental design.' *Archives of Physical Medicine and Rehabilitation 88*, 12, 1581–1592.

Ouellet, M-C., Savard, J. and Morin, C.M. (2004) 'Insomnia following brain injury: a review.' *Neurorehabilitation and Neural Repair 18*, 4, 187–198.

Parcell, D.L., Ponsford, J.L., Rajaratnam, S.M. and Redman, R. (2006) 'Self-reported changes to nighttime sleep after traumatic brain injury.' *Archives of Physical Medicine and Rehabilitation 87*, 2, 278–285.

Ponsford, J.L., Ziino, C., Parcell, D.L., Shekleton, J.L. *et al.* (2012) 'Fatigue and sleep disturbance following traumatic brain injury: their nature, causes, and potential treatments.' *Journal of Head Trauma Rehabilitation 27*, 3, 224–233.

Reid, K.J. and Zee, P.C. (2011) 'Circadian Disorders of the Sleep-Wake Cycle.' In M.H. Kryger, T. Roth and W.C. Dement (eds) *Principles and Practice of Sleep Medicine*, 5th edn. St Louis, MO: Saunders.

Rios Romenets, S., Creti, L., Fichten, C., Bailes, S. *et al.* (2013) 'Doxepin and cognitive behavioural therapy for insomnia in patients with Parkinson's disease: a randomized study.' *Parkinsonism and Related Disorders 19*, 7, 670–675.

Srinivasan, V., Cardinali, D.P., Srinivasan, U.S., Kaur, C. *et al.* (2011) 'Therapeutic potential of melatonin and its analogs in Parkinson's disease: focus on sleep and neuroprotection.' *Therapeutic Advances in Neurological Disorders 4*, 5, 297–317.

Swick, T.J. (2012) 'Parkinson's disease and sleep/wake disturbances.' *Parkinson's Disease 2012*. doi: 10.1155/2012/205471.

Tandberg, E., Larsen, J.P. and Karlsen, K. (1998) 'A community-based study of sleep disorders in patients with Parkinson's disease.' *Movement Disorders 13*, 6, 895–899.

Taphoorn, M.J.B., van Someren, E., Snoek, F.J., Strijers, R.L.M. *et al.* (1993) 'Fatigue, sleep disturbances and circadian rhythms in multiple sclerosis.' *Journal of Neurology 240*, 7, 446–448.

Trenkwalder, C. and Arnulf, I. (2011) 'Parkinsonism.' In M.H. Kryger, T. Roth and W.C. Dement (eds) *Principles and Practice of Sleep Medicine*, 5th edn. St Louis, MO: Saunders.

Verma, A., Anand, V. and Verma, N.P. (2007) 'Sleep disorders in chronic traumatic brain injury.' *Journal of Clinical Sleep Medicine 3*, 4, 357–362.

Wallace, D.M., Ramos, A.R. and Rundek, T. (2011) 'Sleep disorders and stroke.' *International Journal of Stroke 7*, 3, 231–242.

Watson, N.F., Dikmen, S., Machamer, J., Doherty, M. and Temkin, N. (2007) 'Hypersomnia following traumatic brain injury.' *Journal of Clinical Sleep Medicine 3*, 4, 363–368.

Willis, G.L. and Turner, E.J. (2007) 'Primary and secondary features of Parkinson's disease improve with strategic exposure to bright light: a case series study.' *Chronobiology International 24*, 3, 521–537.

Wulff, K.L., Gatti, S., Wettstein, J.G. and Foster, R.G. (2010) 'Sleep and circadian rhythm disruption in psychiatric and neurodegenerative disease.' *Nature Reviews Neuroscience 11*, 8, 589–599.

Zeitzer, J.M., Friedman, L. and O'Hara, R. (2009) 'Insomnia in the context of traumatic brain injury.' *Journal of Rehabilitation Research & Development 46*, 6, 827–836.

16

THE RELATIONSHIP BETWEEN SLEEP AND PAIN

Cary Brown and Andrew Green

16.1 Introduction

If the purpose of pain is to alert us to a threat, and sleep takes place when arousal levels can diminish, it follows that sleep in the context of pain is likely to be difficult. This will be the experience of anyone who has suffered from toothache or the pain of an injury, for example. Unpleasant as those are, the individual will usually acknowledge that the pain is temporary and that sleep will return to normal in due course; however, that may not be the case in chronic pain or where pain is a feature of a long-term condition.

The relationship between sleep problems and chronic pain endures across the lifespan from children to older adults (Breau and Camfield 2011; Chen *et al.* 2011; Finan, Goodin and Smith 2013; Siengsukon, Emmanuel and Sharma 2013; Tang 2008). Unfortunately, a research-to-practice gap in this area persists, and many health care providers assume that sleep disruption is a simple consequence of chronic pain. The assumption is that if only the pain problem could be remedied, then restorative sleep patterns would return. Research, however, points towards a bidirectional relationship between pain and sleep, suggesting that not only does sleep deficiency arise from the experience of pain, but sleep deficiency also appears to be one of the risk factors for developing and maintaining chronic pain (Tang, Wright and Salkovskis 2007). This suggests that it could be important to address sleep problems early in pain intervention, and there is a growing evidence base for a range of pragmatic, non-pharmacological sleep interventions (NPSIs) that can be incorporated into pain management programmes. Additionally, many of these strategies are controlled by the patient and, as such, are congruent with the patient self-management model favoured by many pain services (Reid *et al.* 2008). The patient self-management approach targets the teaching of active coping strategies and facilitates self-efficacy. This is important because many patients with chronic health conditions come to feel that they are powerless to effect change and that the future is largely unknown, with little about which to be hopeful (Anderson *et al.* 1995). An example of how pain affects sleep and daily life is given in Box 16.1.

BOX 16.1 Case example: Jane

Jane had a long history of pain for which there was no clear diagnosis. She had been to various services and had been scanned and tested, and various medications had been tried. She lost her job as a teaching assistant and also became very low in mood. She seldom went out and her husband and children increasingly had to look after her. Her physical function deteriorated and she mainly used a wheelchair both in and out of the house. She was on large amounts of medication that increased her sleepiness but did not completely ease her pain. Her sleep was disrupted and she found herself spending more and more time in bed, but she was not able to sleep effectively.

There is a growing evidence base for self-management approaches to help patients regain feelings of mastery and control (Williams, Eccleston and Morley 2012). Introducing pragmatic NPSIs in pain self-management programmes may provide additional opportunities to enhance patients' sense of control and hopefulness. Occupational therapy's emphasis on an individual's lifestyle and engagement in meaningful and purposeful activity (Hagedorn 2000) can have a key role in a pain management programme. Important elements of pain management programmes and occupational therapy are to promote the understanding of biological processes, including pain and sleep, and to develop ways that individuals can incorporate this knowledge into useful change that leads to increased participation in valued activity in the home and in the community.

This chapter explores the complex relationships between sleep and pain, focusing on adults. There is some discussion of sleep management approaches more specific to people living with pain at the conclusion; however, many of the sleep intervention strategies are consistent with those for clients and patients with other health conditions, and the reader is referred to the other chapters (particularly Chapter 8) for more details.

16.2 Disturbance of sleep by chronic pain

Chronic or enduring pain occurs at a high rate across industrialized countries. A report by the International Association for the Study of Pain concluded that 'chronic pain is among the most disabling and costly afflictions in North America, Europe, and Australia' (Harstall and Ospina 2003, p.1). Their review of published studies showed a prevalence of severe chronic pain in adults of approximately 11%. Chronic pain is complex and involves an interaction of biopsychosocial factors that has proven to be resistant to intervention (Gatchel *et al.* 2007). People experience persistent pain for a multitude of reasons: arthritic conditions, fibromyalgia, sports and workplace injuries, headache, neuropathies and post-stroke pain are all common health conditions where the symptoms of pain can be enduring. Additionally, we now know that a number of children with neurodevelopmental problems (such as autistic spectrum disorder and fetal alcohol syndrome) experience complex sensory processing problems that contribute to an increased likelihood both of having some form of ongoing pain and of this pain being underdiagnosed and undertreated (Finley *et al.* 2005). Similarly, older adults with dementias also experience unrecognized and untreated enduring pain (Brown 2010; Gibson 2006).

Irrespective of the patient's age or diagnosis, a problem with sleep is a common experience of those living with pain (Lavigne *et al.* 2011). A study by Tang *et al.* (2007) determined that, while 3%[1] of the population without pain reported insomnia, the prevalence for those with low back pain was 53%. In a study involving over 1000 orthopaedic patients in Germany, Artner *et al.* (2012) found that 42.2% had sleep deprivation (defined as less than 6 hours of sleep) even after analgesic medication, and that almost half of those had less than 4 hours of sleep. A review of other studies by Alsaadi *et al.* (2011) estimated the prevalence of sleep problems to be higher still at 58.9% (range 43–71%). The differences between studies might relate to variations between study groups and methodology but could also reflect the complexity of the problem.

The complexity of the problem is exemplified by the findings of O'Donoghue *et al.* (2009) who compared subjective measures, including sleep diaries and the Pittsburgh Sleep Quality Index (PSQI)*, with actigraphy* recordings for a group of people with chronic lower back pain (*n* = 15) and a healthy control group. The back-pain group reported a greater degree of subjective sleep disturbance than the control group, and it was also shown that the level of subjective disturbance was significantly higher than the objective level. This accords with evidence cited in Chapter 7 that people tend to overestimate wakefulness; they are mostly unaware that short periods of wakefulness during the course of the night are not unusual or necessarily harmful. A systematic review of 17 studies concluded that, while the methodological quality of the studies reviewed was generally weak, evidence of a negative association between low back pain and sleep was strong enough to warrant a recommendation that sleep problems be routinely included in back-pain assessment and management strategies (Kelly *et al.* 2011).

The importance of managing sleep problems is demonstrated in a longitudinal population study involving 18,976 people in Finland by Ropponen *et al.* (2012). They found that sleep patterns reported at baseline ('fairly poor/poorly' or 'moderately well') helped predict which participants after 23 years would be registered for a national disability pension due to low back pain. The findings suggested that poor sleep is a risk factor for low back pain resulting in pensionable disability.

Independent of each other, pain and sleep researchers have determined that affect can act as a predisposing and perpetuating influence on each respective condition. However, in a study of 292 American adults with both chronic pain and sleep problems, O'Brien *et al.* (2010) found that negative mood mediated the adverse effect poor sleep exerted on self-reported pain intensity. They concluded that addressing either negative mood or sleep, or both, could have a positive effect on patients' experience of pain. Similarly, Chiu *et al.* (2005) found a relationship between depression, poor sleep and reduced pain threshold. Higher levels of anxiety and depression were also noted in participants attending a pain clinic compared with those without pain (Pilowsky, Crettenden and Townley 1985). Although none of these studies demonstrate causality, they illustrate the complex relationships between pain, sleep and emotion.

In summary, the complexity illustrated above demonstrates that sleep and pain are closely interrelated. It follows that they would benefit from the holistic, person-centred approaches that occupational therapists employ. Occupational therapists who work in pain management services are well versed in working with all of the biopsychosocial domains that comprise occupational performance (Rochman and Kennedy-Spaien 2007) and can extend this same perspective to encompass their clients' sleep problems. Taken together, the evidence indicates a bidirectional relationship between pain and sleep (Abernethy 2008) and emphasizes the importance of taking sleep and sleep problems seriously throughout life. An expert panel at the 2008 International Sleep Disorders Forum supported this conclusion in stating in their report that the 'management of the sleep disorder may consequently improve the co-morbid disease process itself' (Roehrs 2009, p.5).

16.3 The influence of sleep on the perception of pain

The experimental data exploring the relationship between sleep and pain at the biological level have been reviewed in depth by Lautenbacher, Kundermann and Krieg (2006), who noted that the mechanism of action is not yet sufficiently clear. However, they concluded that there was strong evidence that sleep deprivation, and particularly rapid eye movement (REM) sleep* deprivation, exerted a hyperalgesic effect and appeared to suppress production and metabolism of both opioid medications and endogenous, naturally produced, opioid-like neurochemicals such as endorphins. This hyperalgesic effect was also found in a German study of 14 healthy young adults who, after only one night of total sleep deprivation, reported higher pain response to heat, cold and blunt pressure (Schuh-Hofer *et al.* 2013). Schuh-Hofer *et al.* (2013) also concluded that, although the exact manner in which sleep and pain influence each other is not yet fully understood, sleep deprivation seems to influence neurotransmitters involved in endogenous pain control.

Neurochemicals that are important to the stress response (e.g. cortisol) and other body functions determined by the neuroendocrine system are largely regulated through interactions between the hypothalamus, the pituitary system and the adrenal gland. The pathway of these interactions is more commonly referred to as the hypothalamic-pituitary-adrenal (HPA) axis. Importantly, in separate lines of study, researchers have identified the importance of the HPA axis to both pain (Aloisi 2011) and sleep regulation (Goodin *et al.* 2012).

The study by Goodin *et al.* (2012) involved 40 healthy volunteers (without a diagnosed sleep disorder) whose tolerance of pain was measured by a cold-pressor task – immersing their dominant hand in cold water (at 4°C) for 2 minutes. Levels of cortisol in saliva were measured before the task (baseline), upon termination of the task and during a 40-minute recovery period. Participants also completed the PSQI and a pain questionnaire. It was found that participants who had poor sleep as measured by the PSQI had higher serum cortisol levels at baseline, lower pain threshold to the cold-pressor task and increased cortisol reactivity to the stress of the cold-pressor task than volunteers whose sleep was rated as good. In other words, participants reporting poor sleep quality in the previous month also reported a more severe pain response than those with better sleep. Goodin *et al.* (2012) make two observations: first, that chronically poor sleep increases cortisol secretion and, conversely, greater levels of circulating cortisol predict arousal and wakefulness; second, that cortisol might have a hyperalgesic effect, but pain itself can act as a stressor which leads to activation of the HPA axis and secretion of cortisol.

The influence of sleep deprivation on the central nervous system's sensitization to pain is a complex process which researchers are only beginning to unpick. While the study by Goodin *et al.* (2012) reveals associations, it does not indicate causation. However, the encouraging 'take home' message appears to be that helping patients achieve restorative sleep has the potential to have two beneficial effects: it could decrease the role of developing chronic pain and it could assist in managing existing pain conditions.

16.4 Managing sleep in the context of pain

The assessment of sleep problems is covered in other chapters (Chapter 8 in particular) and is not considered here. Among the approaches in the management of sleep problems are education, sleep hygiene, cognitive behavioural strategies and lifestyle factors.

Engagement and education

Patients who understand the physiological, psychological, environmental and social forces that influence their sleep are better able to assume a self-management role and build feelings of control – important components in successful pain management outcomes (British Pain Society 2007). It is therefore helpful in a pain management programme to cover the elements of sleep science: that it is important to 'set the body clock' each day by seeing daylight on waking in the morning and to increase the homeostatic drive to sleep by rising at a consistent time and avoiding naps (see Chapter 3). It is also useful to understand that there are different stages of sleep, which occur in cycles, and that waking between cycles is entirely normal (and could be an advantage in providing an opportunity to change position; see Box 16.2). Furthermore, with increased fragmentation of sleep it is more likely that total sleep time will be underestimated.

The difference between objective and subjective assessment of sleep is well documented in the literature, for example, by Means *et al.* (2003). (See also Chapter 7 for a discussion on paradoxical insomnia and for further references.) The point of highlighting the possibility of a difference is not to challenge the patient's experience but to introduce the idea that their sleep might not be quite as bad as they think, because anxiety about poor sleep can contribute to perpetuating insomnia. However, a particular difficulty is that patients with chronic pain often already experience disbelief about their pain – not only from health professionals but also from others in the community – and could feel that a sleep problem is also not taken seriously. (See Newton *et al.* 2013 for an in-depth exploration of disbelief in chronic pain.) Occupational therapists working in pain management are experienced in engaging patients who are used to being disbelieved by health professionals, and will need to make their own judgement as to whether, and when, it would help to discuss the possibility of sleep misperception if it is suspected.

BOX 16.2 Case example: Marie

Marie had poor sleep related to her neck and arm pain. She tried sleep management strategies to good effect and, combined with medication, experienced several nights of 8 hours of unbroken sleep. However, in a later session she concluded that 'a full night's sleep makes the pain worse because I don't move enough; its actually better if I do wake up two or three times a night, and now I know about sleep patterns so I feel more relaxed about it so am getting back to sleep faster.'

Sleep hygiene

In managing sleep problems in chronic pain, all the usual sleep hygiene measures should be discussed with patients. Sleep hygiene is discussed in detail in Chapter 8, where it is also observed that sleep hygiene alone is not the solution for many sleep problems, although directions should be individualized and not simply given as a set of rules. It is as important as ever to ensure that sleeping conditions are comfortable, but there is no particular bed that is recommended for back-pain sufferers; the main thing is that it be comfortable. The idea that a bed should be especially firm probably goes back to times when the quality of the average bed was poor; however, a modern sprung mattress of reasonable quality on a good base should provide adequate support for most people. It may be important, however, that the bed be of sufficient height to make independent access possible so that the individual can get in without exertion and get out easily in the night, if necessary, and in the morning.

Some people with chronic pain find that sharing a bed can cause disturbance – or fear that their difficulty getting comfortable will disturb their partner. People often feel that sleeping separately from a partner is somehow shameful, but it is a personal choice and they may be reassured that it is more common than is often acknowledged (see Chapter 4). The evidence and guidelines for pain management are clear that mobilization is important, and that prolonged bed rest should be avoided (British Pain Society 2007; Hagen *et al.* 2005). However, some patients may spend long daytime periods in bed watching television or engaging in other waking activity. Another possibility is using the bed as a place of retreat and for rest during a flare-up of pain. As explained in Chapter 8, this could create unhelpful associations with the bedroom which, ideally, should be reserved for sleep. Sometimes understanding this and changing habitual behaviours takes time. Occupational therapists can help patients recognize that coping strategies, fear of movement and lack of daytime activity, as opposed to sleep, are wider issues that need to be reframed and then addressed through the graded-activity approach. Box 16.3 shows an example of someone who spent long periods in bed during the day.

BOX 16.3 Case example: Jim

Jim, who has a five-year history of low back pain, spent days at a time in bed, and when he did get up, he would get up in the night. Then, because his sleep had been poor, he would go back to bed. After attending a 12-week pain management course and having to get up for that he said, 'I realized I wasn't getting up because I was avoiding people and things I need to do and blamed lack of sleep.' He found that focusing on things that mattered to him, such as seeing friends and family, caring for his animals and being in natural settings, and then setting very small, achievable daily and weekly goals as part of a supportive group, helped him address this.

Whether patients with chronic pain are prescribed hypnotic medication (or other medication to promote sleep) is a matter for them to discuss with their doctor. However, from the perspective of sleep hygiene it is important to take analgesic medication at the optimum time in order that it has time to work, or that the effects have not worn off, by bedtime. Conversely, any medication that has sedative properties could affect daytime activity, which in turn might affect night-time sleep (see below). Where there is any doubt a patient should be advised to consult their doctor or pharmacist for advice.

Perhaps the most important aspect of sleep hygiene involves limiting the client's exposure to blue-spectrum light in the evening and at night. Blue-spectrum-light exposure (from televisions, laptops, tablets and other electronic devices) suppresses melatonin* production and, as a consequence, sleep onset is often delayed. (There are detailed sections on light in Chapters 9 and 12 where the reader can find recommendations to help clients modify their environment to decrease blue-spectrum light exposure.)

Although detailed discussion of nicotine is beyond the scope of this chapter, there is evidence of an association between smoking and pain. For example, a postal study distributed to 21,201 adults in the UK found that current smokers and ex-smokers had a higher risk for pain than lifetime non-smokers (Palmer *et al.* 2003). The direction of the relationship was unknown, and it may be that smoking was a risk factor for developing pain or that people with pain are more likely to smoke as a form of self-medication. There is some evidence of a potential benefit of nicotine as an analgesic (Powledge 2004), but given the well-known risks of smoking, it would be an unwise strategy for pain relief. Furthermore, as a recent review of 52 sleep and nicotine studies indicated, smoking increases the risk of sleep problems such as delayed sleep onset, frequent night-time awakenings (because of nicotine cravings), respiratory conditions that disturb sleep, decreased slow-wave sleep* and daytime sleepiness (Jaehne *et al.* 2009). There is therefore clear incentive to stop smoking, although individuals must take account of many factors in making a decision whether to quit. Many smokers use nicotine dermal patches as part of giving up smoking and are best advised to see their doctor or a specialist in smoking cessation for advice about their use, in particular whether to use a 16-hour patch or a 24-hour patch. This is not a straightforward issue as it has been well documented that some patients using transdermal patches report that they experience more vivid and disturbing dreams when using the patches than when they were not using a patch (Page, Coleman and Conduit 2006). Some studies suggest that using a 24-hour patch, as opposed to the 16-hour patch, removed at bedtime, may be more effective in reducing sleep disruption because of nicotine craving (Jaehne *et al.* 2009; Staner *et al.* 2006). Smoking cessation researchers also point out that subjective sleep disruption can contribute to an increased likelihood of resuming smoking (Okun *et al.* 2011). So, taken together, the only clear conclusion is that the issue of smoking and sleep is complex and needs to be considered at an individual level. As Derrida said, 'if the answer was that simple, word would have gotten around' (Derrida 1988, p.119). (For further discussion see Jaehne *et al.* 2009 and Staner *et al.* 2006.)

The effect of caffeine on sleep is generally well known, although not everyone realizes how much caffeine is in tea and chocolate (see Chapter 8). Caffeine is often added to headache medication because it counteracts the sedative effect of some analgesics and acts as a vasoconstrictor whereby the decreased blood flow itself has an analgesic effect in certain types of headache (Sawynok 2011). The way that caffeine affects sleep is by blocking the uptake of adenosine, a function of which is to promote drowsiness and sleep. Additionally, as Sawynok (2011) determined in his review of the evidence, research seems to indicate that the analgesic effect of caffeine is actually limited. In headache pain, for example, once the concentration of caffeine in the bloodstream drops off, withdrawal effects can actually compound and intensify headache pain. Other studies cited in the same review suggest that caffeine can cause interactions that decrease the analgesic effectiveness of a number of medications such as paracetamol/acetaminophen and amitriptyline. Furthermore, by blocking adenosine uptake, caffeine might interfere with the analgesic effect of acupuncture and of transcutaneous electrical nerve stimulation (TENS). Habitual use of over-the-counter pain medications that contain caffeine and consumption of caffeine in beverages needs to be explored with clients in order that they can make informed choices.

Although there is a widespread belief that alcohol helps to promote sleep, as Roehrs and Roth (2001) illustrate in their evidence review, the reality is different. Alcohol might initially help a person get off to sleep, but it can significantly interfere with sleep later in the night (when longer periods of REM sleep occur in each cycle). In parallel, the belief that alcohol helps with pain management is also widespread. Once again the reality is that, while alcohol is often used to self-medicate for pain, long-term use of alcohol in this manner can have serious consequences including addiction, gastrointestinal and liver damage, and adverse reaction to opioid and some other forms of analgesic medication (Riley and King 2009). The relationships between pain, sleep and alcohol are complex and, while a blanket directive to 'stop drinking' may prove challenging, excessive use of alcohol is to be avoided. The approach to tackling the issue needs to be considered on a client-by-client basis, referring for further help as required.

Cognitive behavioural strategies

Stimulus control, as explained in Chapter 8, suggests that the bedroom is reserved for sleep (and sex) only, a regular rising time is adhered to, naps are avoided and that an individual should go to bed when sleepy, that is, feeling drowsy or ready to fall asleep, as opposed to feeling tired. All of these 'rules' can be applied in the context of chronic pain, but it might not be appropriate to apply the '15-minute rule' which advises getting out of bed if not asleep after 15 minutes. This rule should not be applied rigidly and may well be best overlooked if the process of getting out of bed causes increased pain (or if there is a risk of falls); equally, if someone can remain relaxed in bed and confident of getting or returning to sleep, there is a case for staying put.

Applying sleep restriction therapy rules (described in Chapter 8) might also be difficult, but again, the principle is important – not to spend excessive time awake in bed and to increase sleep efficiency*. Experience indicates that it might be too much to expect participants in a multi-component pain management programme (where, for example, they are also trying to increase levels of exercise or re-engage with work or other occupations) to focus also on such a difficult strategy. However, building on work by Currie *et al.* (2000) and Edinger *et al.* (2005), Jungquist *et al.* (2010) show that an eight-session CBT-I programme can bring about improvements in sleep. The programme of Jungquist *et al.* (2010) appeared to focus on sleep restriction therapy but also included sleep hygiene instructions, stimulus control and cognitive therapy; it yielded improvement in sleep onset latency*, wakening after sleep onset and sleep efficiency, although total sleep time did not increase significantly. Subsequently, Jungquist *et al.* (2012) showed that improvements were maintained in spite of the persistence of pain. They suggest that such findings support the idea that insomnia co-morbid with chronic pain is not an inevitable consequence of the pain. Jungquist *et al.* (2012) also suggest that CBT-I is something that can be provided by advanced practitioners (nurses in their case) in a multi-disciplinary pain clinic setting.

As noted elsewhere in the book and earlier in this chapter, the perception of sleep among people with chronic pain, as well as others, might not seem to match the objective measurement in a sleep laboratory. One factor that is likely to affect that perception is waking in the night, but it is important to be aware, as noted in Chapter 3, that night-time waking is entirely normal. This might be reassuring for some people to know, but the difficulty is that on waking, the individual may become aware of pain – or might have been disturbed by pain – and, unlike the person who sleeps well, they might remain awake. In some cases, the pain may be such that sleep is not immediately likely, but it is also likely that the mind becomes active and may be overwhelmed by negative thoughts, thereby further increasing arousal. (Measures to calm the mind are described in Chapter 8 and include strategies such as imagery and ensuring that the business of the day has been concluded before winding down for bed.)

One method that might reduce the ruminations that delay sleep was tested in a pilot study conducted by Brown *et al.* (2014). Patients with chronic pain were taught hand self-shiatsu – a form of body work that requires participants to concentrate on using one hand to apply stimulation to a prescribed series of pressure points on the other hand for a set period of time. A trained shiatsu therapist can teach a patient to administer hand self-shiatsu in under an hour. Most participants in the study reported that they felt that it was easier to fall asleep, and that they slept for longer, when they did the self-shiatsu. The researchers speculated that positive outcomes might be a consequence of the cognitive demand of remembering the specific directions to carry out the hand self-shiatsu sequence competing with the cognitive demand of typical pain-related ruminations that delay sleep. Attentional theorists propose that the brain can only attend to one cognitive demand at a time (Styles 2006), and therefore carrying out hand self-shiatsu can interfere with sleep-delaying ruminations. Although the study was small and not conclusive, hand self-shiatsu is a low-cost and practical intervention that holds promise as a means of promoting the transition to sleep. It also raises the possibility that therapists might experiment with other methods (for example, meditation) requiring concentrated attention as well as strategies such as imagery that are suggested in Chapter 8.

Lifestyle factors

Although there is accumulating evidence that CBT-I has a role in managing sleep problems in the context of chronic pain, other measures will remain important. For example, it is observed in several other chapters that a good sleep pattern is supported by engagement in regular activity; this includes exercise. The object of most pain management programmes is to reduce the distress and disability associated with chronic pain (see, for example, Ashworth, Davidson and Espie 2010) and this is likely to include re-engagement with exercise and activity. The level of exercise involved in a pain management programme is unlikely to be sufficient to influence sleep directly as, for example, in studies cited in Chapter 6. However, Chapter 6 also suggests that the establishment of routines, which could include exercise, could contribute to improved sleep. Furthermore, stretching exercises can improve flexibility, reduce stiffness and improve a patient's ability to get comfortable in bed. Sometimes it can be the sleep management that enables an individual to implement the activity management and exercise advice, as seen in the example in Box 16.4.

BOX 16.4 Case example: Tim

Tim was a patient who attended a 10-week outpatient pain management programme. He had ongoing lower back pain which affected all aspects of his life. He had lost his job, his marriage had ended and his mood had been very low. He struggled with the other aspects of the programme, such as setting baselines of regular activity, exercise and ensuring a balance of activity, until he set a regular rising. Although that did not immediately improve his sleep, he found that by having a goal to get up before 10 a.m. every day he felt that he had more time to pace himself and also do more of the things he enjoyed.

One of the cornerstones of pain management is pacing, although the term has been found to be ill-defined (Gill and Brown 2009). It is usually understood to mean balancing rest and activity, and someone experiencing chronic pain is advised to break activities and not to remain in any position too long. Despite that, someone experiencing pain might also aspire to remain in a recumbent position for 7 or 8 hours in order to sleep, and there is therefore an argument for pacing sleep by adopting unconventional sleep patterns. For some people the benefit of having more predictable sleep in more than one period might outweigh the disadvantages of being asleep and awake at unusual times. For example, as shown in Chapter 4, a single period of unbroken sleep is not necessarily the way that humans have always slept. Not only is it natural to wake frequently in the night, as shown in Chapter 3, but a period of wakefulness between two longer periods of sleep is also natural.

Some possible ways that people use a period of nocturnal wakefulness are given in Chapter 4, but others with chronic pain also find their own ways; for example, some people who are able to work flexibly from home choose to spend time at night working and to have more than one period of sleep. Similarly, a shorter night-time sleep with an afternoon sleep, or siesta, could provide a way both to pace sleep and to reduce the frustration of long periods of wakefulness at night. Of course, these patterns are not possible for the majority and it is not suggested that therapists actively advocate them; however, it is important to know that while they may not be practical for most people, they are options and could allow an individual to increase total sleep time in 24 hours.

16.5 Conclusion

Sleep loss is a significant burden for many people living with enduring pain. The fact that insufficient sleep can be both a consequence of, and a risk factor for, persistent pain makes this a complex health issue. Non-pharmacological sleep interventions delivered within a self-management framework can be a means of helping clients develop self-efficacy and sufficient resilience to begin tipping the balance in a restorative direction. Occupational therapists' training and approach to practice makes them well suited to both deliver programmes to promote the management of pain and the improvement of sleep and to lead in developing innovative approaches based on new evidence as it emerges in this challenging area.

Note

1   This is lower than in most studies (for example, Ohayon 2002 gives a prevalence of 6%); however, either way, the difference is substantial.

Acknowledgements

We thank Dr Peter Gladwell (physiotherapist) and Fiona Wright (occupational therapist) at the North Bristol Pain Management Service for helpful contributions to this chapter.

References

Abernethy, A.P. (2008) 'Pain and sleep: establishing bi-directional association in a population-based sample.' *Pain 137*, 1, 1–2.

Aloisi, A.M., Buonocore, M., Merlo, L., Galandra, C. *et al.* (2011) 'Chronic pain therapy and hypothalamic-pituitary-adrenal axis impairment.' *Psychoneuroendocrinology 36*, 7, 1032–1039.

Alsaadi, S.M., McAuley, J.H., Hush, J.M. and Maher, C.G. (2011) 'Prevalence of sleep disturbance in patients with low back pain.' *European Spine Journal 20*, 5, 737–743.

Anderson, K.O., Dowds, B.N., Pelletz, R.E., Edwards, W.T. and Peeters-Asdourian, C. (1995) 'Development and initial validation of a scale to measure self-efficacy beliefs in patients with chronic pain.' *Pain 63*, 1, 77–84.

Artner, J., Cakir, B., Spiekerman, J.-A., Kurz, S. *et al.* (2012) 'Prevalence of sleep deprivation in patients with chronic neck and back pain: a retrospective evaluation of 1016 patients.' *Journal of Pain Research.* doi: 10.2147/JPR.S36386.

Ashworth, P.C.H., Davidson, K.M. and Espie, C.A. (2010) 'Cognitive-behavioral factors associated with sleep quality in chronic pain patients.' *Behavioral Sleep Medicine 8*, 1, 28–39.

Breau, L.M. and Camfield, C.S. (2011) 'Pain disrupts sleep in children and youth with intellectual and developmental disabilities.' *Research in Developmental Disabilities 32*, 6, 2829–2840.

British Pain Society (2007) 'Recommended guidelines for pain management programmes for adults.' Available at www.britishpainsociety.org/book_pmp2013_main.pdf, accessed on 28 November 2013.

Brown, C.A. (2010) 'Pain in communication impaired residents with dementia: analysis of Resident Assessment Instrument (RAI) data.' *Dementia 9*, 3, 375–389.

Brown, C.A., Bostick, G., Bellmore, L. and Kumanayaka, D. (2014) 'Hand self-Shiatsu for sleep problems in persons with chronic pain: a pilot study.' *Journal of Integrative Medicine 12*, 2, 94–101.

Chen, Q., Hayman, L.H., Shmerling, R.H., Bean, J.F. and Leveille, S.G. (2011) 'Characteristics of chronic pain associated with sleep difficulty in the older population: the MOBILIZE Boston Study.' *Journal of the American Geriatric Society 59*, 8, 1385–1392.

Chiu, Y.H., Silman, A.J., Macfarlane, G.J., Ray, D., Gupta, A., Dickens, C., Morriss, R. and McBeth, J. (2005) 'Poor sleep and depression are independently associated with a reduced pain threshold. Results of a population based study.' *Pain 115*, 3, 316–321.

Currie, S.R., Wilson, K.G., Pontefract, A.J. and deLaplante, L. (2000) 'Cognitive-behavioral treatment of insomnia secondary to chronic pain.' *Journal of Consulting and Clinical Psychology 68*, 3, 407–416.

Derrida, J. (1988) *Limited Inc.* Evanston, IL: Northwestern University Press.

Edinger, J.D., Wohlgemuth, W.K., Krystal, A.D. and Rice, J.R. (2005) 'Behavioral insomnia therapy for fibromyalgia patients.' *Archives of Internal Medicine 165*, 21, 2527–2535.

Finan, P.H., Goodin, B.R. and Smith, M.T. (2013) 'The association of sleep and pain: an update and a path forward.' *Journal of Pain 14*, 12, 1539–1552.

Finley, G., Franck, L., Grunau, R. and von Baeyer, C. (2005) 'Why children's pain matters.' *Pain: Clinical Updates 13*, 4, 1–4.

Gatchel, R.J., Peng, Y.B., Peters, M.L., Fuchs, P.N. and Turk, D.C. (2007) 'The biopsychosocial approach to chronic pain: scientific advances and future directions.' *Psychological Bulletin 133*, 4, 581–624.

Gibson, S. (2006) 'Older people's pain.' *Pain: Clinical Updates 14*, 3, 1–4.

Gill, J.R. and Brown, C.A. (2009) 'A structured review of the evidence for pacing as a chronic pain intervention.' *European Journal of Pain 13*, 2, 214–216.

Goodin, B.R., Smith, M.T., Quinn, N.B., King, C.D. and McGuire, L. (2012) 'Poor sleep quality and exaggerated salivary cortisol reactivity to the cold pressor task predict greater acute pain severity in a non-clinical sample.' *Biological Psychology 91*, 1, 36–41.

Hagedorn, R. (2000) *Tools for Practice in Occupational Therapy.* London: Churchill Livingstone.

Hagen, K.B., Jamtvedt, G., Hilde, G. and Winnem, M.F. (2005) 'The updated Cochrane Review of bed rest for low back pain and sciatica.' *Spine 30*, 5, 542–546.

Harstall, C. and Ospina, M. (2003) 'How prevalent is chronic pain?' *Pain: Clinical Updates 11*, 2, 1–4.

Jaehne, A., Loessl, B., Bárkai, Z., Riemann, D. and Hornyak, M. (2009) 'Effects of nicotine on sleep during consumption, withdrawal and replacement therapy.' *Sleep Medicine Reviews 13*, 5, 363–377.

Jungquist, C.R., O'Brien, C., Matteson-Rusby, S., Smith, M.T. *et al.* (2010) 'The efficacy of cognitive-behavioral therapy for insomnia in patients with chronic pain.' *Sleep Medicine 11*, 3, 302–309.

Jungquist, C.R., Tra, Y., Smith, M.T., Pigeon, W.R. *et al.* (2012) 'The durability of cognitive behavioral therapy for insomnia in patients with chronic pain.' *Sleep Disorders.* doi: 10.1155/2012/679648.

Kelly, G.A, Blake, C., Power, C.K., O'Keeffe, D. and Fullen, B.M. (2011) 'The association between chronic low back pain and sleep: a systematic review.' *Clinical Journal of Pain 27*, 2, 169–181.

Lautenbacher, S., Kundermann, B. and Krieg, J.-C. (2006) 'Sleep deprivation and pain perception.' *Sleep Medicine Reviews 10*, 5, 357–369.

Lavigne, G., Smith, M.T., Denis, R. and Zucconi, M. (2011) 'Pain and Sleep.' In M.H. Kryger, T. Roth and W.C. Dement (eds) *Principles and Practice of Sleep Medicine*, 5th edn. St Louis, MO: Elsevier Saunders.

Means, M.K., Edinger, J.D., Glenn, D.M. and Fins, A.I. (2003) 'Accuracy of sleep perceptions among insomnia sufferers and normal sleepers.' *Sleep Medicine 4*, 4, 285–296.

Newton, B.J., Southall, J.L., Raphael, J.H., Ashford, R.L. and LeMarchand, K. (2013) 'A narrative review of the impact of disbelief in chronic pain.' *Pain Management Nursing 14*, 3, 161–171.

O'Brien, E.M., Wazenberg, L.B., Atchison, J.W., Gremillion, H.A. *et al.* (2010) 'Negative mood mediates the effect of poor sleep on pain among chronic pain patients'. *Clinical Journal of Pain 26*, 4, 310–319.

O'Donoghue, G.M., Fox, N., Heneghan, C. and Hurley, D.A. (2009) 'Objective and subjective assessment of sleep in chronic low back pain patients compared with healthy age and gender matched controls: a pilot study.' *BMC Musculoskeletal Disorders.* doi: 10.1186/1471-2474-10-122.

Ohayon, M.M. (2002) 'Epidemiology of insomnia: what we know and what we still need to learn.' *Sleep Medicine Reviews 6,* 2, 97–111.

Okun, M.L., Levine, M.D., Houck, P., Perkins, K.A. and Marcus, M.D. (2011) 'Subjective sleep disturbance during a smoking cessation program: associations with relapse.' *Addictive Behaviors 36,* 8, 861–864.

Palmer, K.T., Syddall, H., Cooper, C. and Coggon, D. (2003) 'Smoking and musculoskeletal disorders: findings from a British national survey.' *Annals of the Rheumatic Diseases 62,* 1, 33–36.

Pilowsky, I., Crettenden, I. and Townley, M. (1985) 'Sleep disturbances in pain clinic patients.' *Pain 23,* 1, 27–33.

Powledge, T.M. (2004) 'Nicotine as therapy.' *PLoS Biol 2,* 11, e404.

Reid, M.C., Papaleontiou, M., Ong, A., Breckman, R., Wethington, E. and Pillemer, K. (2008) 'Self-management strategies to reduce pain and improve function among older adults in community settings: a review of the evidence.' *Pain Medicine 9,* 4, 409–424.

Riley, J.L. and King, C. (2009) 'Self-report of alcohol use for pain in a multi-ethnic community sample.' *Journal of Pain 10,* 9, 944–952.

Rochman, D.L. and Kennedy-Spaien, E. (2007) 'Chronic pain management approaches and tools for occupational therapy.' *OT Practice 12,* 13, 9–15.

Roehrs, T.A. (2009) 'Does effective management of sleep disorders improve pain symptoms?' *Drugs 69,* Suppl. 2, S5–S11.

Roehrs, T. and Roth, T. (2001) 'Sleep, sleepiness, sleep disorders and alcohol use and abuse.' *Sleep Medicine Reviews 5,* 4, 287–297.

Ropponen, A., Silventoinen, K., Hublin, C., Svedberg, P. *et al.* (2012) 'Sleep patterns as predictors for disability pension due to low back diagnoses: a 23-year longitudinal study of Finnish twins.' *Sleep 3,* 6, 891–897.

Sawynok, J. (2011) 'Caffeine and pain.' *Pain 152,* 4, 726–729.

Schuh-Hofer, S., Wodarski, R., Pfau, D.B., Caspani, O. *et al.* (2013) 'One night of total sleep deprivation promotes a state of generalized hyperalgesia: a surrogate pain model to study the relationship of insomnia and pain.' *Pain 154,* 9, 1613–1621.

Siengsukon, C., Emmanuel, N.M. and Sharma, N.K. (2013) 'Relationship between low back pain and sleep quality.' *Journal of Novel Physiotherapies.* doi: 10.4172/2165-7025.1000168.

Staner, L., Luthringer, R., Dupont, C., Aubin, H.J. and Lagrue, G. (2006) 'Sleep effects of a 24-h versus a 16-h nicotine patch: a polysomographic study during smoking cessation.' *Sleep Medicine 7,* 2, 147–154.

Styles, E.A. (2006) *The Psychology of Attention,* 2nd edn. London: Psychology Press.

Tang, N.K.Y. (2008) 'Insomnia co-occurring with chronic pain: clinical features, interaction, assessments and possible interventions.' *Reviews in Pain 2,* 1, 2–7.

Tang, N.K.Y., Wright, K.J and Salkovskis, P.M. (2007) 'Prevalence and correlates of clinical insomnia co-occurring with chronic back pain.' *Journal of Sleep Research 16*, 1, 85–96.

Williams, A.C., Eccleston, C. and Morley, S. (2012) 'Psychological therapies for the management of chronic pain (excluding headache) in adults.' *Cochrane Database of Systematic Reviews.* doi: 10.1002/14651858.CD007407.pub3.

17

CHRONIC FATIGUE SYNDROME, OCCUPATIONAL THERAPY AND SLEEP

Fiona Wright

17.1 Introduction

Chronic fatigue syndrome (CFS), also known as myalgic encephalomyelitis (ME), and commonly abbreviated as CFS/ME,[1] is a condition that affects between 0.4 and 2.5% of people worldwide (Afari and Buchwald 2003; Ranjith 2005). It can present very differently and impact variously on function and quality of life. Occupational therapists are probably the largest profession within specialist CFS/ME services throughout the UK.[2] It is also likely that occupational therapists will come into contact with people with CFS/ME in other settings; for example, community therapists may be asked to advise on environmental adaptations for the more severely affected, and in vocational rehabilitation they may need to advise on a graded return to work or on workplace adaptations. Furthermore, with the high prevalence of CFS/ME, occupational therapists are likely to come across CFS/ME in general medical and mental health settings. Sleep is very often disrupted and a key diagnostic feature of CFS/ME is unrefreshing sleep (Fukuda *et al.* 1994; NICE 2007). While improvement of sleep is not known to 'cure' CFS/ME, establishing a helpful pattern of sleep supports effective management and can improve function thereby aiding recovery from this condition. This chapter looks at current understanding of sleep and CFS in the research and how this translates to a clinical setting. Some of the behavioural management approaches that can be used by occupational therapists in different settings are discussed.

17.2 CFS/ME and its management

According to the National Institute for Health and Clinical Excellence (NICE), CFS/ME is characterized by persistent or relapsing unexplained, disabling chronic fatigue which lasts for at least 4–6 months (NICE 2007). There are no biological markers and the diagnosis depends on self-report, according to various criteria. The diagnostic criteria established by Fukuda *et al.* (1994) are commonly used in clinical services and research: they define the fatigue in CFS/ME as being of new or definite onset, and not the result of an organic disease or of continuing exertion. The fatigue is usually not alleviated by rest and results in a substantial reduction in previous occupational, educational, social and personal activities. In addition to fatigue, other symptoms include impaired memory or concentration, sore throat, tender cervical or axillary lymph nodes, muscle pain, pain in several joints, new headaches and malaise after exertion (Fukuda *et al.* 1994). Of particular relevance to this book, patients often report difficulties with sleep. These difficulties include feeling unrefreshed upon waking despite sufficient or extended total sleep, daytime sleepiness and napping, and other sleep-related symptoms, such as difficulty initiating sleep and disturbed sleep.

There has been some research focusing on the cause of non-restorative sleep and sleep disturbance in CFS/ME, and whether or how these symptoms might relate, or contribute, to fatigue. Sleep abnormalities in CFS have been differentiated from sleep changes in other conditions, such as depression, and have been significant in determining CFS/ME as a distinct condition separate from depression and primary sleep disorders (Jackson and Bruck 2012). Additionally, a recent outcome study of UK services found that anxiety and depression at assessment did not mediate outcome in CFS/ME in young people (Crawley *et al.* 2013).

The cause of CFS/ME remains unknown, but there is often a history of a viral infection and a period of stress (for example, having influenza at a time when needing to care for a sick relative, pushing through without resting appropriately, perhaps also feeling stressed and/or distressed). Between 75 and 95% of people report a viral onset and, historically, CFS/ME has been linked with the Epstein-Barr virus glandular fever. However, many other viruses are now seen to be triggers, and there are many people diagnosed with CFS/ME who cannot pinpoint a particular episode of either distress or illness (Hashimoto *et al.* 1992; Vercoulen *et al.* 1994; Wessely and Powell 1989). There is no evidence that a particular virus is present in the longer term, although people often report feeling as though they have a flu-like virus.

Research continues and it seems that the stress response, with corresponding immune activation, may be overly activated, even at rest and in sleep (Wyller, Eriksen and Malterud 2009). The hypothalamic-pituitary-adrenal axis appears to be disturbed, with some evidence showing that individuals with CFS have abnormally flattened cortisol rates, which are also associated with chronic stress and insomnia (Van den Eede *et al.* 2007). Whether or not this is the cause of CFS/ME or is secondary to other mechanisms remains debatable, although it is thought likely this change contributes to the symptoms of CFS/ME. In clinical practice a pragmatic model of CFS/ME is developing; it describes a disrupted protective (fight-or-flight) system that benefits from being stabilized through behavioural adaptations (Clauw 2010; Rahman *et al.* 2011; Van den Eede *et al.* 2007; Wyller *et al.* 2009).

Evidence from single- and multi-centre controlled trials, with outpatients who can attend clinics regularly, suggests that cognitive behaviour therapy (CBT) and graded exercise/graded activity therapy (GET/GAT) are the most suitable approaches in facilitating management of CFS/ME. These approaches are effective for 40–48% of affected individuals (Price *et al.* 2008; White *et al.* 2011). NICE (2007) guidance also includes activity management as an approach that is helpful, although protocols have not been designed or formally researched as in the case of CBT and GET. A survey of treatment outcomes of six CFS/ME specialist services using the CFS/ME national outcomes database showed that four of them described the treatment offered as activity management or a combination of CBT, GET and/or pacing. The specialist services, while achieving outcomes consistent with research for fatigue and anxiety, are not making the same changes in physical function that randomized trials achieved. Interestingly, services that described themselves as using activity management showed better results than those describing themselves as offering CBT or GET; however, the numbers of services involved were small, and what this meant in practice is undefined (Crawley *et al.* 2013).

17.3 Occupational therapy and CFS/ME

CFS/ME disrupts an individual's occupations, usually across all domains of life: work, leisure and home life are all affected. Significant impact on function is part of the diagnostic criteria (NICE 2007). The case example in Box 17.1 describes onset and the impact on function as typically seen in clinical practice.

The rehabilitative treatment approach of balancing and grading activity, and working with both physical and psychological factors, utilizes all the core skills of the therapist (Cox 2000; Hughes 2009). Occupational therapy specific skills include complex activity analysis and goal setting. Knowledge of the condition is important, as is an understanding of employment and social factors and relevant legislation, social security benefits and possibilities for social and emotional support. The training that occupational therapists have in both physical and mental health is useful because an understanding of the impact of associated problems, such as depression and pain, is important. Occupational therapy's focus on wider goals and a balanced life keeps a broad recovery focus.

Many people with CFS/ME feel that their condition is perceived as 'not real'; many will have had at least one experience with a health professional where they felt they were not taken seriously, or that their symptoms were alleged to be all in their mind (Burgess and Chalder 2004; Prins, van der Meer and Bleijenberg 2006).

Common derogatory names for the condition (such as 'yuppy flu' or 'lazyitis') do not help this perception. Some people find the lack of a conclusive biological marker to be confusing and distressing. These factors mean it can be hard to accept the condition, and therefore the treatment. CBT for CFS/ME has been shown to help this process (Brooks, Rimes and Chalder 2011). Education of other professionals in health and social care can also be important; for example, paediatric specialists could spend time working with teachers of a child who has CFS/ME.

BOX 17.1 Case example: Pauline

Pauline is a teacher in a secondary school. Her partner is a plumber and they have two children (aged 10 and 14 years). She has developed CFS/ME after a viral infection that left her very weak. She was referred to a specialist CFS/ME service 9 months after the initial infection. She had attempted to return to work after 2 months off but had to go on sick leave again after 3 weeks. Her sleep pattern is erratic: she sometimes sleeps for long periods in the day and has difficulty sleeping at night. She manages to do simple things around the house but struggles to do a full supermarket shop, or do heavier housework or gardening. She can drive short distances infrequently, mainly because she also has poor concentration. Her problems with concentration mean that she cannot read for more than a short time and is unable to watch a film. She has had to cut family trips short and cannot have long days (e.g. hill walking with her family). During a camping holiday she had to rest extensively and took 2 weeks to return to her pre-holiday level of function. Her mood has become low and her husband is feeling stressed because he is taking on more of the housework and responsibilities for the children. She is now on half pay but is concerned that she will not be able to return to work before her paid sick leave comes to an end.

Although there are different focuses in the treatment of CFS/ME, the common feature is breaking a 'boom-and-bust cycle' which causes an individual to take excessive rest in order to recover after a period of exertion. Establishing a more regular pattern of behaviour then can enable activity levels to be gradually increased. Setting a baseline of activity is common to all approaches. A baseline is not about reducing activity to a manageable level; rather, it involves establishing a balance of activity that includes exercise, rest, enjoyable, social and productive activities and dealing with any barriers to implementing this, such as thought processes, external pressures and environmental considerations. Treatment of CFS/ME cannot be explored in detail here and readers are directed to the resources in Appendix 17.1. However, the management of sleep problems does not occur in isolation, and it is necessary to touch on other areas of management (Cox 2000; NICE 2007; Pemberton and Berry 2009; White *et al.* 2013).

17.4 Sleep disruption in CFS/ME

Establishing how sleep is affected, and differentiating between primary sleep disorders and CFS/ME, is fraught with complexity. Jackson and Bruck (2012) report in their review of research that the 'consensus from a number of studies is that pathological sleepiness...is not observed in CFS/ME patients despite subjective reporting of sleepiness' (p.723). However, there are studies that confound this conclusion, and Jackson and Bruck (2012) go on to cite the following examples that challenge this consensus:

- There are mixed findings relating to circadian-rhythm disturbances.

- The sleep architecture* of CFS/ME patients may differ from that of healthy individuals.

- Stage 3 sleep or slow-wave sleep (SWS)* is typically observed for approximately a fifth of the sleep period in young, healthy individuals, and a number of studies have reported reduced time in SWS in CFS/ME patients relative to controls.

Whether or not these changes in sleep cause *clinically* significant changes is debatable (Westcombe and O'Dowd 2012). Research appears to be reaching a conclusion that although sleep is troubled in people with CFS/ME, their fatigue is not caused by a sleep disorder. Neu *et al.* (2008) differentiated between fatigue and sleepiness and indicated that different clinical approaches are required for managing fatigue and improving sleep.

It does appear that poor sleep is a problem for the majority of people diagnosed with CFS/ME, and it can exacerbate symptoms. Pain and fatigue symptoms, similar to those reported in CFS/ME and the related fibromyalgia syndrome, have been induced in healthy individuals by disrupting SWS, and from this it has been suggested that 'the physiological arousals that are observed during sleep reflect a vigilant nocturnal state that contributes to daytime fatigue, pain, and hypersensitivity, and subjective feelings of non-restorative sleep' (Jackson and Bruck 2012, p.721). A study by Rahman *et al.* (2011) found that there was a loss of vagal modulation of heart rate in CFS/ME patients during sleep indicating increased sympathetic arousal; the researchers suggest that vagal modulation is required to make sleep restorative and that this difference could account for the reported poor sleep quality. In plain language, this suggests that the protective fight-or-flight system does not relax and the body is on alert even during sleep, which is just how many patients describe it.

The issue is further complicated by research trials of sleep in people who have been diagnosed with CFS/ME by specialist clinics which report that approximately half of the participants diagnosed with CFS/ME actually *do* have sleep disorders, such as insomnia, limb movement disorder and obstructive sleep apnoea (Jackson and Bruck 2012). A recent example is a study by Gotts *et al.* (2013) who conducted polysomnography* on people diagnosed by a specialist service with CFS/ME according to the criteria of Fukuda *et al.* (1994). Although a primary sleep disorder is an exclusion for diagnosis of CFS/ME, the researchers found that a third of participants did in fact have a primary sleep disorder – mainly sleep apnoea or restless limb syndrome. However, as the evidence suggests that treating primary sleep disorders does not improve the fatigue associated with CFS/ME, sleep disorders could therefore be considered as co-morbid rather than necessarily exclusionary (Mariman *et al.* 2013a, 2013b).

Putting aside the complexity of diagnosis, there have been recent attempts to categorize sleep in people diagnosed with CFS/ME. Recent consensus criteria for CFS/ME (Carruthers *et al.* 2011) have described sleep difficulties in two categories: (1) disturbed sleep patterns, which include insomnia, prolonged sleep, naps, frequent awakenings and vivid dreams; and (2) unrefreshing sleep, including excessive daytime sleepiness. Gotts *et al.* (2013) used polysomnography to examine differences in the sleep patterns of people with CFS/ME and postulated that there are possibly four different phenotypes of sleep disturbance in CFS/ME that could be helpful in designing useful therapeutic strategies. The authors concluded that when comparing the symptoms to the DSM-5 (APA 2013), two groups could be classified as having insomnia-type sleep problems, one group had a hypersomnolence problem and the fourth had no overlap with a DSM-5 defined disorder (see Table 17.1).

Table 17.1 Characteristics of sleep phenotypes identified by Gotts *et al.* (2013)

Insomnia-type difficulty	Hypersomnolence difficulty	No DSM-5 sleep disorder
Problems in getting off to sleep but few awakenings once asleep; sleep that is obtained is of normal quality with high amount of deep sleep and less rapid eye movement (REM) sleep	No difficulties in getting off to sleep and few awakenings but feelings of being unrefreshed on waking despite a significant amount of time in bed asleep	No difficulties in getting off to sleep and few awakenings but feelings, or evidence, of 'restless' night-time sleep; high number of arousals and high amount of light stage 2 sleep
Short sleep duration and, although no difficulties getting off to sleep, many awakenings for significant periods of time; also increased feelings of daytime sleepiness; low amounts of slow-wave sleep		

17.5 Management of sleep problems in CFS/ME in a clinical setting

Unfortunately, many of our common-sense responses in trying to solve the problems of fatigue and sleepiness can lead to further problems with a sleep pattern. Beliefs such as 'I am tired – I therefore need to sleep', 'If I sleep for a long time, it must be necessary' and 'If I haven't slept, then I need to catch up' are logical, but they could lead someone to adopt unhelpful sleep habits which perpetuate and exacerbate fatigue. In clinical practice some patients report that they find it impossible to sleep in the day and that they do not fall asleep readily, whereas others find it a challenge to stay awake during the day and can sleep for hours at night as well. In conversations about sleep and fatigue, many patients distinguish the difference between sleepiness as being ready for sleep and fatigue as one of 'relentless exhaustion, untouched by sleep'. The difference between fatigue and sleepiness and tiredness can be hard to distinguish, as discussed by Westcombe and O'Dowd (2012). It is a murky area, as fatigue does not necessarily lead to a need for sleep, or to sleeping, and sleep does not necessarily ease fatigue. Helping people who are troubled by fatigue to explore this usefully is an important aspect of management.

The detailed history-taking and assessment of the symptoms and their consequences can uncover possible alternative diagnoses, and it is useful to be aware of them. Many sleep problems in CFS/ME can be solved by conventional sleep intervention strategies with some adaptation to work with the fatigue and other symptoms. In the remainder of this section some of the typical sleep difficulties are outlined. The emphasis is on how they may present in individuals with CFS/ME in clinical practice, as opposed to research findings, and on areas that an occupational therapist may focus on in the assessment period.

Poor-quality sleep

One of the typical experiences that patients report is feeling unwell and exhausted in the morning, despite having been in bed for a long time. This is one of the primary diagnostic criteria for CFS/ME (Carruthers *et al.* 2011; Fukuda *et al.* 1994).

Hypersomnolence: too much sleep and feeling sleepy

This is often a problem in the first few months of illness where people sleep a lot at night (over 10 hours) and can also fall asleep in the day. The need to sleep is a characteristic of infectious diseases; it can also be a hallmark of depression.

Sleep apnoea

A sleep breathing disorder may be suspected if a person snores, or if he or she, or a bed partner, is aware of them gasping for breath, and the individual is very *sleepy* in the day – as opposed to fatigued – which can show as a high score on the Epworth Sleepiness Scale* (Johns 1991).

Disrupted sleep patterns

An example of a disrupted sleep pattern is when someone goes to bed at 10:30 p.m., does not sleep until 1:30 a.m., wakes regularly and then falls asleep again at 4 a.m. before waking at midday, feeling unwell and napping in the afternoon. In extreme cases there can be night/day reversal. This is often uncovered in diaries or in a conversation about a typical day or week.

Insomnia

Patients frequently report trouble getting to sleep; this can be due to anxiety, discomfort, not enough or too much activity, disordered sleep/wake patterns or going to bed too early. Any of these situations might contribute to waking up and not getting back to sleep, although it can also result from going to bed too early and waking after sufficient sleep but at a time that is too early.

Insomnia may present in the clinic with fatigue but without all the symptoms typically needed for the diagnostic criteria for CFS/ME. It may be suspected if symptoms improve significantly with better sleep. Studies cited by Burgess and Chalder (2005) describe people without CFS/ME (or any other diagnosed condition) who have disrupted sleep patterns and are also experiencing symptoms very similar to those of CFS/ME, including muscle aches, physical weakness, sleepiness and poor concentration. Sometimes the problem can be caused by other factors; for example, in a patient seen in a CFS/ME service, the onset of symptoms occurred when her partner became ill and her sleep reduced from 7 to 5 hours. Her 'CFS/ME' was 'cured' when the therapist helped her find solutions to the problem of her poor sleep.

17.6 Assessment of sleep problems

Assessment is the start of a collaborative understanding of the problems. Engaging the individual in an open conversation is an important part of supporting them in making changes that may be challenging, as Burgess and Chalder (2004, p.32) describe:

> The assessment provides a wonderful opportunity for participants to tell their story. Often it is the first time that they will have been able to go into detail

about their problems. Allowing participants to elaborate on their illness often gives them the feeling that their illness is being taken seriously, often for the first time. Acknowledging the difficulties they have encountered along the way in terms of their illness, whether related to its impact on their life or response from other health professionals, etc, is important... There is no doubt that getting people to change previous routines can be difficult in a number of ways. The participant may be very fearful of changing the way they do things, fearing worsening of the symptoms.

As well as conversation, clinicians will probably wish to use a variety of assessment methods including interviews, self-monitoring and standardized questionnaires, which are considered in turn in this section.

Interviews

Because sleep difficulties are commonly part of the picture of CFS and, as discussed above, daytime fatigue may or may not be related to sleep, it is useful to ask about activity over a 24–48-hour period: 'Are you doing things one day and then struggling to do much at all on the next?' The balance of activity can be considered by asking about what the individual has stopped doing or has reduced. Activity changes can increase stress and can also decrease physical fitness; these are common factors in perpetuating a sleep problem. In discussing sleep in detail, the questions in Box 17.2 can be useful in helping to tease out the differences between sleep difficulties, sleepiness, fatigue and tiredness. Although assessment is covered elsewhere (Chapter 8 in particular), it may be more complex in the case of CFS/ME, and at times a different emphasis may be necessary. It is worth going into some detail and encouraging the individual to reflect on their coping strategies and patterns of behaviour.

Asking someone to talk through a typical day can be illuminating for both therapist and patient. Because of the boom-and-bust cycle, it may be necessary to ask someone to describe a day with more energy as well as a day with low energy, noting how these days are spaced and how they may be related. It can be helpful to consider that people normally do the things they do because they believe them to be sensible and helpful. When we have fatigue it is logical to rest, sleep more and then use energy when we have it, and perhaps to ignore and push though it or to be concerned that it is caused by something sinister and either worry or increase activity levels in order to ignore the symptoms. The work of the therapist at this point is to elicit what helps and what has been tried, highlight patterns and then develop a shared understanding of where imbalance lies; perhaps a more balanced lifestyle could be one of the ways that fatigue and other symptoms would be improved.

BOX 17.2 Assessment of sleep pattern in the context of CFS/ME

Tell me about your sleep. This is an open invitation seeking what is most important to the individual. More specific details can be elicited, if not already given, in a conversation that includes the following:

- *What time do you go to bed?* How long do you sleep? When do you fall asleep (Do not assume that time to bed is time asleep.)

- *What time do you get up?* (Do not assume that this is necessarily the waking-up time, so ask also when they wake up.)

- *Do you do anything specific to help you sleep?* (Winding-down routine, sleeping tablets, relaxation techniques, for example)

- *Do you wake in the night?* If you do, what do you do?

- *How do you feel in the morning?* (Feeling unwell in the morning is a significant symptom.)

- *Do you feel the need to sleep in the day?* How long, when, where? Is it like this every day? Is it a habit, or does it happen on days when there is a particular pattern of activity?

- *How long has your sleep been like this?* What was different before you were ill and at other points in the illness, or on different days of the week, perhaps after a period of overexertion?

- *Any caffeine or medication?* What times are these substances taken? Are you aware of any impact on sleep, sleepiness or energy levels?

- *Pain?* If you have pain, does it affect your sleep, how does it vary? (This is a fairly complex subject, as many people with CFS/ME have significant levels of pain and the therapist may need to explore in more detail; see Chapter 16.)

- *Does your sleep help your fatigue?* Have you noticed any relationship between your sleep and your fatigue? (This is an important question as it starts to open the way to other potential approaches to managing fatigue.)

Self-monitoring

Monitoring activity and sleep over a few weeks can be a useful exercise, particularly when combined with guided reflections in a therapy session. This can be done on paper diary sheets or using actigraphy* or smartphone applications. For example, in the UK the National Health Service has developed an app called ActiveME (see Appendix 17.1), which enables the simple recording of sleep, rest and low- and high-activity levels. Monitoring in these ways can give a clear picture of what is happening day and night. Sometimes it can be reassuring to find that, for example, night-time waking is not as consistent as was thought and help someone to be less tense about what they are dealing with; for others, it can highlight unhelpful activity and sleep patterns that they can begin to address.

Standardized questionnaires

There is not a sleep questionnaire specifically for people with CFS/ME; however, the Epworth Sleepiness Scale (Johns 1991) is sometimes used, mainly to help determine whether a sleep disorder might actually be the primary problem. The Sleep Assessment Questionnaire (Cesta, Moldofsky and Sammut 1999) has also been evaluated by Unger et al. (2004) who found that it was promising and that it identified more of the problems associated with CFS/ME than the Epworth; however, it is not available in the public domain and has not been correlated to polysomnography nor been extensively validated (to date).

17.7 Individualized management plan

Intervention in a specialist CFS/ME service is negotiated with the individual with a range of options including individual appointments, group sessions, telephone consultations and email contact. The number of sessions varies, but the best results seem to be when patients have longer duration of contact (Crawley et al. 2013). Establishing a routine that supports good health management is one of the first things to be considered, and sleep is a primary consideration. Thoughts and beliefs about sleep, rest and the meaning of symptoms are elicited throughout the process, initially creating a dialogue between the therapist and the person with CFS/ME and then moving towards a self-management approach.

Information – knowledge is power

Education about CFS/ME and sleep is an important component of management, providing people with information about CFS/ME, patterns of the illness, baselines of activity, the role of exercise and sleep management. The sleep element of the psycho-educational approach can include information about sleep physiology (stages of sleep, normal sleep patterns and regulation of the body clock) as well as information on sleep hygiene* to maximize a regular pattern and also to reassure that many of the sleep concerns are within the realms of 'normal sleep'. Once the association of 'fixing' fatigue with sleep has been questioned, and people have an understanding of the physiology of sleep, they are often able to make changes that can bring about improvements. Sometimes this is relatively simple as in the case example of Philippa (Box 17.3), but in other cases more support is necessary and a number of strategies might need to be implemented before there is improvement.

BOX 17.3 Case example: Philippa

Philippa, a 42-year-old teaching assistant, slept from 8 p.m. to 7 a.m. and then fell asleep in the day, having a regular afternoon sleep of 3–4 hours. She found that whenever she sat down she fell asleep. She was becoming very worried as the fatigue was increasing. She had stopped work but found that all she seemed to do was sleep and she felt worse and worse.

After receiving information about sleep and fatigue management, she set a rising time before 7:45 a.m. 7 days a week, and decided to do all she could to stay awake by moving around and taking up knitting and crossword puzzles to stay busy when seated. She felt much better, had some symptom reduction and was able to increase her activity levels, being able to do more with her family and commence a phased return to part-time work.

Sleep and activity analysis

For someone whose fatigue is overwhelming, the suggestion to sleep less can at best seem illogical and at worst feel impossible, but grading sleep, like any other activity, is possible. This can be achieved by gradually waking and getting up earlier over a few weeks, perhaps in half-hour stages. If someone is sleeping for more than 11 hours at night, gradually reducing this to 11 hours would be the first step. Then, if daytime sleep is excessive, reducing the amount of time asleep, or in bed, can also be graded slowly. Resting anywhere but the bed can be a good way to start. For some this process itself may have to be graded further by starting on 2 or 3 days a week and gradually decreasing the amount of daytime spent in bed. This has been done to good effect by people choosing to rest on a sofa or in a chair and using relaxation techniques and strategies instead of sleeping. If, for example, falling asleep at 2 p.m. is a habit, then planning to rest earlier may be appropriate (i.e. resting *before* the feeling of exhaustion and setting time limits, with alarms if necessary, for 30 minutes).

In order to make changes like this, a 24-hour approach to sleep and activity can be taken. Activity diaries can be used to identify current sleep patterns as well as the activities, or clusters of activity, that may be perpetuating the problem, for example, periods of high activity without breaks. Analyzing the energy requirements of a week's activities can aid insight. This is described by Cox (2000), who breaks activities into low, medium and high demand. It can be helpful to see them as a continuum with sleep and rest, as in Figure 17.1.

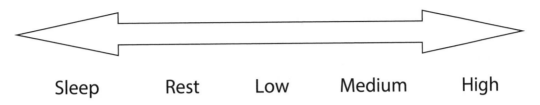

Sleep   Rest   Low   Medium   High

FIGURE 17.1 THE SLEEP–REST–ACTIVITY SPECTRUM
Adapted from Cox (2000).

Balance is encouraged by ensuring a spread of each level of activity throughout the day. This analysis also breaks the link or at least nuances an understanding of the difference in function and experience of rest and sleep.

Rest

Sleep can be enhanced by daytime resting as the body and mind can be calmer and the sleep pattern can be less disrupted due to minimizing daytime sleep. Rest also supports circadian rhythms by enabling people to stay up for longer in the evening.

The boom-and-bust cycle has very little place for rest unless it is just a need to recover from exertion. Even the 'good days' can be fraught ('I need to get everything done before I am ill again'). The bed (and sleep) can become the only place to stop, and then sleep is neither satisfying nor effective. Effective rest is important. It can be used to help adjust to less time in bed and also to spread out and balance activity in the day.

Rest can be at different levels; it could include sitting and listening to a radio play, stretching, listening to music or to birdsong, having a bath or lying down for 20–30 minutes and doing a deep-breathing exercise. Having a variety of ways in which to rest for different purposes can be helpful and can also help calm the system down. Sleep is not generally considered rest, but 'nodding off' for a few minutes during relaxation may be necessary at that moment and should not unduly destabilize the sleep pattern. However, some people find it does disrupt sleep and should avoid dozing off during rest periods by making sure they rest when they are not over-tired, and use alarms as a precaution.

Learning relaxation and meditation exercises can be helpful and many people find calm and gentle stretches to be helpful during one of their rests. Learning very short ways of resting and also gently focusing during an activity is a way of integrating rest into activity so it does not perpetuate the boom-and-bust cycle. Mindfulness-based approaches can be introduced to support this (Rimes and Wingrove 2012). A case example of the use of rests is given in Box 17.4.

BOX 17.4 Case example: Tom

Tom was going to bed at 2 a.m., sleeping until 11 a.m. and for up to two extra hours during the day. After learning more about sleep, and in discussion with his therapist, he chose to set an 8:30 a.m. rising time and have three 30-minute rests: during two rests he would use a relaxation CD, and listen to an audio book in the third. He also added in some small 5–10-minute 'breathers' at different points in the day, for example, when he got into his car and before driving. He found it challenging, but after a month he reported better sleep, being able to fall asleep more quickly. He continued to feel fatigue but found that he had more time to carry out activity and rest and, as a result, was actually able to do more. After 5 months he dropped one of the longer rests, finding the short 'breathers' were adequate. He also became busier and did not have time for the longer rests.

Implementing strategies and working with barriers to change

Once the general principles in management of CFS/ME and the specific sleep issues that may be present are understood, the work of the therapy session is to support the process of change and to deal with potential problems. This section considers ways that therapy sessions can support the individual in deepening their understanding and aid their recovery from CFS/ME. Specifically, the role of wider goal-setting in the context of sleep management is considered, as well as practising specific strategies within a therapy session and a further discussion of the role of cognitions in maintaining or sabotaging change.

Implementing changes using goals

Sleep is an integral part of daily activity and its management is not confined to what happens at night, but is affected by activity throughout the day. Recovery from CFS/ME requires goals that envisage a healthy life (Prins *et al.* 2006). While full recovery may seem some way off, finding a focus for change is essential. Linking sleep management to occupational goals helps the individual incorporate their knowledge into their own life and circumstances. It prevents this potentially directive approach of sleep, exercise and diet from becoming something that the individual 'has' to do and enables changes to be integrated in a meaningful way. For occupational therapists, it can remind us of the role of occupation in maintaining and developing health. Keeping the initial baseline personally relevant, small and manageable means the individual is more likely to be able to achieve it, which then starts a cycle of positive reinforcement (Stahl, Rimes and Chalder 2013). Many people with CFS/ME are excellent at describing what they have not done, or what else needs to happen, rather than acknowledging small gains (Burgess and Chalder 2005). Frequent review of goals, and steps towards them, in the first stages helps the individual to experiment and provides an opportunity for the therapist to give positive feedback and discuss success as well as constructively problem-solve more challenging areas. The case in Box 17.5 is an example of this.

BOX 17.5 Case example: Pat

Pat's sleep pattern was very variable: she sometimes slept until midday and at other times got up at 7 a.m. She had a preferred early rising time because her role as parent was very important to her and she wanted to have breakfast with her children. She sometimes took her youngest child to school on days that she felt better. Because she did not know when she would be unable to take him, it was a source of stress since her husband then had to adjust his work schedule according to her health. In discussing goals she decided to focus on parenting as a main goal with a target of taking her son to school. When establishing a starting point or baseline for this goal she decided to get up with her children every day but not to get dressed until after they had gone to school; this would be her baseline and they could then gradually make changes in a planned way over time. For example, she would then aim to get dressed earlier twice a week and take her son to school on those days. Her husband felt that would help him as he would know how to plan his work.

Practising strategies in session

Practising a short exercise in a therapy session can be very helpful as it can identify any particular benefits or challenges that can be worked with immediately. Relaxation, meditation or stretching can all be used as they are activities we encourage to help improve sleep but which can also lead to a wider conversation. Using a relaxation or meditation exercise as a break in a session models the use of these techniques as part of a normal routine and the effect or change that people can notice after just a few minutes of calm concentration. Enquiring into how it felt to pause or move in that way, what the person noticed during and afterwards, is an important aspect of using an activity like this in a session. It is useful not to assume it is a 'pleasant' experience as some can find the act of stopping alarming, particularly if they are in a high state of sympathetic arousal. Sleepiness can also be increased if someone has been pushing through periods of fatigue so that when they do stop, they feel very tired. Being able to voice these feelings and understand them in a way that supports recovery and constructive behaviour is an important part of the therapy. Eliciting any struggles or feelings of guilt for stopping and examining this in a supportive way can encourage an experiential shift in thinking. Involving partners can be helpful as they can encourage and support practice and may also find it personally beneficial.

Working with unhelpful thinking patterns

The role of thoughts and attitudes has been woven throughout this chapter and other chapters in this book. The changes required to improve management and aid recovery from CFS/ME involve a shift in understanding and require a degree of reflection on habits and beliefs about symptoms, sleep, activity and rest. Eliciting specific thoughts relating to sleep and fatigue and considering how these can impact on the goals and plans that are being developed is an essential component, particularly if there are challenges in implementing changes. Thoughts that hinder the plan to rest for 20 minutes instead of sleeping in the day at a different time could be: 'I must carry on'; 'I'll feel bad later, so I need to get it done now.' Some people in this situation can feel so used to keeping going and then needing to recover that it could feel strange when they stop earlier and they may feel guilty about stopping when they are not exhausted.

Thoughts and worries about the nature and meaning of the symptoms can affect the plan to regulate a sleep pattern; for example, the plan to get up at a set time despite having a bad night can include: 'I can't cope' or 'I need to sleep.' Thoughts like these are likely to be automatic (Beck 1996) and reacted to without awareness of their impact on the changes and actions an individual wishes to make. Once the thoughts are noticed, it is possible to question them and seek alternatives. Once this pattern is noticed, the role and impact of thoughts can be taken further to sometimes profound effect. The example in Box 17.6 demonstrates how someone changed their experience through thought challenging.

BOX 17.6 Case example: Jeremy

Jeremy identified a tendency always to think *I feel terrible in the morning*. He realized that this meant he was always looking for evidence to confirm that he was feeling bad in the morning and decided that was probably not helping. He therefore tried to turn it around and look for things that were tolerable for him in the mornings. 'It took time but after a while I noticed more and more things that were all right and I started to do positive things in the morning, at first just for a few minutes but eventually I found that it didn't matter how I felt, I could still do things by planning and using a baseline.'

17.8 Conclusion

Sleep has a complex relationship with fatigue. In the case of CFS/ME it seems that sleep does not 'cure the fatigue' and individuals can feel they have very little choice but to sleep to try to feel better; however, the sleep is often of poor quality and does not solve the problem. CFS/ME is not a disorder of sleep, but sleep can become disrupted, and sleep management is a cornerstone of CFS/ME management and part of an initial baseline aiming to regulate activity, sleep and rest. Like all elements of CFS/ME management, taking account of individual goals and preferences, and being aware of issues that can affect implementation of the strategies, requires a person-centred approach that emphasizes the self-management of this condition. Occupational therapists with a good understanding of CFS/ME and its paradoxes are well placed to support individuals to recover.

Notes

1   In this chapter the term 'chronic fatigue syndrome/myalgic encephalomyelitis' (CFS/ME) is used. It is acknowledged that some individuals and groups distinguish CFS and ME from each other, whereas others consider the terms interchangeable. There is also a movement to change the order of terms to 'ME/CFS'; however, at the time of writing, the term used in the National Health Service in the UK is CFS/ME.

2   This point was made at the conference of The British Association for Chronic Fatigue Syndrome/ME in 2013.

Appendix 17.1 Further resources

Books

- Cox, D. (2000) *Occupational Therapy and Chronic Fatigue Syndrome.* Chichester: Wiley Blackwell.

- Pemberton, S. and Berry, C. (2009) *Fighting Fatigue.* London: Hammersmith Press. (This is a self-help book for people with CFS/ME written by an occupational therapist and someone with CFCS/ME.)

- Burgess, M. and Chalder, T. (2005) *Overcoming Chronic Fatigue Syndrome: A Self-Help Guide Using Cognitive Behavioural Techniques.* London: Robinson and Constable Ltd.

Online resources

- The Pace trial manuals for CBT, GET and APT are available at www.pacetrial.org/trialinfo. (Occupational therapists should note that although the APT manual was devised by occupational therapists, this was within the confines of the trial and based on work completed by Action for ME and is *not* occupational therapy; the CBT and GET manuals describe the most effective treatments and are consistent with occupational therapy practice.)

- The NICE guidelines also provide guidance on assessment and intervention (http://guidance.nice.org.uk/CG53).

- BACME (www.bacme.info) is the UK clinicians' organization that provides interdisciplinary training.

- Patient charities Action for ME (www.actionforme.org.uk) and Action for Young People with ME (www.ayme.org.uk)

- Active ME app (http://apps.nhs.uk/app/activeme)

- Kings College CFS research unit (www.kcl.ac.uk/innovation/groups/projects/cfs/index.aspx)

All websites were accessed in May 2014.

Acknowledgements

I would like to thank Dr Hazel O'Dowd (clinical psychologist) for reading through and commenting on this chapter and Beverly Knops (occupational therapist), Dr Peter Gladwell (physiotherapist) and Dr Alex Westcombe (clinical psychologist) at North Bristol NHS Trust who have all contributed to my knowledge of sleep and CFS/ME. I should also acknowledge the contribution of Professor Diane Cox of the University of Cumbria whose thoughts and words are embedded in my discussion of the role that occupational therapists play in CFS/ME intervention.

References

Afari, N. and Buchwald, D. (2003) 'Chronic fatigue syndrome: a review.' *American Journal of Psychiatry 160*, 2, 221–236.

American Psychiatric Association (2013) *Diagnostic and Statistical Manual of Mental Disorders*, 5th edn. Washington, DC: American Psychiatric Association.

Beck, A. (1996) 'The past and the future of cognitive therapy.' *Journal of Psychotherapy Practice and Research 6*, 4, 276–284.

Brooks, S.K., Rimes, K.A. and Chalder, T. (2011) 'The role of acceptance in chronic fatigue syndrome.' *Journal of Psychosomatic Research 71*, 6, 411–415.

Burgess, M. and Chalder, T. (2004) *Manual for Therapists: Cognitive Behaviour Therapy for CFS/ME*. Available at www.pacetrial.org/docs/cbt-therapist-manual.pdf, accessed on 9 April 2014.

Burgess, M. and Chalder, T. (2005) *Overcoming Chronic Fatigue: A Self-Help Guide Using Cognitive Behavioural Techniques.* London: Robinson and Constable Ltd.

Carruthers, B.M., van de Sande, M.I., De Meirleir, K.L., Klimas, N.G. *et al.* (2011) 'Myalgic encephalomyelitis: international consensus criteria.' *Journal of Internal Medicine 270,* 4, 327–338.

Cesta, A., Moldofsky, H. and Sammut, C. (1999) 'The sensitivity and specificity of the Sleep Assessment Questionnaire© (SAQ)© as a measure of nonrestorative sleep.' *Sleep 22,* Suppl. 1, 14.

Clauw, D.J. (2010) 'Perspectives on fatigue from the study of chronic fatigue syndrome and related conditions.' *Physical Medicine and Rehabilitation 2,* 5, 414–430.

Cox, D. (2000) *Occupational Therapy and Chronic Fatigue Syndrome.* Chichester: Wiley Blackwell.

Crawley, E., Collin, S.M., White, P.D., Rimes, K., Sterne, J.A. and May, M.T. (2013) 'Treatment outcome in adults with chronic fatigue syndrome: a prospective study in England based on the CFS/ME National Outcomes Database.' *QJM 106,* 6, 555–565.

Fukuda, K., Straus, S.E., Hickie, I., Sharpe, M.C. *et al.* (1994) 'The chronic fatigue syndrome: a comprehensive approach to its definition and study.' *Annals of Internal Medicine 121,* 12, 953–959.

Gotts, Z.M., Deary, V., Newton, J., Van der Dussen, D., De Roy, P. and Ellis, J.G. (2013) 'Are there sleep-specific phenotypes in patients with chronic fatigue syndrome? A cross-sectional polysomnography analysis.' *BMJ Open.* doi: 10.1136/bmjopen-2013-002999.

Hashimoto, N., Kuraishi, Y., Yokose, T., Tajima, N. *et al.* (1992) 'Chronic fatigue syndrome: 51 cases in the Jikei University School of Medicine.' *Nippon Rinsho 50,* 11, 2653–2664.

Hughes, J.L. (2009) 'Chronic fatigue syndrome and occupational disruption in primary care: Is there a role for occupational therapy?' *British Journal of Occupational Therapy 72,* 1, 2–10.

Jackson, M.L. and Bruck, D. (2012) 'Sleep abnormalities in chronic fatigue syndrome/myalgic encephalomyelitis: a review.' *Journal of Clinical Sleep Medicine 8,* 6, 719–728.

Johns, M.W. (1991) 'A new method for measuring daytime sleepiness: the Epworth Sleepiness Scale. *Sleep 14,* 6, 540–545.

Mariman, A., Delesie, L., Tobback, E., Hanoulle, I. *et al.* (2013a) 'Undiagnosed and comorbid disorders in patients with presumed chronic fatigue syndrome.' *Journal of Psychosomatic Research 75,* 5, 491–496.

Mariman, A., Vogelaers, D.P., Tobback, E., Delesie, L.M., Hanoulle, I.P. and Pevernagie, D.A. (2013b) 'Sleep in the chronic fatigue syndrome.' *Sleep Medicine Reviews 17,* 3, 193–199.

Neu, D., Hoffman, G., Moutrier, R., Verbanck, P., Linkowski, P. and Le Bon, O. (2008) 'Are patients with chronic fatigue syndrome just "tired" or also "sleepy?"' *Journal of Sleep Research 17,* 427–431.

NICE (2007) *Chronic Fatigue Syndrome/Myalgic Encephalomyelitis (or Encephalopathy): Diagnosis and Management of CFS/ME in Adults and Children.* London: National Institute for Health and Clinical Excellence.

Pemberton, S. and Berry, C. (2009) *Fighting Fatigue.* London: Hammersmith Press.

Price, J.R., Mitchell, E., Tidy, E. and Hunot, V. (2008) 'Cognitive behaviour therapy for chronic fatigue syndrome in adults.' *Cochrane Database of Systematic Reviews.* doi: 10.1002/14651858. CD001027.pub2.

Prins, J.B., van der Meer, J.W.M. and Bleijenberg, G. (2006) 'Chronic fatigue syndrome.' *Lancet 367*, 9507, 346–355.

Rahman, K., Burton, A., Galbraith, S., Lloyd, A. and Vollmer-Conna, U. (2011) 'Sleep-wake behaviour in chronic fatigue syndrome.' *Sleep 34*, 5, 671–678.

Ranjith, G. (2005) 'Epidemiology of chronic fatigue syndrome.' *Occupational Medicine 55*, 1, 13–19.

Rimes, K. and Wingrove, J. (2012) 'Mindfulness-based cognitive therapy for people with chronic fatigue syndrome still experiencing excessive fatigue after cognitive behaviour therapy: a pilot randomized study.' *Clinical Psychology and Psychotherapy 20*, 2, 107–117.

Stahl, D., Rimes, K. and Chalder, T. (2013) 'Mechanisms of change underlying the efficacy of cognitive behavior therapy for chronic fatigue syndrome in a specialist clinic: a mediation analysis.' *Psychological Medicine.* doi: 10.1017/S0033291713002006.

Unger, E., Nisenbaum, R., Moldofsky, H., Cesta, A. *et al.* (2004) 'Sleep assessment in a population-based study of chronic fatigue syndrome.' *BMC Neurology.* doi: 10.1186/1471-2377-4-6.

Van den Eede, F., Moorkens, G., Van Houdenhove, B., Cosyns, P. and Claes, S.J. (2007) 'Hypothalamic-pituitary-adrenal axis function in chronic fatigue syndrome.'

Vercoulen, J.H., Swanink, C.M., Fennis, J.F., Galama, J.M., van de Meer, J.W. and Bleijenberg, G. (1994) 'Dimensional assessment of chronic fatigue syndrome.' *Journal of Psychosomatic Research 38*, 5, 383–392.

Wessely, S. and Powell, R. (1989) 'Fatigue syndromes: a comparison of chronic "postviral" fatigue with neuromuscular and affective disorder.' *Journal of Neurology, Neurosurgery & Psychiatry 52*, 8, 940–948.

Westcombe, A. and O'Dowd, H. (2012) 'Too Tired to Sleep.' In A. Green and A. Westcombe (eds) *Sleep: Multiprofessional Perspectives.* London: Jessica Kingsley Publishers.

White, P.D., Goldsmith, K., Johnson, A.L., Chalder, T. and Sharpe, M. (2013) 'Recovery from chronic fatigue syndrome after treatments given in the PACE trial.' *Psychological Medicine 43*, 10, 2227–2235.

White, P.D., Goldsmith, K.A., Johnson, A.L., Potts, L. *et al.* (2011) 'Comparison of adaptive pacing therapy, cognitive behaviour therapy, graded exercise therapy, and specialist medical care for chronic fatigue syndrome (PACE): a randomised trial.' *Lancet 377*, 9768, 823–836.

Wyller, V.B., Eriksen, H.R. and Malterud, K. (2009) 'Can sustained arousal explain the Chronic Fatigue Syndrome?' *Behavioral and Brain Functions 5*, 10. doi: 10.1186/1744-9081-5-10.

18

A PLACE TO SLEEP
Environmental Factors

Andrew Green and Eva Nakopoulou

18.1 Introduction

This chapter examines the environmental conditions that influence sleep and, in particular, the challenges posed in the special circumstances in places where the individual has less control over their living conditions and routines: hospitals, prisons and residential care. In each of these environments it is arguable that there are different priorities in play, although a manager of any of them is likely to insist that the welfare of the patient, prisoner or resident is paramount and to acknowledge the importance of sleep. However, in a hospital, for example, there may be life-and-death issues that have to be addressed, whereas in a prison the maintenance of security is a key issue.

It is shown in Chapter 4 how sleeping conditions have changed over the course of history and still vary around the world, and it should be acknowledged again that there are no rights or wrongs about what constitutes the ideal sleeping environment; however, it is necessary to take account of what is customary in Western society and what are the general expectations of most people. It is therefore reasonable first to revisit those expectations, and to review the environmental factors that are discussed in relation to sleep hygiene (see Chapter 8), and then to examine the conventional sleep environment before turning to the particular circumstances of institutional settings.

18.2 Home environment

According to Jones and Ball (2012) 'a western perception of "good" sleep is independent sleep, in a dark, quiet location, in a consolidated night-time bout, with rapid sleep onset at the start of the sleep period, and minimized wakings during the night' (p.89). It might be added that 'independent sleep' would encompass couple sleep. To a great extent we expect to have choices about who we sleep with (although the housing conditions for many people may not permit such choice) and we expect to choose when to sleep. It may not feel like much of a choice if it is necessary to rise at 6 a.m. to get to work on time, or to sleep in the morning after working all night, but adults do not expect to be told *when* to sleep. As discussed in Chapters 3 and 4, when we sleep is affected by a combination of factors: age and, to some extent, gender, our natural sleep duration, the extent to which we are an 'owl' or a 'lark' and some degree of choice. We also expect to choose how we spend our waking time although, again, our responsibilities might limit that choice considerably. However, as discussed in Chapter 6, our daytime activity can affect our night-time sleep. Apart from these social factors, environmental factors that affect sleep are light, temperature (and ventilation) and noise.

Most people probably give little thought to environmental conditions most of the time: we know what our preferences are for darkness, room temperature and bedding, and we know our tolerance of variation of these elements and of noise. We expect to be able to control the conditions we need for sleep, although in practice it can be very difficult to control environmental noise and it may be difficult, or expensive, to heat a room in winter or keep it ventilated and cool in summer. Whereas people work out for themselves their preferred conditions for when they get to bed, it cannot be assumed that everyone is aware of the ideal conditions for others such as children and elderly relatives, and it is possible that sometimes these conditions are overlooked. For example, it has been found in one study (Jones and Ball 2012) that a quarter of the parents involved allowed their 3-year-old children to fall asleep on the sofa when they were tired, which suggests that they remained exposed to artificial light and, very probably, television.

There is a great deal of variation in individual preferences in sleeping environments. It is noted in Chapter 4 that thermal regulation in couples might be different, suggesting a need for different bedding. Some people tolerate little light – in extreme cases, for example, taping over an LED on a smoke detector in a hotel room – and insist on a blackout. (This might be helpful for some people for getting to sleep, but it is uncertain whether a blackout is helpful in the morning when natural light might aid waking.) Similarly, some people are very sensitive to noise, whereas others can sleep adjacent to a busy road without a problem. It is difficult, therefore, to specify conditions necessary for sleep, but, as noted in other chapters, there are some guidelines.

The close and complex associations between thermoregulation, circadian rhythms and sleep are examined by Okamoto-Mizuno and Mizuno (2012) and Van Someren (2006). Okamoto-Mizuno and Mizuno (2012) note that 'excessively high or low ambient temperature…may affect sleep even in healthy humans without insomnia' (p.1). This of course accords with the experience of most of us and hardly needs stating. However, Okamoto-Mizuno and Mizuno (2012) note how humans use clothing and bedding in response to environmental conditions in order to maintain body temperature and create a favourable microclimate in the bed with a temperature of 32–34°C and relative humidity of 40–60% under the covers. According to the website of the National Sleep Foundation (see Appendix 18.1) ambient temperatures above 24°C (75°F) and below 12°C (54°F) will disrupt sleep. A room temperature of 18–20°C (65–68°F) is commonly cited as the ideal.

Light, as mentioned in several other chapters in this book, is an essential regulator of the sleep-wake cycle (see also Cajochen 2007). Darkness is the cue for the production of melatonin* in the evening and light the cue for its suppression in the morning. However, according to Gooley *et al.* (2011), in exposing ourselves to electric lighting after the time of melatonin onset, we alter the timing and duration of melatonin synthesis. Gooley *et al.* (2011) conclude that 'melatonin levels are remarkably sensitive to room light levels' (p.E470). Exposure to artificial light before bedtime causes suppression of melatonin synthesis and we therefore need to pay attention to light in the winding-down period before sleep.

Czeisler (2013) observes that 'many people are still checking e-mail, doing homework or watching TV at midnight, with hardly a clue that it is the middle of the solar night' (p.S13) but, as he points out, artificial light striking the retina between dusk and dawn inhibits sleep-promoting neurons, activates arousal-promoting neurons and suppresses production of melatonin. Czeisler (2013) goes on to note that modern solid state lighting (light-emitting diodes or LEDs) is typically rich in blue light, to which the light-detecting cells in the retina are most sensitive. However, it could be possible to modify technology to reduce light's negative effects if a solid state white light fitting were also to contain multi-coloured LEDs, which could enable control of both intensity and colour of light at different times.

Sleep is susceptible to disturbance by noise because our brains can still process incoming acoustic stimuli (Zaharna and Guilleminault 2010), and noise levels that affect sleep are much lower than levels that would impair hearing. World Health Organization (WHO) guidelines recommend levels of background noise no higher than 30dB and individual noises at a level of less than 45dB (Berglund, Lindvall and Schwela 1999). Zaharna and Guilleminault (2010) note that noise has a variable effect on sleep according to the individual and that among important individual factors are personality and self-estimated sensitivity to noise.

With respect to transport noise (at the same average noise level) Basner, Müller and Elmenhorst (2011) report that annoyance levels of residents are greatest for aircraft noise, ahead of road traffic noise and rail traffic noise. In their study of the effects of transport noise on sleep measured in laboratory conditions with polysomnography*, Basner *et al.* (2011) found subtle effects on sleep structure. There was a slight increase in time before the first period of slow-wave sleep*, a small increase in duration of stage 1 sleep*, and a slight decrease in duration of slow-wave sleep. Road traffic noise led to the most changes in sleep structure and continuity, but it was aircraft- and rail-noise exposure that were *subjectively* more disturbing. It is possible that road traffic noises were not long enough to be perceived consciously compared with longer rail- and aircraft-noise events, and it is suggested that consciously perceived noise is responsible for the subjective assessment of sleep quality. Some habituation to noise was observed over the three nights of monitoring, and a further significant finding was that over 90% of wakenings in response to noise replaced wakenings that would have occurred spontaneously. (For a recent detailed review on the effects of noise on sleep see Hume, Brink and Basner 2012.)

A related problem is 'internal noise' – tinnitus, or the perception of sound in the absence of corresponding sound in the environment. Many people who experience tinnitus find that it is less noticeable when they are doing something; conversely, it is likely to be more troublesome at night. A possible strategy is the use of speakers under the pillow which can play music to mask the sound with minimal disturbance to a partner. (See Appendix 18.1 for the URL to the British Tinnitus Association website.)

The effects on our sleep of what we can see and hear are relatively well researched, but there has been less research on the effect of what we can smell. It is very difficult to get to sleep where there are unpleasant smells in the room but the extent to which an odour can cause arousal from sleep is not clearly understood. It may be the experience of individuals that they have been woken to the smell of someone cooking a very late meal, or an early breakfast, but Carskadon and Herz (2004) demonstrated that humans cannot be reliably woken from any stage of sleep, except stage 1, by olfactory stimuli. Participants in their study were woken from stage 1 sleep in about 90% of trials using peppermint or the chemical, pyridine, but responses in other stages of sleep were limited (less than 50% in stage 2* and rapid eye movement (REM) sleep* and none in slow-wave sleep*); in contrast, participants responded to 75% of auditory stimuli.

It is not surprising that human sleep is relatively undisturbed by smells since the sense of smell is generally less sensitive than the senses of hearing and sight. It is possible that in other species the sense of smell might alert a sleeping animal to danger. However, there is some recent evidence that odours can be arousing in the development of a smoke alarm for use by deaf people. It appears that a very pungent smell may be necessary, and reports of experiments with wasabi (a root used for flavouring in Japanese cookery) have indicated that it can wake people (Buerk 2010).

To summarize, temperature, light and noise all impact on sleep and the impact of smells is limited. Individual tolerance to each of them varies and some habituation to raised noise levels is possible. In the home environment it is possible to a great extent to control these factors – or to find ways to compensate (with blackouts or earplugs, for example) – but it is less easy to control conditions in other settings.

18.3 Hospital environment

Yoder *et al.* (2012) note that noise levels in intensive care units may be as high as 67dB and can reach 42dB in surgical wards; these compare with the WHO recommendation of 30dB for patient rooms (Berglund *et al.* 1999). In their study in the US Yoder *et al.* (2012) found noise levels on a general ward to be markedly higher than the recommended level; this was associated with 'clinically significant sleep loss' (p.69). The difficulty of sleeping in hospital has been reviewed in the UK by Pilkington (2013) who stresses the negative consequences of sleep deprivation; she classifies its causes in hospital as pain, anxiety and stress, and environmental factors. The association of sleep loss and pain is well documented (see Chapter 16) and, as well as any discomfort caused by the injury or illness, there could be consequences on sleep as a result of treatment or management. Hospital admission is bound to be associated with anxiety and stress; not only is it an unfamiliar and often frightening environment, but patients are likely to worry about their illness, or perhaps how the family is managing in their absence. Although single rooms are now much more common, most people will not be used to sleeping in the company of strangers in open wards.

Environmental disturbances in hospital are many; Pilkington (2013) cites studies describing the level of interruption. For example, Freedman *et al.* (2001) showed how intensive care patients had non-consolidated sleep over the course of 24 hours: for the 17 patients in their study the mean number of sleep periods per day was 41, and the mean length of each period of sleep was 15 minutes. Reviewing difficulties in intensive care units, Kamdar, Needham and Collop (2012) cite causes of disturbance as noise, patient care activity, light, mechanical ventilation and medications as well as other causes such as pain and pre-existing illness. Pilkington (2013) also lists noise (staff conversations, telephones and televisions) and light, which can desynchronize the circadian rhythm. Additional factors on a hospital ward that may not help sleep at night are other patients' emergencies, including deaths, and disturbance caused by confused patients. Hospital routines – cleaning, medication, meal times, shift changes – might also be unhelpful. Lastly, as discussed below in relation to care homes, night-time checking by staff can also disturb a patient's sleep (that is, waking patients when checking whether they are sleeping).

After her very thorough review, the recommendations made by Pilkington (2013) are slightly disappointing – although, in reality, they only highlight the insolubility of the problem: switching off main lights at 'an acceptable and regular time every night, with dimmer bedside lights…if required' (p.40). With regard to noise, she cites suggestions of reducing the level of staff conversations and telephone ring tones, as well as minimizing nursing interventions. They are the kind of measures that work: Li *et al.* (2011) showed how sleep-care guidelines could reduce noise and light and improve sleep quality of intensive care patients. The difficulty of patients getting good sleep is a further reason for endeavouring to keep admissions as short as possible.

Can occupational therapists do much to assist? Maybe not in a brief admission, but they should at least be aware of the possibility of patients' performance in assessments being compromised by poor sleep. They can also work with ward staff to reinforce good practices and environmental changes that might enhance sleep, which in turn will assist recovery and improve occupational performance. Perhaps more can be achieved in psychiatry where hospital admissions might be longer and where conditions are different; for example, patients will get up and dress and eat their meals away from their beds.

As noted in Chapter 1, most psychiatric disorders are accompanied by sleep disturbance and, accordingly, insomnia is widespread among psychiatric inpatients. For a qualitative investigation into the experience of insomnia on a psychiatric ward see Collier, Skitt and Cutts (2003), but Donaldson and Chinapanti (2009) reported that 78% of psychiatric inpatients in their sample of 46 had poor sleep as defined by the Pittsburgh Sleep Quality Index*. They also suggest that sleep is disturbed by unfamiliar surroundings, noise, bright lighting and monitoring by, or interactions with, staff; additionally, there are physical and psychological factors such as medication side effects and substance use.

Donaldson and Chinapanti (2009) stress the need for non-pharmacological management of sleep problems. With regard to the ward environment they advocate regular routines, provision of single rooms, and attention to lighting and ambient noise. They also recommend paying attention to medication schedules, and to the use of caffeine, alcohol and other substances, as well as to exercise programmes. Noting the effectiveness of cognitive behavioural management of insomnia they also suggest using the skills of mental health professionals to provide 'lower cost education initiatives to promote good sleep' (p.40). 'Sleep education' would be a good use of time in hospital as clients can gain information and learn skills for use not only in hospital but also in the community. (For reviews of management of insomnia secondary to psychiatric and other conditions see Smith, Huang and Manber 2005, and Stepanski and Rybarczyk 2006. See also Chapter 13 for an outline of a 'sound sleep' course that could be adapted for delivery in an inpatient setting.)

18.4 Prison environment

Conditions in prisons vary greatly around the world and even within the UK, on which this section is based. There are still Victorian gaols where prisoners share cells but, increasingly, large, privately run modern facilities are replacing them. Security levels vary from high-security establishments, intended to hold those prisoners considered most dangerous, to open prisons where low-risk prisoners and others nearing the end of their sentences are held. Conditions in individual institutions vary according to local circumstances, types of prisoner, facilities and staff resources.

Despite such variation, the constant is the lack of freedom with a routine imposed by others. For some prisoners it might be a new experience to have a structured routine, but generally options are limited. Times of meals are fixed, as are times when prisoners are locked in their cells, often from quite early in the evening (or late afternoon) except when there is time for association with other prisoners. Access to a gym might be limited. Social and leisure opportunities are therefore few.

Similarly, opportunities for work, training and education tend to be limited. Participation in training depends first on a prisoner remaining in the same prison for long enough. Some prisoners are able to get regular work shifts – cleaning or in the laundry, for example – and develop a regular work pattern, but even then there are still long periods in the day when they are unoccupied. For those prisoners without work, the tendency to sleep in the day is likely to be greater (see below).

The prison population is also varied, but although some very high-profile individuals (such as former government ministers, celebrities and business executives) sometimes find themselves in prison, the figures suggest that different sections of the population are not equally represented. For example, Table 18.1 illustrates how, on a number of measures that indicate social exclusion, sentenced prisoners are over-represented in comparison with the population at large. This is significant since, as noted in Chapter 4, those who are more socially disadvantaged tend to report worse sleep, even before environmental factors in prison are considered.

There appears to be a lack of research relating to sleep in the prison population. Clinical experience of occupational therapists working in prisons indicates that many prisoners experience sleep problems, and that over 50% identify themselves as having difficulties. The beginning of a sentence can be particularly stressful, and medication might be offered for a few nights. Many prisoners have mental health difficulties and will have the same difficulties with sleep as individuals in the general community who suffer from depression or other serious mental illness.

One study in the assessment unit of a maximum-security prison in New Zealand (Whiteford 1997) found that 'sleeping was mentioned by all inmates as a central occupation' (p.128). It is not clear how many inmates took part (no more than 14), but in interviews they mentioned 'sleeping a lot, sleeping all morning and then feeling crappy, dreading getting up because there is nothing to do' (p.128). Similarly, studies in forensic psychiatry units have indicated that a disproportionate amount of time is spent in daytime sleep (Farnworth, Nikitin and Fossey 2004; Stewart and Craik 2007; Sturidsson 2007; see also Green 2012).

Table 18.1 Comparison between offenders and the general population in terms of factors contributing to social exclusion

Indicator of social exclusion	General population	Sentenced prisoners
No qualifications	15%	52% men 71% women
Unemployed/not working in 4 weeks prior to conviction	5%	67%
Two or more mental disorders	5% men 2% women	72% men 70% women
Drug use in previous year (or year before imprisonment)	13% men 8% women	66% men 55% women
Long-standing illness or disability (males aged 18–49 years)	29%	46%
Hazardous drinking (current or in year before imprisonment)	38% men 15% women	63% men 39% women
Homeless or not in permanent accommodation before imprisonment	0.9% of households	32%

Data from report of the Social Exclusion Unit (2002).

If prisoners sleep as much as the studies in forensic units indicate, it could suggest that they might not in fact have sleep problems; however, the difficulty with such observations is that they are just that, and no objective measurement (e.g. actigraphy*) has been done. It is probable that recorded sleep time in studies includes time at night set aside for sleep as well as daytime sleep, without taking account of time at night spent awake. The most likely scenario is that many prisoners sleep during the day through boredom, in order to pass the time, and that this adds to the other problems that affect night-time sleep.

A number of factors are therefore involved in prisoners' sleep problems:

- stress/anxiety related to being in prison and worry about loved ones outside

- some have never had a structured routine before and struggle with imposed timetables (although prison routines also lack balance)

- limited awareness of sleep hygiene (e.g. when to drink coffee or when to do exercise)

- mental health problems and drugs and/or alcohol problems

- environment: for example, noise levels, smells and general lighting do not promote good sleep.

Prisoners inevitably have limited control over their immediate environment. They have no choice over cellmate, if they share, and they are locked in the cell for long periods. Central lights are put out late in the evening, although prisoners can use personal lamps and televisions well into the night. It is up to prisoners to regulate noise from televisions and music systems, and they may reach agreements between themselves; however, not all individuals cooperate, some become disturbed or upset – and some snore. Noise tends to be amplified throughout the wings because of the large open space, and even a relatively minor movement, such as opening the viewing hatch on the cell door, can be heard throughout the wing.

The question of managing sleep problems in prison is complex. Conditions for sleep are unfavourable and there is scope to debate how much the element of punishment and the deprivation of liberty and opportunities should outweigh other considerations. However, a first line of treatment is often medication, but because of the risk of drug abuse, the taking of medication is supervised and sleeping tablets may therefore be given at a time that is not appropriate (i.e. far too early); other measures are therefore necessary.

Sleep hygiene for prisoners tends to be a challenge because of the restrictive nature of the environment. Cognitive behavioural strategies (see Chapter 8) are not practical where, for example, it is not possible to leave the sleeping space if awake at night (as part of stimulus control), or where a cellmate would be disturbed by someone getting up and putting a light on to read: the self-discipline required to pursue a sleep restriction programme rules that out for nearly everyone in such confined circumstances. More cognitive strategies are difficult; for example, evidence to challenge negative thoughts may be scarce. Possibilities worth investigating are the mindfulness approach and an educational approach that looks at sleep as part of a 24-hour activity cycle.

In any event, there is a need for occupational therapists to be creative, although it will not be easily possible to create better routines. Any kind of physical exercise is to be encouraged. It has been observed in practice that attending the gym can help sleep (as well as physical and mental well-being). Therapists should consider activities that prisoners can do in their cells; this is very limited and, without the availability of tools, tends to be 'paper-based' activities, such as crosswords, Sudoku, origami or creative writing, and therefore may exclude many prisoners. As ever, learning relaxation skills can be useful. As part of an educational approach therapists can help prisoners to structure a better routine for themselves within the constraints of the system. This might also include sleep hygiene education in cases where there is a lack of understanding, for example, of the effects of caffeine or nicotine on sleep. Nakopoulou and Cullen (2012) show how such an approach has been used.

18.5 Residential care of older people

It is established in other chapters that sleep can be disrupted by a number of illnesses that might affect older people, that circadian rhythms are less robust in older people and that if someone is less able to exercise and participate in activity, sleep may be negatively affected. It should therefore not be surprising if the sleep of older people in care homes is often compromised. Two studies illustrate the problem.

Using actigraphy Meadows *et al.* (2010) compared the sleep and activity patterns of 122 non-demented residents in 10 care facilities in south-east England and 52 community-dwelling people (aged over 65 years) with poor sleep. They found that the rest-wake cycle of elderly residents in institutional care was more fragmented than in the elderly people living in the community, and that there was less distinct differentiation between night-time and daytime movement. The difficulties of sleep in care homes, as highlighted by Garms-Homolovà, Flick and Röhnsch (2010), are described in more detail in Chapter 6 but they illustrate a reciprocal relationship between sleep quality and engagement in activity: there could be a vicious cycle whereby people who sleep poorly engage less in activity and those who engage less tend to have worse sleep.

As indicated above, there are many reasons why the sleep of care home residents might be disturbed. In a report on night-time care in residential homes for the Joseph Rowntree Foundation Kerr, Wilkinson and Cunningham (2008) note that UK regulatory guidance provided no explicit direction on night care and that national vocational standards for staff training did not specify education on care needs at night. Their survey revealed that residents found that night staff were less satisfactory (often because of over-reliance on agency workers); many were disturbed by staff checking on them at night, perhaps putting the light on (although others found it reassuring); they complained of noise from staff and other (confused) residents. (Anyone involved in running a care home is advised to look at the full report by Kerr *et al.* 2008, which is available online.) The conflict between staff members' duty of care and the residents' right to an undisturbed night is discussed further by Eyers *et al.* (2012b).

In another piece of revealing research Eyers *et al.* (2012a) investigated the daily life of 145 residents in the 10 care homes involved in the study cited above (Meadows *et al.* 2010). Data collection involved completion of activity diaries, conversations with residents and field observations; home managers were also interviewed. A restriction of choice over bedtime was evident: it was noted, for example, that one resident had to be hoisted into bed and therefore had to be in bed by 8 p.m. because no staff were available later. A new resident in one home was offered the choice to remain downstairs at 7 p.m. or go to her room: the staff preference to go upstairs was implicit and since all other residents were already in their rooms, this resident's 'only choice at 7 pm was between being isolated in the conservatory or in her bedroom' Eyers *et al.* (2012a, p.64). One matron commented:

> I notice when I go out to assess people in their own homes they say 'I stay up until 11 o'clock and I watch TV in bed'. But within a very short period of time [in residential care], they are going to bed at 9 o'clock.

Another report from the same study (Luff *et al.* 2011) shows that the mean length of time in bed for residents was 10 hours and 50 minutes, whereas the mean length of time awake in bed was 2 hours and 25 minutes (a sleep efficiency* of about 78%).

A disquieting observation by Eyers *et al.* (2012a) was that 'the interviews with the Activities Organisers indicated that they were oblivious to residents' opinions about the activities' (p.69), yet some residents complained about the standard of activities offered. Activity organizers might work hours that were not actually in line with residents' routines and they were not replaced when absent for any reason (meaning that formal activities did not go on). Outings (a residents' favourite) were seldom arranged because of the cost of extra staff and the need to carry out a risk assessment. If this research is representative (which it does not claim to be), it would suggest that the constraints of providing care at an affordable cost appear to deny elderly residents the choice about when they go to bed, to limit participation in valued activities and to restrict opportunities to get out. (Other chapters in this book show how it is recommended not to spend long periods in bed if not asleep, and that daytime activity and daylight are important regulators of sleep.)

Particular interventions for people with dementia are discussed in Chapter 14 but a case study by McCurry *et al.* (2009) shows how relatively simple measures can improve sleep – in this instance, for a 93-year-old woman living in a small care home. The bedroom was improved: a lamp that the resident kept on at night was removed, and thicker curtains were fitted. Daytime activity was enhanced to include things she enjoyed as well as involving her in helping in the home. She was taken outside to spend time in the garden, and decaffeinated coffee was substituted. She was given an evening shower as part of a winding-down routine and a favourite chair was moved every evening after the resident went to bed so she did not remain in the living room if she got up in the night. The resident's views on the changes are not known, but objective improvements in sleep were achieved and staff members were able to give her more positive attention during the day. The key to such success appears to be the detailed analysis of the problems, application of scientific principles and, crucially, the active involvement and commitment of the whole care team.

Another institutional factor that affects all elderly people, and especially those with dementia, is lighting. An early study by Van Someren *et al.* (1997) showed that bright light by day could improve circadian-rhythm disturbances in people with severe dementia. This is important because older people typically have reduced exposure to light, although they need three to five times more light because of age-related changes in the eye. More recently Riemersma-van der Lek *et al.* (2008) showed that bright lighting by day can improve mood and cognition as well as sleep, although the effect is modest.

There is much scope for using other technologies (in the home as well as in residential facilities). For example, Ellmers *et al.* (2013) suggest that to save having to check on residents at night, telecare devices that tend to be used in older people's own homes could also be used more in care homes; for example, bed-occupancy sensors, floor-pressure sensors or enuresis sensors could alert staff. Researchers at the Bath Institute of Medical Engineering (Evans, Carey-Smith and Orpwood 2011) describe innovations for use in independent living but which could be adapted for residential settings, including automatic lighting to guide the way to the toilet or the use of recorded messages to suggest getting back into bed if the person has been out of bed for a long time. Other research ideas from Bath include a compartmentalized tray with touch-sensitive illumination for the over-bed table so that a resident can find things at night without needing to leave on a light; a simple device like that can help someone to feel that everything is organized and thereby reduce anxiety (see also Eyers *et al.* 2013 and Carey-Smith, Evans and Orpwood 2013).

18.6 Conclusion

Temperature, noise and light are key factors in creating the right environmental conditions for sleep, and different challenges are posed by the different environments considered here. However, while acknowledging that people's sensitivities vary, the principles remain the same: we need a temperature in the mid-range, darkness and minimal noise in order to sleep well. These conditions can be hard to achieve in some settings (and some homes), and the sleep of hospital patients, prisoners and residents of care homes can be disrupted to a significant extent.

There could be several key roles for occupational therapists in improving conditions. Apart from occasional direct action, such as oiling the wheels of a noisy medicine trolley, they can:

- advocate appropriate organizational practices that respect individuals' routines (such as giving medication at the most appropriate time for the individual), enhanced environmental conditions (such as appropriate lighting) and better training of night staff

- advise individuals on sleep hygiene measures and strategies that might help sleep

- work to increase daytime activity levels[2] – promoting the 'behavioural contrast' that encourages regular sleep

- offer educational packages in mental health units and prisons

- make assessments and prescribe assistive technology devices in care homes.

Notes

1   Many comments relating to activity levels of elderly people in residential homes might equally relate to care of adults with a learning disability.

2   The College of Occupational Therapists has launched a resource, 'Living well through activity in care homes: the toolkit' (see URL in Appendix 18.1).

Appendix 18.1 Further resources

- Alzheimers's Association (www.alz.org/index.asp)

- Alzheimer's Australia, Sleeping (www.fightdementia.org.au/services/sleeping.aspx)

- British Tinnitus Association (www.tinnitus.org.uk)

- College of Occupational Therapists' free resource, 'Living well through activity in care homes: the toolkit' (www.cot.co.uk/living-well-care-homes)

- Joseph Rowntree Foundation: *Supporting Older People in Care Homes at Night* (www.jrf.org.uk/sites/files/jrf/night-care-older-people.pdf)

- National Sleep Foundation: *Inside Your Bedroom: Use Your Senses!* Advice on the bedroom environment (http://sleepfoundation.org/bedroom)

- SomnIA: *Sleep in Aging: Optimising quality sleep among older people in the community and care homes* (www.somnia.surrey.ac.uk/finalconference.html)

- Sundowning (www.alz.org/care/alzheimers-dementia-sleep-issues-sundowning.asp)

Acknowledgements

The authors thank David Davies and Kristel Davies (Adult Forensic Community Team, ABM ULHB, Swansea, UK) for their contribution to the section on prisons.

References

Basner, M., Müller, U. and Elmenhorst, E.M. (2011) 'Single and combined effects of air, road, and rail traffic noise on sleep and recuperation.' *Sleep 34*, 1, 11–23.

Berglund, B., Lindvall, T. and Schwela, D.H. (1999) 'Guidelines for Community Noise.' Geneva: World Health Organization. Available at http://whqlibdoc.who.int/hq/1999/a68672.pdf, accessed on 31 October 2013.

Buerk, R. (2010) 'How the stimulating smell of wasabi can save lives.' Available at http://news.bbc.co.uk/1/hi/world/asia-pacific/8592180.stm, accessed on 16 December 2013.

Cajochen, C. (2007) 'Alerting effects of light.' *Sleep Medicine Reviews 11*, 6, 453–464.

Carey-Smith, B.E., Evans, N.M. and Orpwood, R.D. (2013) 'A user-centred design process to develop technology to improve sleep quality in residential care homes.' *Technology and Disability* 25, 1, 49–58.

Carskadon, M.A. and Herz, R.S. (2004) 'Minimal olfactory perception during sleep: why odor alarms will not work for humans.' *Sleep 27*, 3, 402–405.

Collier, E., Skitt, G. and Cutts, H. (2003) 'A study on the experience of insomnia in a psychiatric inpatient population.' *Journal of Psychiatric and Mental Health Nursing 10*, 6, 697–704.

Czeisler, C.A. (2013) 'Perspective: casting light on sleep deficiency.' *Nature.* doi: 10.1038/497S13a.

Donaldson, L. and Chinapanti, P.K. (2009) 'Mental illness and comorbid insomnia: a cross-sectional study of a population of psychiatric in-patients.' *British Journal of Medical Practitioners 2*, 2, 36–41.

Ellmers, T., Arber, S., Luff, R., Eyers, I. and Young, E. (2013) 'Factors affecting residents' sleep in care homes.' *Nursing Older People 25*, 8, 29–32.

Evans, N., Carey-Smith, B. and Orpwood, R. (2011) 'Using smart technology in an enabling way: a review of using technology to support daily life for a tenant with moderate dementia.' *British Journal of Occupational Therapy 74*, 5, 249–253.

Eyers, I., Arber, S., Luff, R., Young, E. and Ellmers, T. (2012a) 'Rhetoric and reality of daily life in English care homes: the role of organised activities.' *International Journal of Ageing and Later Life 7*, 1, 53–78.

Eyers, I., Young, E., Luff, R. and Arber, S. (2012b) 'Striking the balance: night care versus the facilitation of good sleep.' *British Journal of Nursing 21*, 5, 303–307.

Eyers, I., Carey-Smith, B., Evans, N. and Orpwood, R. (2013) 'Safe and sound? Night-time checking in care homes.' *British Journal of Nursing 22*, 14, 827–830.

Farnworth, L., Nikitin, L. and Fossey, E. (2004) 'Being in a secure forensic psychiatric unit: every day is the same, killing time or making the most of it.' *British Journal of Occupational Therapy 67*, 10, 430–438.

Freedman, N.S., Gazendam, J., Levan, L., Pack, A.I. and Schwab, R.J. (2001) 'Abnormal sleep/wake cycles and the effect of environmental noise on sleep disruption in the intensive care unit.' *American Journal of Respiratory and Critical Care Medicine 163*, 2, 451–457.

Garms-Homolovà, V., Flick, U. and Röhnsch, G. (2010) 'Sleep disorders and activities in long-term care facilities – a vicious cycle?' *Journal of Health Psychology 15*, 5, 744–754.

Gooley, J.J., Chamberlain, K., Smith, K.A., Khalsa, S.B.S. *et al.* (2011) 'Exposure to room light before bedtime suppresses melatonin onset and shortens melatonin duration in humans.' *Journal of Clinical Endocrinology and Metabolism 96*, 3, E463–E472.

Green, A. (2012) 'A Question of Balance: The Relationship Between Daily Occupation and Sleep.' In A. Green and A. Westcombe (eds) *Sleep: Multiprofessional Perspectives.* London: Jessica Kingsley Publishers.

Hume, K.I., Brink, M. and Basner, M. (2012) 'Effects of environmental noise on sleep.' *Noise & Health 14*, 61, 297–302.

Jones, C.H.D. and Ball, H.M. (2012) 'Medical Anthropology and Children's Sleep: The Mismatch Between Western Lifestyles and Sleep Physiology.' In A. Green and A. Westcombe (eds) *Sleep: Multiprofessional Perspectives.* London: Jessica Kingsley Publishers.

Kamdar, B.B., Needham, D.M. and Collop, N.A. (2012) 'Sleep deprivation in critical illness: its role in physical and psychological recovery.' *Journal of Intensive Care Medicine 27*, 2, 97–111.

Kerr, D., Wilkinson, H. and Cunningham, C. (2008) *Supporting Older People in Care Homes at Night*. York: Joseph Rowntree Foundation. Available at www.jrf.org.uk/sites/files/jrf/night-care-older-people.pdf, accessed on 6 November 2013.

Li, S.-Y., Wang, T.-J., Wu, S.F.V., Liang, S.-Y. and Tung, H.-H. (2011) 'Efficacy of controlling night-time noise and activities to improve patients' sleep quality in a surgical intensive care unit.' *Journal of Clinical Nursing 20*, 3–4, 396–407.

Luff, R., Ellmers, T., Eyers, I., Young, E. and Arber, S. (2011) 'Time spent in bed at night by care-home residents: choice or compromise?' *Ageing and Society 33*, 7, 1229–1250.

McCurry, S.M., LaFazia, D.M., Pike, K.C., Logsdon, R.G. and Teri, L. (2009) 'Managing sleep disturbances in adult family homes: recruitment and implementation of a behavioral treatment program.' *Geriatric Nursing 30*, 1, 36–44.

Meadows, R., Luff, R., Eyers, I., Venn, S., Cope, E. and Arber, S. (2010) 'An actigraphic study comparing community dwelling poor sleepers with non-demented care home residents.' *Chronobiology International 27*, 4, 842–854.

Nakopoulou, E. and Cullen, S. (2012) 'Our time in prison.' *OTnews 20*, 4, 30–31.

Okamoto-Mizuno, K. and Mizuno, K. (2012) 'Effects of thermal environment on sleep and circadian rhythm.' *Journal of Physiological Anthropology*. doi: 10.1186/1880-6805-31-14.

Pilkington, S. (2013) 'Causes and consequences of sleep deprivation in hospitalised patients.' *Nursing Standard 27*, 49, 35–42.

Riemersma-van der Lek, R.F., Swaab, D.F., Twisk, J., Hol, E.M., Hoogendijk, W.T.J. and Van Someren, E.J.W. (2008) 'Effect of bright light and melatonin on cognitive and noncognitive function in elderly residents of group care facilities: a randomized controlled trial.' *Journal of the American Medical Association 299*, 22, 2642–2655.

Smith, M.T., Huang, M.I. and Manber, R. (2005) 'Cognitive behavior therapy for chronic insomnia occurring within the context of medical and psychiatric disorders.' *Clinical Psychology Review 25*, 5, 559–592.

Social Exclusion Unit (2002) *Reducing Reoffending by Ex-Prisoners*. London: Office of the Deputy Prime Minister. Available at www.nobars.org.au/downloads/Reducing-Reoffending-Report.pdf, accessed on 14 February 2014.

Stepanski, E.J. and Rybarczyk, B. (2006) 'Emerging research on the treatment and etiology of secondary or comorbid insomnia.' *Sleep Medicine Reviews 10*, 1, 7–18.

Stewart, P. and Craik, C. (2007) 'Occupation, mental illness and medium security: exploring time-use in forensic regional secure units.' *British Journal of Occupational Therapy 70*, 10, 416–425.

Sturidessen, K. (2007) 'Measures in forensic psychiatry: risk monitoring and structured outcome assessment.' PhD Thesis, Karolinska Institutet. Available at https://publications.ki.se/xmlui/bitstream/handle/10616/39524/thesis.pdf?sequence=1, accessed on 14 February 2014.

Van Someren, E.J.W. (2006) 'Mechanisms and functions of coupling between sleep and temperature rhythms.' *Progress in Brain Research 153*, 309–324.

Van Someren, E.J.W., Kessler, A., Mirmiran, M. and Swaab, D.F. (1997) 'Indirect bright light improves circadian rest-activity rhythm disturbances in demented patients.' *Biological Psychiatry 41*, 9, 955–963.

Whiteford, G. (1997) 'Occupational deprivation and incarceration.' *Journal of Occupational Science: Australia 4*, 3, 126–130.

Yoder, J.C., Staisiunas, P.G., Meltzer, D.O., Knutson, K.L. and Arora, V.M. (2012) 'Noise and sleep among adult medical inpatients: far from a quiet night.' *Archives of Internal Medicine 172*, 1, 68–70.

Zaharna, M. and Guilleminault, C. (2010) 'Sleep, noise and health: review.' *Noise & Health 12*, 47, 64–69.

19

WAKING UP
Concluding Comments

Andrew Green and Cary Brown

19.1 Introduction

This book presents evidence drawn from a wide range of disciplines, and from occupational therapy, in the hope that occupational therapists might take a greater part in managing the sleep problems of their clients and patients. The diversity of approaches described is exciting because diversity affords therapists rich opportunities to build and advance practice in this important area. With those opportunities comes the responsibility to research and evaluate and build the evidence base. After summarizing some of the key points of the book, this brief concluding chapter reviews the roles that occupational therapists might take on and outlines areas of research that could be pursued.

19.2 Key messages and roles for occupational therapists

Among the key messages from the first half of the book are the following:

- Sleep does not occur in a single unbroken period, and waking several times during the night is natural.

- Sleep varies throughout the course of life: some people need more sleep than others, or naturally sleep at different times (and are known as 'owls' or 'larks').

- Different sleep patterns are possible and none is any more or less 'natural' than any other.

- Without adequate sleep, performance of daytime occupation is compromised.

- Long-term sleep deprivation affects physical and mental health and well-being.

- Daytime occupation can influence sleep.

- The environment plays an important role in how, and how well, people sleep.

Furthermore, it is proposed that occupational therapists are well placed to identify sleep problems, often having close and continuing involvement with patients. It is argued that, like other health professionals, they have a responsibility to assess for sleep problems that accompany medical and psychiatric conditions; however, unlike many other professionals, occupational therapists are also in a position to assist in the management of sleep problems in a variety of ways, as may be seen in the chapters dealing with a range of conditions.

First, occupational therapists are used to assessing the environment of their patients and clients and advising on adaptations. With increased awareness of the environmental conditions that promote sleep, therapists can take account of factors such as lighting and noise, as well as use of space (for example, minimizing the influence of waking activity, such as television viewing, in the sleeping area).

Second, they are used to looking in detail at individual daily routines and can easily review factors that could be categorized under the heading of sleep hygiene. For example, a therapist can advise on relatively simple changes such as reduction of use of caffeine, or on more complicated matters such as the timing of exercise or bathing, or other aspects of a winding-down routine, especially where other measures necessary in managing an illness have to be taken into account.

Third, occupational therapists frequently work with people with chronic conditions (for example, in pain and fatigue management) to facilitate behaviour change using cognitive behavioural principles. With appropriate training and supervision it is a relatively small step to advise on the strategies that comprise cognitive behavioural therapy for insomnia (CBT-I).

Fourth, with increased knowledge of the rudiments of sleep science, occupational therapists can advocate and advise at the organizational level on practices to improve sleep. For example, where involved in a residential home for the elderly, a therapist should use evidence-based knowledge of sleep to argue against practices such as those that see residents being put to bed early in the evening in order to fit with staff shift patterns.

The fifth way in which occupational therapists can involve themselves in promoting good sleep is the one that draws particularly on their training and ethos and relates to occupation. It is shown in Chapters 3 and 6 that engagement with the environment can enhance sleep by increasing the amount of restorative, deep sleep (stage N3 or slow-wave sleep). If good health is closely related to good sleep, this seems to be clear evidence that occupation is good for health – what occupational therapists, and most people, know instinctively – and reminds us of the importance of balance (as discussed in Chapter 2). Modern science provides clues as to why balance is so important, in ways that the founders of occupational therapy could not know.

19.3 The challenge (or opportunities) for occupational therapy

Sleep science informs us of the importance of sleep and of its structure. The synaptic homeostasis hypothesis offers a plausible explanation for some of the functions of sleep, as seen in Chapter 3, and in doing so offers evidence for the beneficial effect of occupation. It also offers a scientific rationale for the concept of balance. The related science of chronobiology is developing rapidly and shows the importance of living in synchronization with the body clock. Both of these branches of science illustrate how what we do, and when we do it, influences our health – directly, or indirectly through the medium of sleep. They both offer opportunities for occupational therapy, in addition to other possibilities.

Occupational engagement

Whether the synaptic homeostasis hypothesis will be substantiated will be seen as time goes on, but the research it generates is interesting nevertheless. For example, Chapter 6 outlines an experiment by Huber, Tononi and Cirelli (2006) that shows how the sleep quality of laboratory rats was related to the extent to which the animals were allowed to interact with their environment – or to engage in exploratory behaviour. It is much more difficult to control variables in experiments with humans, but Huber, Ghildardi *et al.* (2006) were able to show that if an arm is immobilized for 12 hours, there is a reduction in slow-wave electrical activity in the corresponding contralateral sensorimotor cortex during subsequent sleep. This might seem to be a highly specialized experimental finding, but it provides further evidence that waking activity (or lack of it in this case) can have a measurable effect on the activity of the brain during sleep.

Other research described in Chapter 6 suggests a need to develop our understanding of the diverse and less easily quantified forms of physical and social activity that can promote sleep. The role of physical activity in promoting sleep appears to be well established, but the evidence that should be of more interest to occupational therapists is that which shows that engagement in other activities can also improve sleep. For example, Garms-Homolovà, Flick and Röhnsch (2010) conclude that the link between low activity levels of older people in residential care and sleep disorders 'seems obvious' (p.751). However, it can be difficult to tease apart the factors that could help sleep. Just being busy is not enough: in clinical practice it is possible to meet people who say that they have tried doing so much in a day in order to tire themselves out but they still cannot sleep. The study involving elderly nuns (Hoch *et al.* 1987) described in Chapter 6 did not show that being *busy* was the key to their good sleep: regularity (see below) was probably an important factor, but it is possible that their vocation, or sense of purpose, was also significant.

The idea that the 'quality' of what we do – or the way and extent to which we engage with our environment – might affect sleep quality ties in with the philosophy of occupational therapy. Kielhofner and Burke (1980) asserted that 'all of human occupation arises out of an innate, spontaneous tendency of the human system – the urge to explore and master the environment' (p.573). Although this assertion is not attributed, it seems to originate in the work of White (1959, 1971) who proposed a competence motivation (known as effectance). White (1971) suggested that occupational therapists were already aware that 'an urge towards competence' (p.273) is an inherent human characteristic, and that providing clients with opportunities for performance is beneficial for them. It could now be added that there could be extra benefit in the improvement of sleep.

Regularity

The importance of regularity is also considered in Chapter 6; drawing on literature from chronobiology, it offers evidence of the beneficial effects of routine for sleep. The importance of habits and routine has long been recognized by occupational therapists – at least since the conception of the Model of Human Occupation (Kielhofner and Burke 1980), which included the habituation subsystem – and there is now even more reason to investigate the concept of regularity. Not only does regularity appear to enhance sleep, but Wulff *et al.* (2010) suggest that stabilization of sleep-wake patterns should have a positive effect on a number of psychiatric and neurodegenerative conditions. They cite evidence for the roles of light and melatonin* in entraining the circadian system and suggest that social cues are (or zeitgebers*) also useful (p.597):

> Timed activities can influence daily patterns of light exposure and can modify the timing of behaviour through associative learning and reinforcement. Meal timing, for example, is a strong stimulus for the synchronization of peripheral circadian rhythms in animals and humans and could prove valuable if incorporated into cognitive behavioural therapy (CBT) paradigms.

Time-use studies cited in Chapter 18, and other studies (Aubin, Hachey and Mercier 1999; Shimitras, Fossey and Harvey 2003), suggest that people with severe mental illness are often inactive and spend long periods in sleep or rest, either in hospital or in the community. In such studies it is often uncertain that there is clear delineation between sleep, time in bed in the hope or expectation of sleep, daytime rest and daytime sleep, and it may appear that individuals sleep a lot. Sleep duration and quality, however, are not always known, but what does seem certain is that lifestyles are restricted – what Whiteford (1997, 2000) describes as occupational deprivation. Enhancing daytime activity (restoring balance) would not only enrich the lives of people with severe mental illnesses, but keeping regular hours could also improve sleep and health. Occupational therapy is therefore poised to take a key role in applying the knowledge that research in chronobiology is generating, if it chooses to take it.

Other opportunities and challenges

A developing area of work for occupational therapists is in the field of occupational health where Cookson (2014) describes challenges for workers in maintaining a work-life balance and the effects of work and the workplace on health. A further occupational challenge to health, not mentioned by Cookson, is shift work. The consequences of shift work on sleep and health are complex, and people who work night shifts will appreciate the challenges of managing sleep and the competing demands of life in general. This area, although covered only briefly in this book (see Chapters 5 and 12), deserves increased attention from occupational therapy and occupational science. Foster and Wulff (2005) illustrate the range of increased health risks associated with long-term shift work and associated sleep disruption (including, for example, effects on mental health and increased risks of cardiovascular disorders, gastrointestinal disorders and cancer); they note possible counter-measures and express surprise 'that long naps have not been incorporated into shift-work schedules' (p.411). To take account of balance in the lives of their patients, occupational therapists need to appreciate, first, that shift work is the reality for thousands of people and that balance is all the more important for them and, second, that a greater understanding of the normal sleep-wake cycle is necessary in order to offer help.

Disruption to the sleep-wake cycle can occur naturally, as seen in Chapter 7, in the case of circadian-rhythm disorders. Delayed sleep phase syndrome is not a problem that affects a large number of people – the prevalence being estimated to be of the order of 0.17% with about a quarter of those having a severe case (Schrader, Bovim and Sand 1993) – but to those affected it is a significant and disruptive problem. Even more disruptive is free-running where sleep-wake cycles do not synchronize with the 24-hour cycle. It could be argued that as disturbances of the activity cycle, these are exactly the kind of problems that an occupational therapist should take an interest in: apart from medication, management of circadian-rhythm disorders involves paying close attention to daily activity cycles in order to reinforce environmental and social zeitgebers.

A final way that knowledge of sleep science can be incorporated into occupational therapy practice relates to learning (see Chapter 5). The importance of sleep in learning is well established, and Siengsukon and Boyd (2009) argue that, in the case of stroke rehabilitation, sleep should be encouraged between physiotherapy sessions in order to promote off-line learning of the skill that had been practised in therapy. They recommend therapy later in the day, or having a nap after a therapy session. There is no reason to suppose that it would be different for occupational therapy patients or patients with other conditions. Therapists and students might, incidentally, apply the principles to their own lives and ensure that they allow enough sleep to permit learning; for example, there is no point in staying up all night revising for an exam without subsequent sleep in which to consolidate learning.

19.4 The future

It is noted in Chapter 1 that training and education on sleep and sleep disorders have been inadequate in all health professions; however, there is now clear evidence that sleep is too important to overlook any longer. Occupational therapists, as well as colleagues from other professions, need to begin to learn more about sleep. Much of the advice given in the chapters in the latter part of this book is based on sound research evidence from sleep science, but as yet there is little evidence of the effectiveness of such advice in practice in occupational therapy: the research has not been carried out. A further challenge for occupational therapists is therefore to undertake that research – to try out in clinical practice pragmatic interventions that are indicated by the evidence base, record outcomes and publish results. The increasing availability of actigraphy* as an objective measure will facilitate this.

In terms of more formal research, others are looking at the application of CBT-I in a wide range of medical conditions, but occupational therapists should be researching the benefit of occupation (if not occupational therapists or occupational scientists, who else?). The possibilities are limitless – investigating the effect of environmental conditions such as lighting on the timing or quality of sleep, for example, or looking at ways in which activity levels relate to sleep quality, or whether different routines can enhance the process of getting to sleep: any of these can be researched with different age groups, client groups with a variety of disorders, and in a variety of situations (home, hospital or residential care, for example). There is a further benefit in researching sleep and occupation. Occupational therapists have for decades been extolling the benefits of occupation for health, although it is difficult to quantify any benefit. If daytime occupation can have a positive (or negative) effect on sleep, and it is accepted that sleep has a direct effect on health, the extent to which sleep varies in response to changes in occupation offers the possibility of a quantifiable outcome measure in research into the links between occupation and health.

This book argues that, engagement in research aside, occupational therapists should attend more to the need of their patients and clients for adequate sleep. It shows the importance of sleep for health and performance and indicates ways in which sleep might be enhanced. Occupational therapists have, or could have, the means (knowledge and skills), motive (increasing the health and welfare of patients and clients) and the opportunity (existing therapeutic relationships) to take on the task of improving sleep. Sleep improves with health and health improves with sleep. Sleep is an occupation that is an essential part of the 24-hour activity cycle and cannot be ignored.

References

Aubin, G., Hachey, R. and Mercier, C. (1999) 'Meaning of daily activities and subjective quality of life in people with severe mental illness.' *Scandinavian Journal of Occupational Therapy 6*, 2, 53–62.

Cookson, K. (2014) 'Occupational therapy in occupational health: Is it working?' *OTnews 22*, 4, 28–29.

Foster, R.G. and Wulff, K. (2005) 'The rhythm of rest and excess.' *Nature Reviews Neuroscience 6*, 5, 407–414.

Garms-Homolovà, V., Flick, U. and Röhnsch, G. (2010) 'Sleep disorders and activities in long-term care facilities – a vicious cycle?' *Journal of Health Psychology 15*, 5, 744–754.

Hoch, C.H., Reynolds, C.F., Kupfer, D.J., Houck, P.R., Berman, S.R. and Stack, J.A. (1987) 'The superior sleep of elderly nuns.' *International Journal of Aging and Human Development 25*, 1, 1–9.

Huber, R., Ghilardi, M.F., Massimini, M., Ferrarelli, F. *et al.* (2006) 'Arm immobilization causes cortical plastic changes and locally decreases sleep slow wave activity.' *Nature Neuroscience 9*, 9, 1169–1176.

Huber, R., Tononi, G. and Cirelli, C. (2006) 'Exploratory behavior, cortical BDNF expression, and sleep homeostasis.' *Sleep 30*, 2, 129–139.

Kielhofner, G. and Burke, J.P. (1980) 'A Model of Human Occupation, Part 1: Conceptual framework and content.' *American Journal of Occupational Therapy 34*, 9, 572–581.

Schrader, H., Bovim, G. and Sand, T. (1993) 'The prevalence of delayed and advanced sleep phase syndromes.' *Journal of Sleep Research 2*, 1, 51–55.

Shimitras, L., Fossey, E. and Harvey, C. (2003) 'Time use of people with schizophrenia living in a North London catchment area.' *British Journal of Occupational Therapy 66*, 2, 46–54.

Siengsukon, C.F. and Boyd, L.A. (2009) 'Does sleep promote motor learning? Implications for physical rehabilitation.' *Physical Therapy 89*, 4, 370–383.

White, R.W. (1959) 'Motivation reconsidered: the concept of competence.' *Psychological Review 66*, 297–303.

White, R.W. (1971) 'The urge towards competence.' *American Journal of Occupational Therapy 21*, 6, 271–274.

Whiteford, G. (1997) 'Occupational deprivation and incarceration.' *Journal of Occupational Science: Australia 4*, 3, 126–130.

Whiteford, G. (2000) 'Occupational deprivation: global challenge in the new millennium.' *British Journal of Occupational Therapy 63*, 5, 200–204.

Wulff, K.L., Gatti, S., Wettstein, J.G. and Foster, R.G. (2010) 'Sleep and circadian rhythm disruption in psychiatric and neurodegenerative disease.' *Nature Reviews Neuroscience 11*, 8, 589–599.

GLOSSARY

Actigraphy: measurement of rest and activity using an accelerometer, or actigraph, usually worn on the wrist or ankle to detect movement. Although people are not totally still in sleep or continually moving in wakefulness, when used in conjunction with a simple log the pattern of sleep-wake cycles can be discerned over the course of a few weeks.

Electroencephalogram (EEG): a recording of the minute electrical potentials generated by neurons in the brain.

Epworth Sleepiness Scale: a widely used self-rated measure of sleepiness or likelihood of falling asleep (see Chapter 8).

Melatonin: a hormone that is secreted by the pineal gland which is important in the regulation of the body's natural rhythms including the sleep-wake cycle. More melatonin is produced when it is dark, whereas production diminishes in the light. It is produced synthetically as a medicine for some sleep disorders.

Microsleep: an episode of light sleep lasting a few seconds, usually an involuntary response to sleep deprivation and a significant risk to drivers.

Multiple sleep latency test (MSLT): an assessment which times how long a person takes to go to sleep and to enter rapid eye movement (REM) sleep. It is an objective measure of sleepiness and is used particularly in the diagnosis of narcolepsy.

Non-REM (NREM) sleep: the stages of sleep (N1, N2 and N3) which are not REM sleep.

Pittsburgh Sleep Quality Index (PSQI): a self-rated questionnaire widely used to measure sleep quality in research and clinical practice (see Chapter 8).

Polysomnography (PSG): recording of multiple physiological variables during overnight sleep, especially the EEG, used to measure the stages of sleep for the purpose or diagnosis of sleep disorder or research.

Rapid eye movement (REM) sleep: the stage of sleep in which dreaming occurs. The body is effectively paralyzed, apart from the muscles involved in respiration and eye movement. As far as electrical activity in the brain is concerned, it resembles wakefulness.

Sleep architecture: the pattern of sleep stages throughout the night. When the succession of different stages of sleep is shown graphically the picture resembles a city skyline.

Sleep efficiency: a figure, expressed as a percentage, reached by dividing total sleep time by the amount of time spent in bed. A good sleeper's efficiency is usually over 85–90% (see Chapter 8).

Sleep hygiene: lifestyle modifications to promote sleep (see Chapter 8).

Sleep onset latency (sleep latency): the time it takes to get to sleep after settling down.

Slow-wave sleep (SWS) (stage N3, or stages 3 and 4 sleep): deep sleep. It is called slow-wave sleep because of the characteristic pattern on the EEG. It is considered to be the most restorative stage of sleep (see Chapter 3).

Stage 1 sleep (stage N1): the lightest stage of sleep or a transitional stage between wakefulness and deeper sleep (see Chapter 3).

Stage 2 sleep (stage N2): light sleep in which we normally spend about half of the night (see Chapter 3).

Suprachiasmatic nucleus (SCN): the 'body clock' – a small group of cells in the hypothalamus directly above the optic chiasm which regulates circadian rhythm.

Zeitgeber: literally 'time giver' – a cue that resets the body clock to keep it entrained with the 24-hour cycle of light and dark, the chief one of which is daylight.

CONTRIBUTORS

Chris Alford is Associate Professor in Applied Psychology at the University of the West of England (UWE), Bristol. He began sleep research at Aston University studying beta-blockers and later set up the sleep laboratory at the University of Leeds, where he completed his PhD and undertook research for the pharmaceutical industry. He was a senior research fellow at Surrey University before moving to UWE and collaborating with groups at Bristol, Loughborough and Oxford investigating sleep and fatigue in transport operations. He is a founding member of the British Sleep Society and an invited expert on the British Association for Psychopharmacology sleep disorders treatment guidelines panel. Current international collaborations include Australia, Netherlands and the US evaluating pharmaceutical and natural hypnotic products.

Anna Aishford holds a Bachelor of Kinesiology from the University of Calgary and recently completed her Master of Science in Occupational Therapy at the University of Alberta. She is a practising occupational therapist working with the geriatric population in a long-term care setting in the area of Calgary, Canada. She has been involved with conducting sleep research since 2012 and continues to utilize the most recent research findings in her everyday practice and is committed to life-long learning, pursuing further education and professional development.

Julie Boswell received her Masters of Science in Occupational Therapy from the University of Alberta, and her Bachelors of Human Kinetics from the University of British Columbia. Julie believes that experiencing is fundamental to learning and development. This has inspired her to take on endeavours such as living in Japan, completing a practicum in India and currently developing paediatric occupational therapy at a private clinic in British Columbia, while also working in an Occupational Rehabiliation 2 programme.

Cary Brown has practised as an occupational therapist and department manager in Canada and Saudi Arabia. She received her PhD at the University of Liverpool and has held academic appointments in Canada and the UK. She is currently an associate professor in the Occupational Therapy Program at the University of Alberta. These diverse experiences underpin her programme of research into sleep deficiency, chronic pain, knowledge translation and health literacy. She publishes and presents regularly at national and international conferences on these topics. Her work in knowledge translation strategies received the Canadian Pain Society's Pain Awareness Award 2010.

Claire Durant gained her PhD in 2012, focusing on sleep and novel treatments for refractory depression. She has a specific interest in the effects of different drugs on sleep and holds a research associate position at the Centre for Neuropsychopharmacology, Imperial College London. She also supports a range of sleep studies at the University of Bristol, more recently focusing on the effects of opiate medications on sleep parameters in patients with chronic pain.

Jillian Franklin is a practising paediatric occupational therapist at Renfrew Educational Services in Calgary, Alberta. With a Bachelors of Science in Human Kinetics and a background in personal training, she is passionate about health promotion. While completing her Master of Science in Occupational Therapy at the University of Alberta, she became fascinated by the occupation of sleep and its impact on day-to-day functioning. Writing the chapter on sleep problems in children inspired her to pursue a career in paediatrics and spread her knowledge about the role of occupational therapy and sleep among parents, caregivers and health professionals.

Katherine Gaylarde qualified as an occupational therapist in 2004 and works in a specialist community neurorehabilitation service in North London with clients with progressive and acute neurological conditions. She has a special interest in sleep and fatigue management and has promoted the inclusion of sleep assessment in the therapy process through development of a sleep management pathway within her service.

Andrew Green trained in occupational therapy in York, having previously gained a degree in Geography at CCAT, Cambridge, and began working in psychiatry in 1986. Since 1992 he has worked in neuropsychiatry in Bristol at the Burden Neurological Hospital – subsequently the Burden Neuropsychiatry Centre, and now the Rosa Burden Centre – and during this time gained further degrees from the University of Exeter and the University of Southampton. He first worked with sleep disorders on being asked to contribute to a therapy group for patients with insomnia in 1999 and now spends most of his time working with patients with a range of sleep disorders. He has several publications related to sleep.

Dietmar Hank is a Consultant in Learning Disability Psychiatry and has also worked in neuropsychiatry in Bristol. He trained in psychiatry in South Wales and Bristol and gained an MSc in Psychological Medicine at Cardiff University and a post-graduate diploma in Neuropsychiatry at the University of Birmingham. His special interests are neurodevelopmental disorders and sleep disorders.

Jane Hicks originally trained in general practice but is now a liaison psychiatrist with an interest in sleep disorders. She was involved in the writing of national guidelines for narcolepsy and completed her MD thesis on the pharmacological and behavioural management of insomnia. She has worked in neuropsychiatry in Bristol at the Burden Neurological Hospital – subsequently the Burden Centre for Neuropsychiatry, and now the Rosa Burden Centre – for over 15 years and was instrumental in developing a successful CBT-I group. This has become a clinical service for patients with chronic insomnia and has been effectively trialled in primary care.

Diana Hurley qualified as an occupational therapist in 1979. In her first post at Greenwich District Hospital mental health unit she researched relaxation techniques in the treatment of anxiety disorders, resulting in 1989 in the publication (under her maiden name, Keable) of *The Management of Anxiety: A Manual for Therapists* with an expanded edition in 1997. She is now the lead occupational therapist for Harrow Mental Health Service. Her recent clinical specialties have focused on the promotion of health and well-being in mental health settings. She has developed various interventions to tackle sleep problems and promote physical activity and, in particular, has produced a specialized smoking cessation support programme for those with stress and mental health problems.

Katie MacQueen qualified in 2005 and has worked since then for Central and North West London NHS Foundation Trust in a rehabilitation unit for adults and older adults with long-term mental health conditions. For the past 6 years she has worked as a specialist occupational therapist in a day assessment unit for older adults with functional and organic mental health conditions. She is particularly interested in working with people who have dementia, and their carers, to promote occupational performance and participation, with a key focus on how the environment may support or restrict either factor.

Eva Nakopoulou gained a degree in fine art before graduating with a Bachelor of Science in Occupational Therapy at the University of West of England (Bristol). During her degree course she spent 2 months with the primary health care centre of an adult male prison with an aim to scope the potential for occupational therapy in that setting and to set up a sleep group for prisoners. After qualification in 2011, she began working with learning disabilities and neurodevelopmental disorders in the Bristol area, and recently moved to a specialist autism service in South Gloucestershire.

Jillian Smith-Windsor graduated with a Bachelor of Science in Kinesiology from the University of Saskatchewan. This degree was followed by a Master of Science in Occupational Therapy from the University of Alberta in Edmonton. She is currently working as a paediatric clinician in Saskatchewan, Canada.

Nicola Stubbs is a graduate of the Bachelor of Science in Biological Sciences and Master of Science in Occupational Therapy programmes at the University of Alberta, Canada. She currently lives in Edmonton, Alberta, and has an interest in military and veterans issues.

Jennifer Thai, currently employed at the Sturgeon Community Hospital, Alberta, is a graduate of the Bachelor of Science in Kinesiology and Master of Science in Occupational Therapy programmes at the University of Alberta. Her clinical occupational therapy experience includes acute care, geriatric mental health, developmental paediatrics and neurology. She has also been involved in research projects in adapted physical activity, information communication technology and capacity assessment.

Megan Wale graduated with a BSc in Occupational Therapy at Coventry University. Her clinical experience is primarily with adults with learning disabilities, in community and in secure settings. She is currently a practising occupational therapist in Oxford in a medium-security unit for adult males.

Sue Wilson is a senior research fellow in neuropsychopharmacology at Imperial College London and has been studying sleep for over 20 years. She has used the measurement of sleep patterns in the EEG to characterize the effects of drugs in the brain and has published on drug effects on sleep in depression, anxiety, addiction and sleep disorders such as insomnia and parasomnias. She participates in a sleep and psychiatry clinic in Bristol, assessing sleep in patients with insomnia, parasomnias and other sleep disorders. She recently coordinated a national consensus group on treatment of sleep disorders.

Emma Wood graduated from Coventry University in 2005 with a BSc Degree in Occupational Therapy, then later completed a post-graduate certificate in Forensic Mental Health Studies at the University of Birmingham. Her clinical experience spans community adult learning disability services, secure forensic services and secure mental health services. Emma is currently practising occupational therapy in community paediatric services in Coventry and is pursuing an interest in sensory integration.

Fiona Wright took a degree in African studies and history before working abroad and completing a post-graduate diploma in occupational therapy at Brighton in 1997. She worked in community and mental health in East London before working in the CFS Service at Oldchurch Hospital, Romford. She has since worked with people with chronic fatigue syndrome in specialist services and as part of mental health and community rehabilitation in London and in south-west England. She worked for Action for ME on residential courses and started working in the Bristol CFS service on the PACE trial in 2007. She is currently registered for an MSc in Mindfulness Based Approaches at Bangor University.

SUBJECT INDEX

AUTHOR INDEX